GROUP DYNAMICS

IN OCCUPATIONAL THERAPY

THE THEORETICAL BASIS AND PRACTICE

APPLICATION OF GROUP TREATMENT

SECOND EDITION

Marilyn B. Cole, MS, OTR/L
Associate Professor of Occupational Therapy
Quinnipiac College
Hamden, Connecticut

SLACK Incorporated, 6900 Grove Road, Thorofare, NJ 08086-9447

Publisher: John H. Bond
Editorial Director: Amy E. Drummond
Senior Associate Editor: Jennifer J. Cahill
Creative Director: Linda Baker

Cover illustration originated by Marilyn B. Cole, MS, OTR/L

This book has been bound with a revolutionary adhesive process called lay flat binding. Using this binding results in a book with a free-floating cover and a flexible spine, allowing the book to open flat for greater ease of use.

Cole, Marilyn B.
    Group dynamics in occupational therapy: the theoretical basis and practice application of group treatment/Marilyn B. Cole--2nd ed.
        p. cm.
    Includes bibliographical references and index.
    ISBN 1-55642-382-9
    1. Occupational therapy. 2. Group psychotherapy. 3. Small groups. I. Title.
RC487.C65 1998
616.89'165--dc21   98-16670

Printed in the United States of America

Published by: SLACK Incorporated
                 6900 Grove Road
                 Thorofare, NJ 08086-9447 USA
                 Telephone: 856-848-1000
                 Fax: 856-853-5991
                 Website: www.slackbooks.com

Contact SLACK Incorporated for more information about other books in this field or about the availability of our books from distributors outside the United States.

Authorization to photocopy items for internal or personal use, or the internal or personal use of specific clients, is granted by SLACK Incorporated, provided that the appropriate fee is paid directly to Copyright Clearance Center, 222 Rosewood Drive, Danvers, MA 01923 USA, 978-750-8400. Prior to photocopying items for educational classroom use, please contact the CCC at the address above. Please reference Account Number 9106324 for SLACK Incorporated's Professional Book Division.

For further information on CCC, check CCC Online at the following address: http://www.copyright.com.

Last digit is print number: 10 9 8 7 6 5

Contents

Acknowledgments ix

About the Author xi

Introduction to the Second Edition xiii

Introduction to the First Edition xvii

Section One: Acquiring Group Skills 1

Chapter 1: Group Leadership 3
Seven-Step Format for Activity Groups
Group Motivation
Setting Limits
Leadership Styles
Co-Leadership
Conclusion

Chapter 2: Understanding Group Dynamics 27
Group Process
Group Development
Group Norms and Roles
Special Patient Problems
Termination of Groups
Summary

Section Two: Group Guidelines From Seven Frames of Reference . . .57

Chapter 3: A Humanistic Approach 61
Focus
Basic Assumptions
Function and Dysfunction
Change and Motivation
Group Treatment
Group Leadership

Chapter 4: A Psychoanalytic Approach 99
Focus
Psychoanalytic Theory
Basic Assumptions
Function and Dysfunction
Change and Motivation
Review of Occupational Therapy Perspective
Group Treatment
Group Leadership

Chapter 5: The Behavioral Cognitive Continuum 131
Focus
Basic Assumptions
Function and Dysfunction
Change and Motivation
Group Treatment
Group Leadership

Chapter 6: Allen's Cognitive Disabilities Groups 177
Focus
Basic Assumptions
Function and Dysfunction
Change and Motivation
Group Treatment
Group Leadership

Chapter 7: A Developmental Approach 205
Focus
Basic Assumptions
Function and Dysfunction
Change and Motivation
Group Treatment
Group Leadership

Chapter 8: Sensory Motor Approaches 239
Focus
Basic Assumptions
Group Approaches
Function and Dysfunction
Change and Motivation
Group Treatment
Group Leadership

Chapter 9: A Model of Human Occupation Approach 267
Focus
Basic Assumptions
Function and Dysfunction
Change and Motivation
Group Treatment
Group Leadership

Section Three: Planning an Occupational Therapy Group 291

Chapter 10: Writing a Group Treatment Protocol 294
Identifying Your Patient Population
How to Select a Frame of Reference
Selecting What Aspect of Treatment to Address
Group Treatment Plan Outline
Group Session Outline
Instructions for Preparing Protocol

Chapter 11: A Group Laboratory Experience 323
            Group Treatment Plan Outline

Appendix A: The Task-Oriented Group as a Context for Treatment 346

Appendix B: The Concept and Use of Developmental Groups 355

Appendix C: Summary of Mosey's Adaptive Skills 361

Appendix D: Uniform Terminology for Occupational Therapy,
            Third Edition 363

Appendix E: Comparison of Group Leadership Guidelines in
            Seven Occupational Therapy Frames of Reference 375

            Index 379

Acknowledgments

For help with the revision of my group dynamics course that led me to write this book, I'd like to thank my colleagues and part-time instructors Roseanna Tufano, Sigita Banevicius, and Betsey Smith, and my department chairperson, Muriel Lerner.

For painstaking review of my chapter drafts and for keeping me in touch with reality, I'd like to thank Valnere McLean, Mildred Ross, Barbara Neuhaus, Karen Macdonald, Ona Killough, and Claudia Allen.

For the group protocol concept, I owe thanks to Anne Scott of SUNY Downstate Occupational Therapy Department in Brooklyn, who convinced me of its importance and encouraged me to write this book.

For ongoing moral and emotional support and for keeping my writing on schedule (almost), I'd like to thank Anne Golenwsky, Amy Mims, and Mary Rose Preston. For trying out the learning exercises presented in this text and for providing so many fine examples, I'd like to thank my occupational therapy students at Quinnipiac.

For help with word processing and encouraging smiles, I'd like to thank my daughter, Charlot.

For the Second Edition, special thanks to Claudia Allen, Joan Toglia, Janice Burke, and Mildred Ross for their feedback and creative ideas on application of updated theoretical developments to group treatment through personal communication.

About the Author

Marilyn (Marli) B. Cole, MS, OTR/L, is a tenured associate professor of occupational therapy at Quinnipiac College, Hamden, Connecticut, and an occupational therapy consultant. She holds a bachelor's degree in English from the University of Connecticut, a graduate certificate in occupational therapy from the University of Pennsylvania, and a master's degree in clinical psychology from the University of Bridgeport. She is licensed by the state of Connecticut to practice occupational therapy and is certified by the Center for Study of Sensory Integrative Dysfunction to administer the Southern California Sensory Integration Tests. The author's clinical experience includes 16 years in mental health, 3 years in pediatrics, and 5 years in geriatrics.

The author has more than 24 years of experience, including Eastern Pennsylvania Psychiatric Institute in Philadelphia, Pennsylvania; Middlesex Memorial Hospital in Middletown, Connecticut; Lawrence and Memorial Hospitals in New London, Connecticut; and Newington Children's Hospital in Connecticut. She has also served as consultant for the West Haven VA Medical Center, the Portland Public Schools, Fairfield Hills Hospital, and St. Joseph's Manor, all in Connecticut.

This is Marli's 16th year of full-time teaching. She has taught courses in psychiatric clinical media, group leadership, group dynamics, frames of reference, Fieldwork I and II, psychopathology, sensory motor integration, computer technology lab, research, and geriatrics.

Marli has published eight professional journal articles and a chapter in *Group Process and Structure* edited by Gibson (1988). She has presented papers and workshops at professional conferences on many different topics.

Marli has also delivered professional presentations to Yale psychiatric residents, the Connecticut Occupational Therapy Association, the New York State Occupational Therapy Association, the American Occupational Therapy Association, and the World Federation of Occupational Therapy.

Currently, she is involved in research investigations of the cognitive aspects of time management in women and the status of the therapeutic relationship in occupational therapy.

Introduction to the Second Edition

The Second Edition of *Group Dynamics in Occupational Therapy: The Theoretical Basis and Practice Application of Group Treatment* updates the theory section, and brings the group leadership and protocol sections into step with today's practice. The changes include additions, deletions, and some reorganization of the First Edition. The following is a summary of the changes made and some of the reasons why.

Chapter 1, *Group Leadership*, remains unchanged, except for an important addition. A co-leadership section was added, giving a review of generally accepted theory along with guidelines for managing some potential co-leadership problems. Both fieldwork students and experienced professionals are expected to co-lead therapy groups in today's practice. Knowing the pros and cons of co-leadership can help therapists to plan effectively and use the situation to gain valuable feedback and learn from one another. Chapter 2, *Understanding Group Dynamics*, is unchanged.

Section 2, *Group Guidelines From Seven Frames of Reference*, has been reorganized rather extensively. A quick glance at the Table of Contents will reveal that a new chapter has been added (*Allen's Cognitive Disabilities Groups*), a chapter has been eliminated (*An Acquisitional Approach*), and three chapters have been renamed (*A Humanistic Approach, The Behavioral Cognitive Continuum*, and *Sensory Motor Approaches*). All of the frames of reference chapters have an additional section, called "Focus," in which the appropriate applications for occupational therapy groups are briefly summarized. Additionally, several new group activity examples have been added to each of the frame of reference chapters to illustrate new applications of theory.

In this Second Edition, the acquisitional and cognitive chapters have been combined. There are several reasons for this. First, Toglia's and Abreu's cognitive rehabilitation theory, which is one of the major components of the "acquisitional" approach, has developed beyond the strictly acquisitional category. According to them, it has become more cognitive by moving away from separate and distinct cognitive subskills and toward a "dynamic interactional approach." Cognitive rehabilitation defines coping strategies for both perception and information processing to be used in a variety of contexts. This approach is intended to maximize each strategy's generalizability over the broad spectrum of life's daily activities. The ways in which this theory has been developed make it ideally suited to group treatment. The practice of compensatory and adaptive strategies applied to the six areas of cognitive functioning (e.g., orientation, visual processing) are best done in groups where persons can create realistic contexts for application for each other. Metacognition, or self-knowledge about one's own capacities and deficits, is another newly developed concept which offers a host of applications in group treatment settings (Toglia, 1997).

Another reason for the combination of acquisitional and cognitive is a conceptual one. The many "cognitive" and "rehabilitative" frames of reference which exist in the occupational therapy literature have a tendency to confuse students and practitioners alike. *The Behavioral Cognitive Continuum* (Chapter 5) represents an attempt to organize the many concepts and techniques occupational therapists use in group treatment, which relate to behavioral and cognitive theory. This very long chapter begins "reductionistic" and ends up "holistic." First, the useful techniques from behaviorism, such as setting behavioral objectives or using practice and rehearsal or role modeling, are newly reviewed and attached to the "frames of reference" which use them. Biomechanical and rehabilitative frames are reviewed, with group treatment approaches that connect physiological concepts with their application in functional performance. Some of these include Trombly and Denton (rehabilitation), Mosey (role acquisition), and Fidler (lifestyle performance). Toglia's and Abreu's cognitive rehabilitation approach (described previously) comes next on the continuum. This frame seems to bridge the gap between the physiological and cognitive aspects of functional rehabilitation. Finally, the cognitive behavioral frame of reference, which was reviewed in the First Edition, is newly defined within the context of occupational therapy. The psychoeducational approach, and its expanded uses, such as Linehan's *Dialectical Behavior Therapy* (1993), Moyers' *Substance Abuse* (1992), and Precin's *Living Skills for Recovery* (1996), are just a few of the newly developed group approaches appropriate for occupational therapy groups. The continuum shows that some of the familiar occupational therapy groups, such as stress management and assertiveness training, are more behavioral in nature, while other groups, like community re-entry, health maintenance education, and interpersonal effectiveness, are closer to the cognitive end. Several new activity examples have been added to clarify the application of theory across the continuum.

If Allen's cognitive disabilities frame of reference seems glaringly missing from Chapter 5, that's because it is! This theory has been so extensively developed over the past decade that it now has a chapter of its own. Chapter 6, *Allen's Cognitive Disabilities Groups*, is the newly added chapter. It covers the precise guidelines Allen has developed for group assessment and treatment in occupational therapy, based on the six cognitive levels in a more detailed manner than the First Edition. Allen's detailed analysis of crafts, and their equivalence in routine daily tasks, gives occupational therapy one of its best guidelines for planning groups and interpreting outcomes.

The chapters on humanistic, psychoanalytic, developmental, and sensory motor approaches are changed only slightly. Several new activity examples have been added to each of them. A "Focus" section has been added to highlight potential uses for these approaches, and some new learning activities have been added.

Chapter 9, *A Model of Human Occupation Approach*, has been revised substantially to reflect new theoretical developments and research. MOHO's contributions to group treatment now acknowledge the importance of occupational choices, habit maps and habitats, and roles and role scripts in the context of one's social group and culture. What really sets MOHO apart as a group approach is its goal of defining and practicing roles for disabled and recovering individuals, which establish for them a meaningful place in society.

Group treatment in occupational therapy shows no signs of diminishing as we enter the next millenium. The Second Edition of *Group Dynamics in Occupational Therapy* continues to provide guidelines for designing and leading theory-based groups in our many areas of practice.

Introduction to the First Edition

This book presents a unique point of view about occupational therapy group treatment: that all group treatment, whether we know it or not, is theory based. Traditionally, group dynamics have been taught as a body of knowledge more or less separate from occupational therapy theory. Group dynamics are the forces that affect the interaction of group members to produce an outcome. The issues of group process, group development, leadership styles, and group norms and roles were a focus of social psychology research in the mid-20th century. The outcomes of this early group research, including the work of Lewin, Bion, Tuckman, Benne and Sheats, and many others, form the basis of what occupational therapy curriculums have defined as group dynamics theory.

Furthermore, the format for leading groups, such as that suggested by Howe and Schwartzberg (1986), has traditionally been generic, that is, presented without an acknowledged bias toward any particular occupational therapy theory.

A theory defines the relationship between occurrences and explains why things happen. A theory is not a fact until it has been substantiated through research. A single theory can include many concepts or ideas. Occupational therapy uses many practice theories, or frames of reference. A frame of reference departs from pure theory when it applies the theory to a specific situation, such as patient treatment. The terms "practice theory" and "frame of reference" will both be used in this text to refer to this application to patient treatment.

The premise of this book is that neither group dynamics nor group format can be understood and used apart from theory. Both reflect a point of view, which has a definite, although often unacknowledged, theoretical basis. All of the group techniques we know of patient treatment are influenced by the larger theoretical trends in our culture, such as in psychology, business management, and medical research. This does not mean that we, the occupational therapy profession, have not developed our own theories. It simply means that we have not developed them in isolation. In this book, I have attempted to acknowledge the origins of many of the group techniques we have come to know as a part of occupational therapy.

My original concept in writing this text was to create a group dynamics workbook for my group dynamics classes. My need was to provide occupational therapy students a guidebook in the application of group dynamics theory, and I wanted to make theory more concrete and usable in the clinic. Thus, this text begins by addressing the need for technique. Chapter 1, *Group Leadership*, suggests a concrete, seven-step method of leading a group. This is a place to begin learning what occupational therapy group treatment is all about.

Likewise, in Chapter 2, *Understanding Group Dynamics*, the traditional body of knowledge about group dynamics is addressed in practical terms. The contributions of early research in social psychology and the writings on application of group psychotherapy by Irvin Yalom are acknowledged. However, these basic concepts are further developed and expanded in ways that are unique to occupational therapy group treatment.

Only when we reach Chapter 3 do we discover that both the seven-step group technique and many of the principles of group dynamics have their roots in the existential/humanistic frame of reference. This context is not intended to limit our use of the techniques, but rather to expand it. The linking of the concepts of humanism and existentialism with an approach to group treatment is a good example of how occupational therapists can apply theory and use it as a guideline for treatment.

My approach to the seven frames of reference tends to be historical, and the concepts collected are often from the original authors/theorists. However, it should be emphasized that the chapters on practice theories (frames of reference) are not intended to be complete; rather, I have selected from these frames of reference those concepts that are most useful to us in planning and leading occupational therapy groups. I have attempted also to show how groups differ in each of the seven frames.

All of the chapters on group format, group dynamics, and frames of reference (Chapters 3 through 9) will hopefully prepare the student for the final phase of occupational therapy group planning—writing a group protocol. The group protocol is a complete plan for group treatment, beginning with defining the population and ending with outlines of the specific group sessions to be included.

Guidelines for how to select a frame of reference and how to use Uniform Terminology for occupational therapy are a part of the group planning process outlined in Chapter 10. Chapter 11 offers an example of a group protocol, a group laboratory experience for students entitled "Developing Your Professional Self." This series of group exercises serves three purposes: besides giving an example of the protocol assignment, it suggests a professional growth experience for occupational therapy students and it gives students group experiences in which to observe and learn about group dynamics.

Hence, this text begins and ends with technique. Throughout the book are individual exercises intended to facilitate learning. The central portion on frames of reference represents an attempt to derive from theory what is useful when planning and leading occupational therapy groups. In this way, what I hope students will see is that applying theory is not a burden, but a way to guide our planning and make it easier. This book helps occupational therapy students to organize their thinking about our multiple practice theories and to apply them systematically to occupational therapy group treatment.

Bibliography

Howe, M., & Schwartzberg, S. (1986). *A functional approach to group work in occupational therapy.* Philadelphia: J.B. Lippincott.

SECTION ONE
Acquiring Group Skills

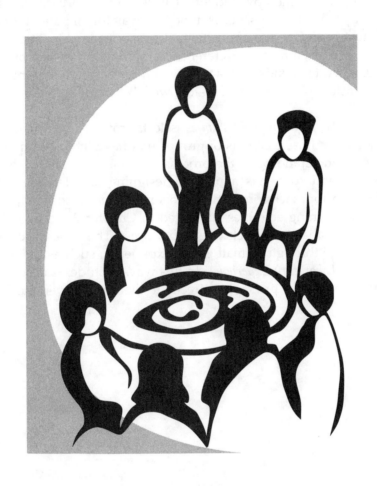

Chapter 1: Group Leadership

Chapter 2: Understanding Group Dynamics

Introduction to Section One

This section begins with experiential learning. Chapter 1, *Group Leadership*, is basically in a how-to format, which is intended as an introduction to therapeutic group leadership for beginning occupational therapy students. This is not to imply that the seven-step format is the only way to lead groups, nor is it the best way for all patient groups. The basic premise of this text is, in fact, the opposite: that group leadership, structure, goals, and activities all vary with each frame of reference as therapy groups are matched to different patient needs. Chapter 1 ends with a review of three occupational therapy leadership styles—director, facilitator, and adviser—followed by guidelines for co-leadership of groups.

Chapter 2, *Understanding Group Dynamics*, selects from the vast body of knowledge about group dynamics those elements of groups that have the most impact for occupational therapy. An understanding of the process of groups, group development, leadership styles, norms, and roles has a part in designing and leading activity groups. Guidelines on how to approach common member problems are also helpful to the beginning therapist. The learning activities suggested in Chapter 2 are intended to increase awareness of the more abstract aspects of group process. This is best accomplished when students personally go through a small group experience, such as the one described in Chapter 11, *A Group Laboratory Experience*. In this way, as students absorb the content of Chapter 2, they can apply the principles directly to their own experience.

Chapter 1

Group Leadership

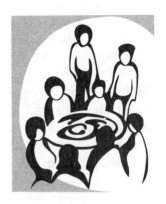

It has been my observation that students learn best by experience. They are anxious to know how to "do" occupational therapy. They are both eager and afraid to begin working with patients. To the beginning student, occupational therapy is just a label. Only when students are put in the role of a professional do they become aware of what needs to be learned.

Acting like a professional is often difficult for students, whose only experience in group leadership is usually with groups of their peers. Part of making the transition to a professional role is learning that it is different from a social role. Professionalism carries with it an authority and a directness of purpose which will need to be practiced by students before they begin interacting with patients.

This book begins with a technique that is a concrete form of group leadership training. This allows students to practice the role of a professional. It is as generic as any technique can be, and is intended as a beginning experience for students enter-

ing the profession. As the educational process continues, it is expected that the technique will be modified many times over to match the needs of each unique group. It is changed in content to meet new goals and address different age groups and disability areas. It is changed in process and structure to align with different frames of reference. But learning has to begin somewhere. Just as motor development precedes cognitive awareness in the infant, a concrete experience in group leadership becomes the forerunner of the knowledge and understanding of its purpose and application in treatment.

Seven-Step Format for Activity Groups

These seven steps can meet the needs of the highest level groups, and thus are very appropriate for student groups. They are chosen for maximum integration of learning by the members. It is clear that this format will not fit every need, goal, or patient population. However, the format is easily adapted to meet the goals of any group. How and why it will be modified will be described later. The steps in group leadership are:

1. Introduction
2. Activity
3. Sharing
4. Processing
5. Generalizing
6. Application
7. Summary

The original idea for this format comes from Pfeiffer's and Jones' *Reference Guide to Handbooks and Annuals* (1977), which presents a five-step format that is expanded and adapted for occupational therapy here.

Step 1: Introduction

Let us assume the occupational therapist is leading the initial session of a group. The therapist does not know the members well, although it is presumed she knows who they are, something about their disability, and the reasons they have been assigned to the group. (In many settings, the therapist would select the members herself.) The members may not know one another. Once the group is gathered, the occupational therapist introduces herself to the group. This introduction includes the therapist's name, title, and the name of the group that is about to begin. Then, even if people know one another, the therapist asks the members to greet the group by saying their names in turn. This procedure does more than just help the members learn one another's names, it acknowledges their membership in the group and invites them to be a part of it. In subsequent groups, it may not be necessary to say names around the room, but acknowledgment of each member's presence should still be done. A friendly "hello" or "welcome back" from the therapist may accomplish this.

Warm-Up

The next thing the leader should be concerned with is the receptivity of the members. How alert are they? How preoccupied are they? How are they feeling? Are members ready to begin a new experience, or do they need to be "warmed up?" A warm-up is an exercise that captures the group's attention, relaxes members, and prepares them for the experience to follow. Warm-ups can be structured or casual and impromptu. A nice collection of structured warm-up activities can be found in Rider's and Gramblin's *The Activity Card File* (1987). An example of a structured warm-up is "Grandma's Trunk." Each member says, "Grandma has an old trunk up in the attic and in it I found _____." Members fill in the blank by saying the name of something that begins with each letter of the alphabet in order. All items must be repeated each time. For example, the first person says she found an Acorn, the second found an Acorn and a Bonnet, etc. If there are eight members to the group, the eighth one must remember the seven items preceding his contribution.

This warm-up obviously requires members to have a good short-term memory. The occupational therapist should choose a warm-up that challenges members enough to hold their interest, but is not beyond their capabilities. Warm-up activities accomplish several important goals. The game creates an atmosphere of spontaneity and fun. It also refocuses members' thoughts from whatever they came to the group thinking about to this group right here, right now. If a warm-up works properly, it gets the members listening for what will come next, and encourages their cooperation in the group experience to follow.

All groups do not need a formal warm-up. Sometimes the best warm-up is just a casual conversation about how members are feeling today. If the group is to engage in a discussion, just getting the members talking may prepare them adequately. If the agenda is more creative in nature, an imaginative warm-up may be in order. Remembering what happened last week may be an appropriate warm-up to an activity that will be the next step in a sequence. It is important to make the warm-up relevant to the activity to follow. One does not set a mood of fun and games when the agenda for the group is a serious issue like coping with loss or finding new employment.

Setting the Mood

Setting an appropriate mood is an important objective in choosing the most appropriate warm-up, however, setting the mood for a group is not only accomplished with a warm-up. The environment, the therapist's facial expression and manner of speaking, and the media used all contribute to the mood. Care should be taken before the group begins to set up the environment accordingly; this includes proper lighting; getting rid of clutter; setting out equipment, supplies, and the correct number of chairs; and avoiding distractions as much as possible.

Expectation of the Group

The therapist's manner and expression should generally reflect her expectation of the group. A therapist cannot expect group members to take an activity seriously if the therapist does not appear to do so. The therapist will always be a role model to members, whether or not it is her intention. If the therapist begins by saying,"OK you guys, listen up!," the members will be expecting a pep talk before a football game, rather than a serious discussion about managing their time. A direct and authoritative presentation of the group is one of those skills that make up the role of the professional that students must learn.

Explaining the Purpose Clearly

Clearly explaining the purpose of the group is a primary task in the introduction phase. How this is done depends on the type of group and the patients' level of understanding. This is a step that should never be left out. The intent of the group has undoubtedly been explained individually to each member why he was assigned to this particular group. But it should not be taken for granted that the patients remember, or even fully understand, the purpose of a group from a previous explanation. The purpose should be reiterated by the occupational therapist in a way the patients are likely to understand. A higher level group of patients will want to know why they are being asked to do a particular activity. If they are asked to do calisthenics, it will be helpful to tell them that physical exercise has been known to change brain chemistry, to relieve stress, to elevate their mood, and to energize their muscles. Patients who understand and believe this will be much more willing to cooperate.

Lower cognitive level patients are unlikely to understand such abstract explanations of purpose. For them, a modified explanation, such as "These exercises will make you feel better so you can do more for yourself," may suffice. With severely ill patients, a friendly expression and a gentle touch that says "Trust me, this will help you" may enlist their cooperation.

We started out assuming that the occupational therapist is introducing a new group experience to a new set of patients. In an initial session, more time is taken in explaining the purpose than in subsequent sessions. In describing the purpose of the group, the goals of the whole series of group sessions should be outlined in the initial session. If possible, the goals should be spelled out in concrete terms. For example, money management is an activity of daily living that occupational therapists often help patients work on improving. In a money management group, members may be expected to plan and carry out a realistic budget for 1 month and keep accurate records in a notebook. Therapists often use behavior change as a measure of progress in their patients. When patients are informed about the behavior that is expected to change, they can keep track of their own progress. This becomes motivating when patients in groups start measuring each other's behavior change (or lack thereof). Peer pressure is a powerful motivator of change in human behavior.

Describing the purpose of each session will not take as much time as the initial explanation. However, the goals for each activity should always be stated clearly at the beginning of each session. Patients need to be reminded of how the group is expected to help them. As the therapist gets to know the members better, explanations can be more individualized and related to the problems each member presents. For example, in introducing a stress management session, the therapist might mention that, "In the previous sessions, you've been complaining about how difficult it is to carry out daily activities when you're feeling so much stress. Today's activity will give you some new strategies for reducing the stress in your lives." Generally, when patients are told exactly how an activity will help them, they are much more interested in doing it.

Brief Outline of the Session

Finally, the introduction ends with a brief outline of the session to immediately follow. The timeframe, the media, and the procedures are told. For example, if the activity for a 1-hour session is to "Draw Yourself," the therapist might say, "We will be using the paper and markers pro-

vided to do a drawing for the next 20 minutes. After we are finished, I will ask each of you to explain your drawing to the group and we will discuss the activity for the last half of the session." This explanation serves several purposes. It tells the patient how long he has to complete the activity. A complex artistic drawing cannot be done in 20 minutes, so if he is to finish, he knows he must keep it simple. The explanation also warns him that he probably should not draw anything he does not wish to discuss. Although this may be seen as inhibiting the patient's creativity, it also allows him to control the image of himself he projects to the group. How the therapist handles this will depend on the goal of the activity. If self-awareness is more important than social awareness, the patients may be given the option not to explain everything about their drawing. They need only say as much as they are comfortable sharing.

As well as understanding the purpose of the drawing activity, patients will want to know what is to be done with it afterward. When they know they will be expected to talk about their work, their drawing may be more focused, and they will be more prepared to speak when it is their turn. It may be helpful to tell patients ahead of time whether their drawings will be kept by the therapist or if they can keep them. The disposition of drawings produced will differ depending on the goals and the frame of reference used. However, stating the procedures ahead of time is most respectful to the patient and may also prevent difficulties later in the session.

The brief outline of the session also gives members a clue to the session's focus. The example given tells patients that the activity portion is relatively short (20 minutes) compared with the discussion portion (at least 30 minutes).

Members will see that the focus is on the discussion rather than the drawing and on learning and interaction rather than artistic talent. The outline helps patients and the therapist get the whole session in perspective.

The introduction is one of the steps that is consistently kept in every frame of reference and every type of group. The structure may become less formal, with practice, but the essential elements must remain. An introduction can make or break a group, and each element plays a part in the effectiveness of group outcome.

Step 2: Activity

Many factors should be considered when planning the activity. In a professional setting, this is, in fact, a tremendously complex process. It incorporates all we know about patients, diseases, and their corresponding dysfunctions, assessment, treatment planning, activity analysis, and synthesis and group dynamics. Selecting a therapeutic activity involves the entire process of clinical reasoning that takes occupational therapists 2 or 3 years of academic training to learn. One of the problems in learning group technique before the theory is that the process will seem oversimplified and incomplete. However, students should have a positive experience in trying out the role of an occupational therapist, even though there is much more to be learned before they can adequately do it in the clinic.

Designing the group experience is a very complex process and many issues should be considered. All of them cannot be addressed here. For the purposes of simplification, the following issues will be presented for consideration in selecting a therapeutic activity: timing, therapeutic goals, physical and mental capacities of the members, knowledge and skill of the leader, and adaptation of an activity.

Timing

With five more steps to go, (sharing, processing, generalizing, application, and summary), it should be evident that the activity to be experienced should be kept fairly simple and short. This will vary of course, but for our purposes in learning to plan and lead groups, the activity portion should last no longer than one third of the total session. For example, in this seven-step process for a 1-hour group, the activity used must be adapted to fit a timeframe of 15 to 20 minutes and to meet a preset therapeutic goal.

Therapeutic Goals

It is impossible to plan an activity without first planning and structuring the goals. Goals are desired outcomes, something patients and therapists strive together to accomplish. Setting therapeutic goals for patients involves assessing their needs and applying our knowledge of their abilities and disabilities. The referral source, such as the hospital treatment team, doctor, or nursing home staff, may have already defined the problem (i.e., "This patient needs to develop adequate social skills" or "Help patient to learn joint protection and energy conservation techniques"). In planning our practice groups for peers, students might first think about what goals might be useful for themselves. Perhaps coping with stress, setting priorities, clarifying values, managing money, managing time, and asserting oneself in social situations may be troublesome areas for students. The group goals should be chosen to meet the needs of most of the members. Once the goal is defined, an activity is designed or selected to help members achieve that goal. For example, when goals have to do with personal growth, creative activities such as drawing, sculpture, dramatics, and storytelling can be helpful. Through the creative process, many parts of the self can be revealed and explored. If goals are more socially oriented, structured group tasks involving interaction of the members are appropriate (i.e., communication exercises or group decision-making and problem-solving).

Physical and Mental Capacities of the Members

Selection of the activity or experience is further determined by the physical and mental capacities of the members. If members are college students around age 20, without physical or mental handicaps, the possibilities are almost unlimited. The challenge would be to find an activity that holds their interest and from which they can learn something new and meaningful. When members of the group are geriatric patients, the physical and fine motor components of the activity may be limited. A game of balloon volleyball or a lively discussion about a topic of interest might be suitable. When group members are mentally retarded, their cognitive limitations must be taken into account, and the activity will need to be more physical and concrete (not abstract) in nature. Cooking and simple crafts and games are often useful activities with the mentally retarded. Assessment of the physical and mental functioning of an individual is the subject of other textbooks in occupational therapy, and thus will not be covered here. In the clinical setting, assessment would be done on each member prior to starting the group.

Knowledge and Skill of the Leader

Another factor in the activity selection process is the knowledge and skill of the leader. What activities are familiar to the leader that can be adapted to this group experience? Student leaders usually choose activities for the group that they themselves are comfortable with or have done before. A student who has had dance lessons may feel very comfortable introducing a movement activity; a leader with artistic talent may choose a drawing activity. Crafts, games, and educational or social experiences may be sources of familiar activities to be adapted. There are a wealth of resource books available offering ideas for structured experiences in human relations. An example is Rider's and Gramblin's *The Activity Card File*, which is updated every few years. When using these references, it should be kept in mind that most of the exercises cannot be done as written, but will have to be adapted to the specific goals set by the occupational therapist.

Adaptation of an Activity

Adaptation of an activity requires some knowledge of activity analysis and synthesis. Activity analysis is the "Process of examining an activity to distinguish its component parts. Activity synthesis is the process of combining component parts of the human and nonhuman environment so as to design an activity suitable for evaluation or intervention relative to performance" (Mosey, 1981, p. 114). The analysis of activities is the subject of other textbooks and will not be fully described here. This is yet another example of the complex process of clinical reasoning in occupational therapy, in bringing together concepts from many bodies of knowledge to influence our treatment choices.

Activity analysis is the breaking down of an activity into its component parts and matching each part with the human functions required to accomplish it. For example, playing "Bingo" may be analyzed as shown in Figure 1-1.

In this oversimplified illustration, the therapist must know how to play "Bingo," and what physical and mental skills are

Playing Bingo	
Activity components	**Skills needed**
A letter and number are called	Patient must hear the call and associate it with written letters and numbers
The bingo card is scanned	Patient must read and understand written letters and numbers
A marker is placed on the number called	Patient must have eye-hand coordination, fine motor skills and grasp-release
When a row of five is marked	Patient must have good visual perception
Patient calls out "BINGO"	Patient must be able to speak loudly

Figure 1-1. Activity analysis.

required to play. Knowing this, the patient's skill is matched with what is required to do the activity. Modifications can then be made in the activity to suit the patient's abilities. This is activity synthesis. For example, a group of patients with poor vision may need Bingo cards with larger letters and numbers and bright-colored markers. A hearing-impaired group will need to have the calls written on a blackboard or flashed on a screen. Patients with poor motor control may need a Bingo card with magnetic markers that will stay in place even if the card is moved. Higher functioning groups may need more challenging requirements to win, such as markers all around the edge or in the shape of an "H" or an "S." Additional motivation may be built in by offering appealing prizes.

Once selected, the therapeutic activity should be presented in a systematic way. First, the activity should be explained as directly and simply as possible. Procedures and instructions are given in language appropriate to the level and background of the group.

The therapist should get feedback from the group as to whether they understood the directions, and should answer any questions before proceeding. Materials and supplies, if needed, should be hidden from view until they are actually needed. As the activity is in progress, the therapist may choose to participate in order to avoid making members feel self-conscious or watched. However, a leader should not allow his participation to detract from making relevant observations of the group to be discussed later.

When the activity portion of the group is finished, any materials used, such as pencils or paints, should be collected and placed out of sight before moving to the discussion stages. This will avoid having some members continue working after time is up or be distracted by the extraneous items. It may be necessary to stop some individuals before they are finished in order to keep the group moving along. The leader needs to be prepared to continually adapt and structure the group.

Step 3: Sharing

After completing the activity, each member is invited to share her own work or experience with the group. The structure and process for sharing may vary with each activity. If the activity involves drawing or writing something individually, members would show the drawing and explain it to the group or read to the group what was written. In activities involving interaction, members share what the experience was like for them or what it meant to them. In either case, the therapist is responsible for making sure each member has a chance to do this. Another important responsibility in this phase is to make sure each member's contribution is acknowledged. Acknowledgment may be done verbally or nonverbally. Sometimes just a smile and a nod may be all that is necessary. Members often want to respond to one another's sharing, but the therapist may need to model this to be sure the responses show caring and concern. Empathy is an important factor here. This means the therapist responds to the patient in a way that communicates understanding of how the patient feels. Empathy will be discussed in more depth in a later chapter.

Some members may be reluctant to share for various reasons. The therapist may need to support and encourage patients to share, or to reassure them that they can do it without negative consequences. However, if a patient refuses to share, this must be accepted; patients should not be unduly pressured to disclose anything about themselves that they do not feel comfortable sharing.

Generally, it does not matter in what order the members share, but often it is easier to keep track if members just go in order around the circle. It is usually best to ask for a volunteer to start the process, so that patients feel some control over the group. However, the therapist can start to role model for the group what is expected to be shared. For example, in the "Best Friend" exercise from Pfeiffer and Jones (1973), the therapist might begin by getting up and standing behind a chair and saying, "This is my best friend, Beth (indicating an invisible self in the empty chair). She's a person who likes cooking healthy food, doing creative projects, and helping other people. Her pet peeve is people who

smoke. She has always wanted to write a book..." The therapist models the format the members will use in sharing.

There are a few activities for which sharing is not a separate step, but is incorporated into a discussion activity. For example, "Moral Decisions" is a group decision-making task which involves extensive discussion as part of the activity. Expressing one's opinion on a given issue is built into the actual task. In this case, the therapist may be more involved during the activity to make sure all of the members participate and express their views and that their responses to one another are respectful and courteous.

Step 4: Processing

This is often the most difficult step for students to learn. Inexperienced group leaders often skip this step entirely. Processing involves expressing how members feel about the experience, the leader, and each other. Feelings guide our behavior more than we know, and they certainly influence patients' behavior in occupational therapy groups. If these emotions remain unexpressed, the outcome of the group can never be fully understood. Expressing feelings is not so difficult when the experience has been positive. But if there are negative feelings, people often wish to avoid expressing them, and this includes both the group members and the leader.

If done correctly, processing can reveal some important and relevant information. If members felt anxious, embarrassed, or belittled while doing an activity, this will help to explain some of their responses when sharing and discussing it. Perhaps they felt intimidated by the leader or angry with some of the other members. Feelings like this can override any possible benefit the activity may have if they are not expressed before the group ends.

When they are expressed, the therapist has the opportunity to incorporate them into the subsequent discussion and to help the patients understand the significance of the feelings related to the group experience.

Processing also includes a discussion of the nonverbal aspects of group. Underlying issues (e.g., struggles for power and control, subgrouping, scapegoating, conflict, attraction, and avoidance) are dynamics that may never be verbalized, but will have a powerful influence on the group. These issues are highly complex for the beginning student, however, they should be well understood by the beginning therapist. Underlying dynamics such as those mentioned can and do occur naturally in all groups. They will strongly influence the outcome of our occupational therapy groups, both positively and negatively, and must be handled openly and skillfully. More will be discussed about the underlying process of groups in Chapter 2.

Step 5: Generalizing

This step addresses the cognitive learning aspects of the group. Here the therapist mentally reviews the group's responses to the activity, and tries to sum them up with a few general principles. If the activity has gone as expected, some of the general principles derived from the group should closely resemble the original goals. However, few groups go exactly as planned. The general principles discussed in the group should not be preplanned, but should come directly from the response of the members. For example, an occupational therapist did an activity called "Incomplete Sentences" with a group of emotionally disturbed adolescents. The goal of the group was to clarify their values, and in fact, the group did accomplish this. However, some additional principles were brought up during the processing phase, which are important to note.

Following are the principles of the "Incomplete Sentences" group:

1. The members generally value making decisions independent of their parents.
2. The most valued activities were those the members chose to do themselves, such as sleeping late on Saturdays or buying their own clothes.
3. Although wishing to be independent, members generally needed and wanted to be accepted by their parents as autonomous adults.

The third principle is the one not planned. During the processing phase, a member pointed out how good it was to be able to ask the leader to complete the sentences, too. The group felt positive toward this leader, who, unlike their parents, seemed to accept them as equals. The comment brought forth many spontaneous stories of parental non-acceptance and it was evident that this was the important issue for the group.

General principles may be arrived at in several ways. The leader can look at the patterns of response among members. What opinions do they have in common? What were the common elements of their drawings or stories? For example, a group of alcoholics may see their drinking as the obstacle to reaching their vocational ambitions—bottles or glasses may appear in their drawings, or they may talk about highly unrealistic vocational ambitions. These common elements are easily seen as general principles.

Another way to distinguish general principles is to look at areas of disagreement. What are the conflicted areas in the group? Some members, for example, may see stress as a motivator to get moving, while others may find it overwhelming and the cause of their inaction.

A third important clue to the general principles is the group's energy. The therapist should follow up on issues that seem to energize the group and stimulate spontaneous conversation. An example is the third principle in the "Incomplete Sentences" activity mentioned earlier. This is one of those unpredictable aspects of groups that makes them continually exciting and interesting.

Step 6: Application

The application phase closely follows the generalizing phase, but takes it one step further. The therapist helps the group to understand how the principles learned during the group can be applied to everyday life. The goal is for each member to understand how he will apply the results of this group experience to help make his own life more functional outside the group.

To begin this process, the therapist should attempt to verbalize the meaning or significance of the experience, such as, "Now that we know how important it is to have our parents' respect and acceptance, each of us needs to find a way to communicate this need to our parents." Application answers the question, "Now that you know how things are, what are you going to do about it?"

The answer to this question will be different for each individual. Knowledge of each patient's background is helpful. The therapist discusses with each member how the principles learned in the group relate to problems or issues each has expressed earlier. For example, Sue will have a hard time explaining to her father, who thinks of her as a child, that she needs for him to trust her judgment about whom she dates and where she goes on Saturday nights. Laura, whose mother travels extensively on business, will have difficulty just getting her mom's attention long enough to talk about it. She sometimes wonders if her mother cares about her enough to take the time. Both girls will have difficulty in communicating with their parents, but in very different ways. Application may sometimes resemble a kind of group problem-solving; members help each other find ways to apply the newly learned information.

One way the therapist can help the group with application is through limited self-disclosure. The therapist can role model application by saying, "When I need to discuss something with my mother and there never seems to be a good time, sometimes I suggest we make a date to go out to dinner together. She has to eat anyway and so do I, so that plan works well for both of us. How do you see that?" The self-disclosure is not so personal as to be distracting, but offers a possible method of getting parents' attention for the group to consider. It gives the group a concrete example and opens the door for them to make their own suggestions.

Step 7: Summary

The final phase of the seven-step group is the summary. The purpose of the summary is to verbally emphasize the most important aspects of the group so that they will be understood correctly and remembered. Like generalizing, there is really no way to preplan a summary. The points to emphasize should come directly from the group's responses. A good summary may take 4 or 5 minutes. It reviews the goals, the content, and the process of the group. Sometimes the therapist asks the group members to help summarize by remembering the activity and giving their ideas about what was learned. The general principles are almost always included in the summary. Having members explain their own views of the group and how it can be applied often reinforces the learning that took place.

The emotional content of the group is also important to summarize. Especially when the group feels positive or the mood has changed for the better, verbal recognition of the good feelings by the therapist will help members remember the group as a positive experience.

One way for the therapist to acknowledge feelings is to thank the members for their participation in the group. While this is not a formula, addressing and thanking individuals for their openness, honesty, and willingness to share or trust in the group is always welcomed.

A final responsibility of the therapist is to end the group on time. If the group is well planned and led, this will mark the completion of all seven steps. If, for some reason, all the steps have not been completed by the end of the session, the missing parts and the reasons for this can also be discussed within the summary.

Before leaving the "how to" section, four additional factors of leadership need to be explored:

1. Group motivation
2. Setting limits
3. Leadership styles
4. Co-leadership

All are the responsibility of the leader and should occur throughout the seven steps as they are needed.

Group Motivation

Ideally, the therapist will have a group that comes to meetings with enthusiasm and interest to participate. Such a group will be eager to listen to the therapist and take direction. A group that is motivated will interact freely with one another, will share with one another easily, and will spontaneously seek to know the meaning of the group activity and how it can be applied. Such a group is probably too healthy to need therapy.

Therefore, the leader needs to develop skills in how to motivate groups that may not be so eager.

Confidence in the Leader

An important factor in the group's motivation is the members' confidence in the leader. If the leader takes charge of the group with some authority and sounds like she knows what to do, the leader will inspire the group's confidence and trust. This confidence is further enhanced by the support and encouragement offered to the members. If patients feel that the therapist empathizes with them and understands their situations, they will tend to be more cooperative in accepting leadership. Trust is the important issue here.

Patients need to feel that the leader is sensitive to them and that she can and will respond to their needs. They also need to know the leader is in control in order to feel safe.

Encouraging Enthusiasm

A leader also motivates the group members by encouraging their enthusiasm. This can be done in a number of ways. First, the leader can show enthusiasm for the group both verbally and nonverbally. A leader who smiles and speaks in a lively tone, makes frequent eye contact, and demonstrates energetic movements often passes on enthusiasm to the group. Talking to members individually and encouraging them to participate may be effective. The approach to patients has to be adapted to the cognitive level of the patients. An explanation of how the group will make a difference in their lives will work for higher level patients. A more immediate benefit may need to be offered to lower functioning patients (i.e., "Doing this activity will make you feel more relaxed"). Activities such as games or creative efforts chosen for the group may stimulate enthusiasm. Some activities will have built-in rewards (i.e., cooking groups and craft groups).

Encouraging Interaction

A final motivating factor is encouraging group interaction. It has been said that people get as much out of a group activity as they put into it. When group members are interacting with one another, they are not only participating, but also taking over some of the responsibility for the group. Interaction should be encouraged, especially in the sharing, processing, generalizing, and application phases of the group. A good leader allows the group members to share the leadership to the extent that they are capable. If they can support one another during sharing, express how they feel about one another during processing, notice similarities and differences during generalizing, and offer ideas to each other about application, they will then learn a lot more than if the leader does all these things for them. The leader can get the group members to interact by indirectly encouraging them or by asking them to do so directly (e.g., the leader might ask, "Susan, what do you think of Peter's drawing?" or "Peter, what do you think the group had in common?"). Often, the leader only needs to ask questions a few times in order for the group to understand what is expected.

A leader who does all the talking in this seven-stage group is working too hard. It benefits both the leader and the group by getting the group to talk more. Members who interact, respond, and ask questions are showing their enthusiasm and helping others to become enthusiastic also. With the leader's guidance, the group can help accomplish many of its goals through interaction.

Setting Limits

This has to do with how the leader exerts authority over the group. The goal is to achieve a balance between control and leniency.

Assuming Appropriate Authority

The leader should assume appropriate authority, guiding the group through all its stages, while giving members the freedom to express their thoughts, feelings, and opinions. A good leader will guide the group assuredly, but will not dominate or intimidate its members. Neither does a good leader allow herself to be dominated by the group. If the group goes its own way unguided, the members will not learn and make therapeutic change, and the group may never reach its goals.

Equal Time

Another part of setting limits is allowing sufficient time for each member to contribute. There are always a few members of a group who seem to take up more time and attention than the others. It is up to the therapist to see that all the members have a chance to participate. The leader controls the pace of the group and lets members know when they are taking more than their share of the time available. In this way, the group can be guided through each stage and can end on time.

Limiting Inappropriate Behavior

Limiting inappropriate behavior is perhaps the most difficult for students to learn. It generally requires that the leader interrupt the process going on in order to request that it be changed. If Joe has embarked on a lengthy discussion about a staff member who has treated him unfairly, but the issue has nothing to do with the goals of the group, it may be necessary for the leader to stop him and redirect the group back to the task at hand.

Respectful Limit Setting

Limits are best set with respect, and without anger, so that the group members will not become defensive. The therapist should develop skill in empathizing with the offending patient. When the leader asks Joe to stop his tirade about the staff member, it is more likely to be heard if she first acknowledges his anger: "Joe, it sounds like you're very angry at ____, and I'd be happy to listen to you tell me about it after the group. But for now, I'd like to hear what all the members have to say about leisure planning." Other types of inappropriate behavior might be members showing disrespect for or disinterest in one another or physical expressions of emotion.

One important principle to keep in mind is always put the good of the group first. When individuals behave in ways that distract the group from benefiting in an occupational therapy activity, the leader is obligated to intervene on behalf of the group. Techniques for dealing with specific patient behaviors that are difficult will be discussed in the next chapter.

Leadership Styles

The leadership style a therapist uses will profoundly affect the outcome of the group. Furthermore, different frames of reference require very different leadership approaches. Knowing the characteristics of several approaches and their likely effects on the group allows us to be flexible and use our skills more effectively to achieve desired outcomes.

According to Lewin and colleagues (1938, 1939), there are three fundamental leadership styles: autocratic, democratic, and laissez-faire. Autocratic leadership implies complete control of the group with little or no input from the members. Democratic leadership allows members to make choices and to have a say in what the group does and becomes. Laissez-faire is a French expression meaning literally "to let do" or to let the people do as they choose. Laissez-faire leadership implies a minimum of control and a deliberate non-inter-

ference in the natural forces of a group or the freedom of individuals within it. Lewin studied the effects of these three styles of leadership at a boys' summer camp. He found that autocratic leadership resulted in the greatest productivity, but created hostility and resentment, poor quality of work, and dependency on the leader. Laissez-faire leadership produced independence in the members, but morale was not very high. It was democratic leadership that resulted in the highest morale and the most group cohesiveness. However, Lewin's study should be understood in the context of the boys' camp. The democratic style that worked best for campers may not work for other populations of subjects, and other styles may be more appropriate.

Three types of occupational therapy group leaderships will be presented in this text: director, facilitator, and adviser. All may be defined democratic in spirit, but with varying amounts of member input. Each is appropriate in different situations and for different levels of patient functioning.

Directive Leadership

In politics, an autocratic leader rules a dictatorship; he fashions the nation according to his own vision, setting up the structures of government and making all the decisions. In therapy, it would not be ethical or desirable to hold this much control over a group of patients. However, as a director, the occupational therapist defines a group, selects activities, and structures the group in ways which she knows to be therapeutically appropriate for a specific group of patients. The director uses authority sparingly, only as necessary to make the group therapeutic for its members. Used inappropriately, too much direction can cause members to feel infantilized, treated like children who cannot think for themselves; it can stunt the growth and development of a group by crushing attempts to question or challenge the leader.

However, directive leadership is absolutely necessary for the lower functioning patients who do not have the cognitive capabilities to make decisions or solve problems. These patients do not feel safe when the therapist is not in control. In a sense, the therapist is always in control, even in the more democratic approaches. The leader sets the goals, the level of structure, the media used, and the extent to which leadership responsibilities are shared with the group. The therapist's decisions about how to lead are, hopefully, based not only on her own preference or style, but on the therapist's expert assessment of the needs of the group. For example, Allen (1985) suggests that the therapist structure the environment and the task demand, but within that context, allow patients to do as much as they can for themselves. If the therapist is knowledgeable about Allen's theory, she will be able to predict fairly accurately how much assistance the patients will need to accomplish a task, and will plan the structure of the group accordingly. (Note: the term "directive" as used here does **not** relate to Kaplan's "directive group," which is discussed in Chapter 9.)

Facilitative Leadership

The next style of leadership on the control vs. freedom continuum is democratic. Just as the democratic leader is voted into power by the citizens, a facilitator gathers support from constituents. The leader must convince the members of the group that she is on their side and represents their best interests. The facilitator earns the support of the members by allowing them to make choices and showing care and concern. Decisions are made by the

group with the facilitator's guidance. The therapist is a resource person, providing the group with needed information, needed structure, and needed equipment and supplies. The occupational therapy facilitator openly discusses the purpose and goals of the group. Just as a democratic government presumes and requires a certain level of education in its citizens in order to work effectively, democratic leadership in therapy requires that the members have a certain level of knowledge and skill. Without the required knowledge, members cannot make good decisions or share the leadership effectively. Thus, the role of a facilitator is also that of an educator. The therapist explains the therapeutic aspects of activity so that the group can choose tasks that are likely to be of benefit to them.

Lewin said that democratic leadership is the most likely to lead to group cohesiveness. This is confirmed in reviewing the group developmental process (further described in Chapter 2). As a group reaches the "control" phase, members must challenge the leadership, the structure, and/or the group task. A facilitator can allow herself to be challenged, use reason and logic to explain the way things have been, and give the group choices about changing them in ways that are not destructive to the group's integrity.

Group facilitation also has its limitations. It is not suitable for patients functioning at a low cognitive level. It presumes a certain level of self-awareness, intelligence, and insight or self-understanding. It is most useful in frames of reference that make personal direction and choice a priority. The humanistic, psychoanalytic (ego functions), and model of human occupation approaches depend on a facilitative leadership style to facilitate a certain level of independent functioning and decision-making in patient group members. However, when the goals of treatment are to develop specific skills and abilities or to promote neurophysiological or cognitive development, a democratic approach may not be appropriate.

Facilitation is the most useful in motivating patients and getting them involved. It is a widely recognized phenomenon that people tend to be more committed to pursuing goals which they have a part in choosing. The more cognitively aware they are, the more they resent goals that are imposed on them. Therefore, discussions that precede a group may use a facilitative approach as a motivator, even when the group itself is more directive.

Group Leader as Adviser

The adviser is the most passive of the leadership styles. Its use in therapy is limited to the highest functioning groups working on goals like problem-solving or attitude change. An occupational therapy leader/adviser may be appropriate in prevention or health maintenance. Clients who seek assistance with specific problems may need an occupational therapist to advise them on issues such as coping with stress on the job, conserving energy in the home, or eliminating architectural and social barriers. The adviser offers expertise as needed or requested, but does not provide structure or goals. Motivation comes from the group itself, and change is produced intrinsically as a result of the internal processes of each member. Frames of reference for which adviser leadership is most appropriate are psychoanalytic, humanistic, and the model of human occupation.

General Principles of Group Leadership

Leaders of therapy groups, whatever their particular style, have certain obligations to the group. Designing the group is the most obvious of these. This planning phase involves choosing the members, setting or acknowledging the goals, setting the time and place, organizing the environment, and choosing the activity or media (sometimes with help from members). The group protocol described in Chapter 10 serves as a guide for how to design a therapy group. Decisions about the best leadership style to use within a given patient setting are often complex. Table 1-1 may be helpful in choosing the best leadership style for certain member and activity characteristics.

The ongoing functions of the leader are to help the group achieve its goals (task function) and to maintain the group's integrity (maintenance function). The therapist may need to focus the group on the task to prevent it from getting sidetracked. She may have to adapt the activity or task along the way. Maintaining the group can involve the use of many leader skills. Setting group norms, like confidentiality and mutual respect, can be important. Modeling behaviors to be learned or effective interaction skills can help the group communicate and resolve its conflicts. The counseling skills Egan (1986) writes about are all useful in leading a therapeutic group (e.g., accurate empathy, concreteness, genuineness, confrontation, and self-disclosure). These are elaborated on in Chapter 3. Giving members feedback and helping members to give and receive feedback is an important function of the leader. Keeping the communication channels open is vital to the survival and growth of groups. These norms and roles are elaborated on in Chapter 2.

A Leadership Experience for Students

To practice the seven-step group leadership, students may be divided into groups of eight members. Each student should plan and lead a group of his peers for 45

Table 1-1.
Leadership Style Guidelines

Member Characteristics	Directive Leadership	Facilitative Leadership	Advisory Leadership
cognitive level	low	medium-high	high
insight capacity	minimal	fair-good	very good
group maturity	immature	medium-high	mature
verbal skills	poor	average	high
motivation	low	medium	high
Activity Characteristics			
structure	therapist selects activity	therapist and members select activity	members select activity
goals	accomplish task	learn skills from experience	understand process
instruction	therapist demonstrates/ teaches	therapist and members teach process	members seek advice as needed
group maintenance roles	mostly done by therapist	members share in leadership	members lead themselves
feedback	given mostly by therapist	members encouraged to give each other	natural consequences from environment

minutes, followed by a 15-minute feedback session from the instructor (and members). Students who are beginning their professional training should not attempt to play the roles of patients. There are plenty of goals students will find useful to work on in these groups. To help the student plan a group, the Practice Group Plan (Worksheet 1-1) is suggested. Students' leadership skills may be evaluated by using Worksheets 1-2 and 1-3.

Co-Leadership

While leadership skills are best learned individually for practice purposes, students may feel more comfortable facing patient groups in the company of a co-leader. Having a co-leader in an occupational therapy group with six to eight patients has a number of advantages. Some of these are mutual support, increased objectivity, collective knowledge, modeling for each other, and taking different roles.

Advantages of Co-Leadership

1. Mutual support. Even if your co-leader is an inexperienced peer, you will be able to encourage one another and cover for each other's weaknesses. One of you is bound to remember what the other one forgets. Overcoming one's fear of coping with difficult patients and situations in the

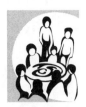

1. Title of group:

2. Purpose of the group:

3. Brief description of activity:

4. Supplies and equipment needed:

5. Goals of the group:

6. Questions for discussion in (at least three in each section):
   - Processing

   - Generalizing

   - Application

7. Points for summary:

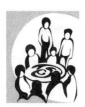

Student Name: _____ Date:_____ Time:_____

Group Title: _____

_____ **Written Group Plan (10 points)**

_____ **Introduction (10 points)**
Explains purpose clearly
Asks for feedback from the group
Uses warm-up to relax/prepare group
Communicates expectations
Outlines timeframe/structure of group

_____ **Activity (10 points)**
Adequately prepared
Directions clearly given
Timing appropriate
Materials appropriate
Environment appropriate

_____ **Sharing (10 points)**
Invites each member to share
Uses appropriate verbal and nonverbal communication
Empathizes and acknowledges feelings of members

_____ **Processing (10 points)**
Elicits members' feelings about the experience
Elicits members' feelings about each other
Elicits members' feelings about the leader (when appropriate)
Helps group understand its own processes

_____ **Generalizing (10 points)**
Points out like or similar responses
Points out contrasts or differences
Develops one or two principles learned

_____ **Group Motivation (10 points)**
Inspires confidence of group
Encourages enthusiasm
Encourages group interaction

_____ **Limit Setting (10 points)**
Allows sufficient time to each member
Limits inappropriate behavior
Assumes appropriate authority (but not too controlling)

_____ **Application (10 points)**
Verbalizes meaning of this experience (significance)
Shows how this experience can relate to everyday life
Relates this experience to issues/problems of members
Uses concrete examples and/or self-disclosure

_____ **Summary (10 points)**
Chooses most important points to emphasize
Verbally reinforces group learning
Acknowledges contributions of members
Ends group on time

_____ **Total Leadership Score**

Member Evaluation Summary (from Worksheet 1-3)
Average leadership score: _____

Summary of strengths:

Summary of weaknesses:

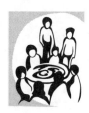

Worksheet 1-3
Member Evaluation of Leader

Directions: This form may be used to obtain reactions of student members prior to discussion of student leader's performance in practice groups. The forms are then collected by the instructor and are considered when rating the student leader. Member evaluations are anonymous.

Date and Time: _____ Title of Activity:_____

How satisfied were you with the way the group was planned and led? (Please check one of the following.)
- ❑ 1 Not at all satisfied
- ❑ 2 Somewhat satisfied
- ❑ 3 Satisfied
- ❑ 4 Very satisfied
- ❑ 5 Extremely satisfied

Please comment on how you found this group experience.

What did you see as the leader's strengths?

What did you see as the leader's weaknesses?

group will be easier when you have a partner to fall back on.

2. Increased objectivity. Much more can be learned by the group when there are two leaders who can compare observations and give each other feedback. An objective understanding of the process of the group will be easier to achieve using both leaders' points of view. This is especially advantageous during supervision.

3. Increased knowledge. Two leaders means twice as much knowledge and experience are available for the group. Both leaders will be able to contribute ideas in the planning stage, as well as providing skilled interventions and leadership during the group itself. A discussion between co-leaders after the group is over is an important learning tool for novice leaders. Yalom (1995) writes that discussion is an "essential ingredient" of a good co-therapy team. He suggests at least 5 minutes before each meeting and 15 to 20 minutes after each meeting be reserved for planning strategy and sharing reflections about each other's behavior during the group. If there are differences of opinion about how to handle difficult patients or interactional problems, this post-group discussion would be the time to work them out. Co-leaders who cannot come to terms with their differences would be well advised to seek out supervision before they re-enter the group arena for another session.

4. Models for each other. Peer co-leaders have much to learn from each other. Every leader has different strengths and weaknesses, as well as different styles of intervention. Co-leader teams can help each other best by taking turns being active or directive and being attentive listeners and observers. In the clinic, students may have practicing therapists as co-leaders; beginning therapists may have experienced co-leaders as models. Each has its obvious advantages. However, ongoing co-leadership teams should eventually equalize their roles so that both are contributing and sharing the responsibility.

5. Different roles. Good co-leadership teams learn to take advantage of each other's strengths by taking on different leadership roles. Some leaders are especially effective in setting limits when group members lose control. Other leaders are better at giving empathetic support. Co-leaders should take turns doing the confronting and rescuing so that no one has to play the "bad guy" all the time.

A much discussed issue in co-leadership is whether or not the group leaders should air their disagreements openly during the group or save them for the post-group discussion. Yalom (1995) points out that timing is the deciding factor here. Newly formed groups should not be exposed to disagreement between the leaders. However, more stable and cohesive groups have much to learn from observing two mature leaders model the open discussion and respectful consideration of their differences of opinion.

Male/female co-leadership can be particularly enlightening to group members when they model different roles. Their interaction during the group generally brings up issues relating to the primary family. They are also prone to the stereotyping of gender roles. That is, typically the female leader is expected to take on supportive and nurturing roles, while the male leader is perceived as critical and judgmental. Male/female co-therapy teams are well advised to share a variety of confrontive and harmonizing roles, so that both are perceived as capable leaders with mutual respect for one another's professional strengths.

Occupational therapists in the clinic may be asked to co-lead groups with professionals from other disciplines. Physicians, psychologists, social workers, nurses, recreation therapists, and dietitians are some of the many possibilities. An OTR and a registered nurse may co-lead a medication education group. A COTA may co-lead a sensory awareness group with a recreation therapist. Each profession brings a different knowledge base and a different point of view. Teams such as these require careful planning to be sure the goals and leadership roles are clear and their attitudes are compatible. Interdisciplinary collaboration has many potential advantages, but also pitfalls for the inexperienced occupational therapist. A well-established professional identity should be in place before attempting to co-lead a group with a person from another discipline. It is not recommended for students.

Disadvantages of Co-Leadership

Although there are many advantages to co-leading groups, the are a few common difficulties to be wary of. These difficulties must be overcome if the co-leadership is to be effective.

1. Splitting. When there are two leaders, group members have a tendency to favor one over the other. Patients often put pressure on one co-leader to take sides against the other. Like children, who, when they are criticized by one parent, turn to the other for refuge, so patients in groups will try to get the co-leaders to disagree or to form alliances with subgroups. Co-leaders should be watchful for such attempts, and openly discuss them in

the group. Not doing so can divide the group and create power struggles, which usually have non-therapeutic consequences.

2. Competition. A certain amount of competition in co-leading a group is normal. Leaders seek to establish themselves as competent therapists, and the approval of others does much to enhance their self-esteem. Student leaders or beginning therapists may be looking for high marks from a supervisor as well. While all competition is not a bad thing, open communication about the feelings it evokes between co-leaders is necessary in order to avoid destructive consequences.

3. Unequal contribution. This disadvantage occurs when one leader does most of the work, while the other sits back and watches. Resentment is bound to develop on both sides. Students have often complained of this problem during supervision of fieldwork experiences. In resolving this dilemma, it must first be acknowledged that both parties are to blame. Once again, the problem must be openly discussed and supervision sought as needed. The partner who is more active may not see the situation as problematic. It is usually the silent partner who feels uncomfortable and increasingly afraid to speak up. Often the passive leader feels dominated by her partner, prevented from doing her part in leading the group, and deprived of the opportunity for needed experience. This problem does not resolve itself and only grows worse as time goes on. Considerable effort and determination on both sides must be given to set aside the blame and to equalize the balance of leadership in fairness to the group members.

Stages of Co-Leadership

Lessler, Dick, and Whiteside (1979) studied the development of the co-therapy relationship. They identified four developmental stages, which parallel the group's development (described in Chapter 2).

1. Formative stage. In this stage, co-leaders are preoccupied with their feelings of self-worth as a leader and plagued by fears of inadequacy. These feelings naturally lead co-leaders to compete with one another. By trying too hard to be "good" leaders, they could end up in a power struggle with one another or a popularity contest with the group members.

2. Development stage. The process of getting comfortable with one another requires much interpersonal discussion and the recognition of differences. This stage must be resolved if the co-therapy team is to work effectively together.

3. Stabilization. After having their fights and talking it out, co-therapists view each other as individuals and recognize each other's strengths and weaknesses as well as their own. They are able to capitalize on their differences by taking on different leadership roles and discussing their perceptions openly during the group as well as afterwards.

4. Refreshment. From the process of the first three stages, a relationship between co-leaders forms that allows each to grow in his role as leader. Their interaction results in renewed enthusiasm for the group experience and its potential to help others. They may experiment with new ideas, do research together, or present their group experiences at professional meetings. They take pride and enjoyment from working with each other, and this energizes the group members

with a sense of hope and anticipation. The lesson from this classic research outcome is that competition in co-leadership can lead to a positive outcome when it is openly discussed and dealt with constructively. However, some leaders may find that after a few sessions they are incompatible as partners. If mutual respect cannot be achieved through discussion of differences, it is best to find another co-leader. The focus of the group should be therapy for its members, not training for the co-leaders.

Co-leadership has many advantages in practice. However, co-leaders should be chosen carefully and matched for compatibility. Students are advised to master individual leadership first, before attempting co-leadership of groups. Those who take on the co-leadership should be prepared to work hard, be open to feedback, and take time to discuss the issues of working together on a regular basis.

Conclusion

Although the seven steps of group leadership are described without reference to theory, it should be noted that no approach is entirely atheoretical. The theoretical basis for this approach has some elements of the humanistic, as well as the behavioral cognitive, frames of reference. It has a sequence of steps that may be seen as developmental in their hierarchical order. These frames of reference (humanistic, behavioral cognitive, and developmental) and their application to occupational therapy groups will be discussed in later chapters. The seven-step approach is not intended to meet all needs for all patients. It can be adapted in many ways to reflect differing patients, goals, and frames of reference.

Section Two will review several frames of reference occupational therapists have used to guide them in planning and leading groups. However, students often understand theory best when it relates to their experience. Therefore, it is suggested that students learn to lead groups first. They can practice their skills by leading groups of their peers. To accomplish this, a seven-step sequence in leading groups has been described. This approach assumes a fairly high level of function among members. Members must be able to communicate with each other, trust and relate to each other, and think abstractly. A high degree of cooperation and motivation is assumed. The approach is well suited to college students, as well as physically disabled patients, substance abuse patients, patients with eating disorders, and many other groups who are operating at a fairly high cognitive level.

Bibliography

Allen, C. (1985). *Occupational therapy for psychiatric diseases: Measurement and management of cognitive disabilities.* Boston: Little, Brown and Co.

Egan, G. (1986). *The skilled helper* (3rd ed.). Monterey, CA: Brooks/Cole.

Johnson, D., & Johnson, F. (1987). *Joining together: Group theory and group skills* (3rd ed.). Englewood Cliffs, NJ: Prentice-Hall.

Korb-Khalsa, Azok, & Leutenberg. (1989). *Life management skills* (Vols. I through IV). Beachwood, OH: Wellness Reproductions Inc.

Lessler, K., Dick, R., & Whiteside, J. (1979). Stages of cooperation: Co-therapy viewed developmentally. *Transactional Analysis Journal, 9,* 1, 67-73.

Lewin, & Lippitt. (1938). An experimental approach to the study of autocracy and democracy: A preliminary note. *Sociometry, I,* 292-300.

Lewin, Lippitt, & White. (1939). Patterns of aggressive behavior in experimentally created social climates. *Journal of Social Psychology, 10,* 271-299.

Mosey, A. (1981). *Occupational therapy: Configuration of a profession.* New York: Raven Press.

Pfeiffer, J., & Jones, J. (1973). *Reference guide to handbooks and annuals.* La Jolla, CA: University Associates.

Pfeiffer, J., & Jones, J. (1977). *Reference guide to handbooks and annuals* (2nd ed.). La Jolla, CA: University Associates.

Posthuma, B. (1989). *Small groups in therapy settings: Process and leadership.* Toronto: Little, Brown & Co.

Raths, L., Harmin, M., & Simon, S. (1978). *Values and teaching* (2nd ed.). Columbus, OH: Merrill.

Rider, B. (1995). *Activities card file.* (2nd ed.). Available from Barbara Rider, 2618 Winchell Ave., Kalamazoo, MI 49008, 616-344-6471.

Simmons, P., & Mullins, L. (1981). *Acute psychiatric care: An occupational therapy guide to exercises in daily living skills.* Thorofare, NJ: SLACK Incorporated.

Simon, S., Howe, L., & Kirschenbaum, H. (1972). *Values clarification.* New York: A&W Publishers.

Stevens, J. (1971). *Awareness.* Moab, UT: Real People Press.

Yalom, I. (1995). *Theory and practice of group psychotherapy* (4th ed.). New York: Basic Books.

Understanding Group Dynamics

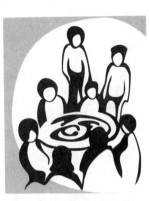

The large body of knowledge regarding group dynamics developed by behavioral scientists over the past 50 years offers a great deal of help in our understanding of how groups work. This body of knowledge comes from a variety of theoretical bases, most commonly, humanistic, behavioral, and psychoanalytic. Because of the verbal nature of the groups being researched, some assumptions have been made about the populations upon which these theories are based. Although even the most dysfunctional groups achieve some level of social organization, members of a group who have verbal skills and are capable of interaction can more easily demonstrate the dynamics described. Another assumption is that when there is enough freedom within the group structure for members to initiate and make choices, the dynamics will be more obvious. A third assumption is that the members are intrinsically motivated to self-improve through self-understanding and by increasing their interaction skills. All of these assumptions are similar to those in

the humanistic frame of reference in Chapter 3.

In general, group dynamics are the forces that influence the interrelationships of members and ultimately affect group outcome. It is important for occupational therapists to understand these forces when planning and implementing treatment groups. Groups have predictable stages of development and will respond best to different activities at different stages. As leaders, our recognition of our group's stage of development should influence our selection of activities. How we design and lead groups also depends on our recognition and understanding of the various dynamics. Some of the "dynamics" that will be included in this chapter are: group process, group development, leadership styles, norms and roles, special problems, and termination.

Group membership experiences are emphasized in this chapter so that students can gain an appreciation for what patients might be experiencing under different group conditions. It is hoped that

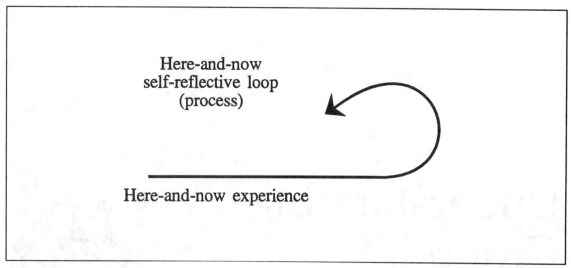

Figure 2-1. Yalom's self-reflective loop.

Group Process

We have already discussed processing as one step in group leadership. An awareness of the underlying process of groups is essential to our approach as therapists. It gives us many clues as to the feelings and motives of members and helps the therapist to make patients aware of these and their impact on wellness and on group function. Irvin Yalom (1985) has written a great deal about the process of psychotherapy groups.

Process is often first understood by what it is not. It is not content. The content of a group is what is done and what is said. For example, the group did pencil drawings and topics discussed were the jobs members had and how they liked them. Bob said he likes being a carpenter, but Sarah hates being a teacher. Process does not include past history or even recent history of the members. Its thrust is what is happening in the group, between and among members, right now. Process concerns the interpersonal relationships of the participants with each other.

There are two parts to process in groups, according to Yalom: "If the powerful therapeutic factor of interpersonal learning is to be set into motion, the group must recognize, examine, and understand process. It must study itself, it must study its own transactions, it must transcend pure experience and apply itself to the integration of that experience" (Yalom, 1985, p. 136). So the process is experienced first, and then it "performs a self-reflective loop," examining what just occurred. The "processing" step in the preceding chapter represents a simplified self-reflective loop (Figure 2-1). Members are asked to reveal how they felt about the activity they just experienced, as well as how they felt about the leader and each other. So the process commentary begins. Its emphasis is often on emotion and its purpose is to establish a cognitive framework that permits members to retain the group experience so that it can be generalized and applied.

The process comments are largely the responsibility of the therapist. She can and should request member participation, but she chooses the direction of intervention according to the needs of the group.

membership experiences will help occupational therapy students to be more observant and empathetic group leaders.

Example

In a task group, the occupational therapist had taken considerable time in helping the group plan their next activity. They were going to construct kites. The plan for Monday was to walk to a craft store (about four blocks from the hospital) to buy paper, string, sticks, and paint. The kites would be constructed during the next two sessions. The seven members of the group assembled with jackets and sneakers ready for the walk. Hannah, age 63, the eldest member of the group, was not feeling well and refused to go. Dave, a 23-year-old member, bluntly asked the therapist if Hannah was too sick to walk. The reply was that she was fine medically. So Dave proceeded to call Hannah a "lazy, do-nothing complainer." The other members verbally attacked Dave for his rudeness and insensitivity to the elder member, and a heated argument ensued until it was too late to carry out the plan.

Content

As an occupational therapy leader, how would you process this group? First, it is helpful to identify content. What was the overt experience? The group came prepared to walk to the craft store as planned. The plan was not carried out because Hannah refused to go. What was verbalized? Dave was verbally abusive to Hannah. The other members verbally attacked Dave for being abusive, and he defended himself with counterattacks, shouting loudly at the group. The virtue of courtesy to one's elders was discussed.

Process

The process involves what is implied by the content. The therapist might consider the following possibilities.

1. Hannah wanted some attention and chose to pursue it by her passivity. Perhaps her refusal was her way of exerting control over the group, or perhaps illness is her usual way of getting attention.
2. The other group members were frustrated at not being able to carry out their plan and were looking for someone to blame.
3. Hannah was to blame, but she seemed too frail and vulnerable to be verbally accused.
4. Dave was impatient and expressed his frustration aggressively. Perhaps aggressiveness is his usual way of coping with frustration, a habit that often gets him in trouble. Perhaps he feels guilt and is looking for a way to be punished.
5. The group's frustration, diverted from Hannah by her vulnerability, was vented on Dave instead. Dave was made the scapegoat of the group. A scapegoat is something that symbolizes all the badness of the group, or someone who is blamed for its problems. The scapegoat generally serves the purpose of allowing the group to avoid its own responsibility for what has occurred.
6. Perhaps the group wanted to avoid either the walk or the activity. Dave and Hannah gave them an excuse to avoid doing any task-oriented problem-solving.

Needs to Be Addressed

Which hypothesis is correct? Any or all of them are. How, then, should the therapist intervene to help the group understand its process? The first thing a leader should ask herself is "What does this group really need?" Here are some possible needs to be addressed:

1. The foremost need is to get Dave off the "hot seat." He may have been rude and aggressive, making him an easy target for the group, but he is

certainly not the direct cause of their frustration. If Dave is not rescued, he will probably be forced out of the group and will be left feeling angry and hurt. Being scapegoated is not a therapeutic experience.

For Dave, the therapist might point out how his behavior tends to elicit this kind of response from others, and how he set himself up to be the scapegoat. For the members of the group, the therapist might discuss their feelings about Hannah. They need to understand why they avoided blaming her, how they ended up in a struggle with Dave, and what they themselves were avoiding by pursuing the argument.

2. The therapist might then want to examine the issue of Hannah's control. What are her real needs (e.g., attention, respect), and how might they be pursued more appropriately? An awareness of her pattern of controlling others with her illness, real or otherwise, might be very helpful as a beginning step toward therapeutic change. The group's collusion with her in achieving her goal to keep the group from acting is another important issue. Why did they allow her to exert such control? What purpose did it serve for them? Why did they not exclude her instead of Dave?

3. The final issue of importance is the group's relationship to the task. How did they feel about the activity they chose? Were they really that invested? Or were they looking for an excuse not to pursue it? What were the group's choices? Could they have found an alternative way to get their supplies? Could they have reorganized their roles so that Hannah would not have to go on the walk, without excluding her from the group

as a whole? If walking is important to them in getting out of the hospital to enjoy the spring weather, perhaps Hannah could have been wheeled in a wheelchair, or she could have walked part of the way and then waited with another member.

If the group is to learn from this rather frustrating and upsetting experience, it is evident that members need the occupational therapist's guidance in problem-solving. Finding alternative solutions and compromising are essential if the group is to accomplish its task. Steps should be taken before the end of this group session to avoid a recurrence of frustration in the next session.

Discovering the Process of Groups

The best way for students to learn about group process is to experience it. Therefore, a real example taken from a student group experience is best used for this exercise. However, if that is not available, the student may use the following example. Use Worksheet 2-1 to evaluate the experience.

The group was engaged in doing an assertiveness exercise. All the members had anonymously written down situations on a card and put them in a basket in the center of the table. Members had to draw a card, read it, and tell what they would do to assertively handle the situation described on the card. Mary drew a card and read it to the group. It said, "On my fieldwork experience, I was working with two patients and one of them started to cry. I didn't know why she was crying so I ran down the hall to find a nurse, leaving the two patients alone in the clinic. I couldn't believe that my supervisor, Miss Hunt, failed me for leaving the patients alone." Mary looked bewildered. "How could the supervisor expect you to know

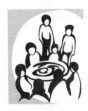

Worksheet 2-1
Content-Process Reaction

Directions: Write the answers to these questions after you have participated in the group session.

I. Content
   A. Give a brief description of the activity.

   B. Identify three major participants and what topics they discussed. If there were more than three, choose the three you think were most important.
      1. Person:
         Topic:
         Others offering feedback:
         Approximate length of time:
      2. Person:
         Topic:
         Others offering feedback:
         Approximate length of time:
      3. Person:
         Topic:
         Others offering feedback:
         Approximate length of time:

II. Process
   A. Name three feelings you personally experienced during the group. To whom or what were the feelings directed?
      1.
      2.
      3.

   B. Based on your observations of verbal and nonverbal behavior, what are some hypotheses (possible explanations or interpretations) about the process of the group?
      1.
      2.
      3.
      4.
      5.

   C. Based on the above hypotheses, what therapeutic intervention(s) would you make as a leader and why?

Table 2-1.
Summary of Group Development Theories

	Stage 1	Stage 2	Stage 3	Stage 4
Tuckman (1965)	Forming	Storming	Norming	Performing
Bion (1961)	Flight	Fight	Unite	
Schutz (1958)	Inclusion	Control	Affection	
Yalom (1985)	Orientation	Conflict	Harmony	Maturity

what to do? You're just a student." Maureen, another member said, "How could the student be so stupid? If she doesn't know what to do, she shouldn't be in occupational therapy." Susan added, "But I had Miss Hunt, too. She's really a hard nose." Several others commented on Miss Hunt's inadequacy as a supervisor. Laurie agreed with Maureen, "Yes, but the student should have known better." Roberta listened silently to this debate, looking more and more distressed as the end of the session approached.

Group Development

Group development refers to the stages groups go through as they progress from initiation to termination. Several theorists have contributed to this aspect of groups, including Tuckman, Bion, Schutz, and Yalom (Table 2-1). Knowing the characteristics of each stage helps the therapist know what to expect. It helps him predict how the group will respond to certain activities, and therefore plan appropriately.

Research shows that all groups progress through a series of predictable stages. Many theories have been suggested as to what these stages are, and in fact, all seem to have similar characteristics. There is an initial stage of orientation, with its search for structure, goals, and dependency on the leader. Next, there is a stage of conflict with its struggle for dominance and rebellion against the leader. Then there is a growth of interpersonal harmony and intimacy, sometimes called cohesiveness. The final outcome is a mature working group characterized by high cohesiveness and commitment to the goals of the group-therapeutic learning.

Our knowledge of group development comes from a collection of studies including observations of therapy groups, training groups (educational), natural groups, and laboratory groups.

Tuckman

Tuckman (1965) published the first major review of these studies from which he abstracted a theory of four stages of group development:

1. Forming
2. Storming
3. Norming
4. Performing

Tuckman believed that all the stages occur in some way regardless of the duration of the group (i.e., shorter length groups impose the requirement of the problem-solving stages to be reached quickly), therefore, the rate of development tends to adjust to the time available.

Tuckman's initial stage, forming,

involves orientation and testing regarding the group task and a dependence on the leader for guidance. Storming involves conflict among group members as they challenge the task, the rules, and the leader. In the norming stage, harmony prevails and members accept and trust one another while conflicts are avoided. The last stage, performing, goes beyond cohesiveness to a point where conflict can be openly discussed and resolved. A performing group can effectively work together in a supportive emotional environment that encourages growth and therapeutic change.

Bion

Bion's work is also frequently quoted, especially with the easy-to-remember titles of the stages:
1. Flight
2. Fight
3. Unite

Bion (1961) looked at the behavior of groups at conferences, having a task rather than a therapeutic focus. Flight represents an avoidance of some problem or threat. Members tend to turn to each other in pairs for more intimate emotional response in this stage. The fight stage represents the challenge of the leader (and possibly scapegoating a rival member-leader). Uniting follows these two emotional states; it settles down the members to a stable working group with relatively little emotionality. Bion's work, although emerging from the corporate and industrial arena, has many parallels in the therapeutic group. This may be especially applicable to the occupational therapy group, which, although therapeutic in its goal, tends to be more task focused.

Schutz

Schutz's (1958) theory, while similar to those previously described, tends to have the clearest interpersonal focus. He says that every individual has three interpersonal needs:
1. Inclusion
2. Control
3. Affection

These needs parallel those of a child in the family, and are generalized to any interpersonal relationship among two or more individuals. In other words, groups follow the same sequence of interpersonal concerns as individuals do. Schutz's stages are shown to have both individual and group characteristics.

Inclusion Stage

In the inclusion stage, the individual is concerned with being accepted: "Where do I fit in? Will I be important? Respected? Can I be myself? How will the leader respond to me?" The group behaviors observed are overtalking, attention seeking, territoriality, and individual self-centeredness. Members listen but do not really hear what others say. They tend to look to the leader when they speak rather than each other. In this initial phase the rational approach is dominant; emotions do not flow freely. The group explores the goals, rationale, and structure. The leader is looked to for the answers. There are multiple attempts at sizing each other up. Members look for similarities and tend to downplay differences. There is concern over those who have not made a contribution, and rightly so; if members are continually passive, they can become blockers to the progress of the group as a whole.

Control Stage

Schutz's control stage also has individual and group concerns. The individual now questions "Where do I stand in relation to power and authority? How much influence do I have? Will I have too much responsibility?" The group is generally, at some point, engaged in a leadership struggle. The once "all-powerful-and-all-knowing leader" (therapist) is now viewed with skepticism and mistrust.

If the leader abdicates, that is, gives up the leadership, a struggle among members ensues to fill the void. Scapegoating of a would-be leader is common, and attempts to lead are often met with severe criticism or are ignored. Members often disagree about how much structure is needed or how the group should be led, and subgroups may arise. There is ambivalence about the leader; like a 2-year-old child, the group at once wants to be autonomous but needs the leader's support and protection.

The importance of all this for occupational therapists is in knowing that rebellion and challenge among group members are normal and necessary to the healthy development of the group. Be prepared to be challenged, and do not take it as a personal affront. How then, should we as occupational therapists handle the challenge? There are three choices.

1. An adviser as leader would tend to back down, to abdicate leadership. To do so invites intragroup conflict which could be more stressful than patients can handle.
2. A director would subdue the rebellion. In this case the therapist remains the leader and encourages further dependency of the group. Such an approach has been known to stifle group development.
3. The democratic leader would not abdicate all the control, but would encourage the group to share the leadership.

The third is Yalom's approach. He states that the group needs to experience the freedom and the responsibility for the group outcome. He suggests the leader not abdicate, but allow expression of dissension and acknowledge it. The therapist should "take the blows" and not allow any group members to become a scapegoat. Ideally, the therapist will make some changes in response to the group to allow the conflict to resolve while preserving the integrity of the group.

Affection Stage

If the conflict in leadership is resolved successfully, the group progresses to the affection stage. This is the stage of group cohesiveness when attention focuses on "How do others feel about me?" and then "How do we feel about each other?" The group is characterized by expression of positive feeling and emotional investment in the group. Members are able to really listen to each other and even direct hostility may be expressed without devastating consequences.

The affection stage is the goal for any therapy group. Here is where members feel safe, cherished, and trusting in one another. This allows members to explore new behaviors and to grow. They value one another, therefore, they value themselves. There is real altruism and consensual validation; members want to help each other and accept feedback from each other to validate their own self-perceptions. It is part of our role, as occupational therapists, to help our groups to reach this stage.

Nevertheless, there are some real barriers to achieving the affection stage. Schutz tells us that groups tend to regress easily, even after they have reached this stage. Events such as the arrival of a new member, leaving of an old member, leadership changes, and long holidays will all cause a group to regress. Furthermore, patients who are lacking in social and interpersonal skills and/or who are unable to trust others may be incapable of reaching the affection stage. Anticipation of termination of the group inevitably causes the development to reverse. A cohesive group may sink once again into conflict in preparation for breaking the ties and moving on.

How Groups Reach Maturity

Why should occupational therapists study group development? There are several reasons. First, understanding the progression to maturity in groups gives us something to strive for; it shows us the true capacity of a mature, cohesive group. As therapists we should do whatever we can to help the group reach a mature, working stage. Corey, Corey, Callanan, and Russel (1988) suggest one way to speed up the process is to prepare members to get the most from a group. These guidelines are helpful to students participating in a group lab and may be kept in mind as suggestions for our higher functioning patients. Some of the suggestions are summarized as follows.

Have a Focus

Think about what you would like to get from the group, what issues you would like to explore, and changes you would like to make. Writing down your goals prior to each group is often helpful.

Pay Attention to Feelings

Groups are an opportunity to explore personal issues that are often heavily laden with emotion. Many times it is the emotions that emerge that offer important insights and an opportunity for personal growth. The group is not a place to censor expression of emotions, but rather to let them flow. Feelings that are bottled up session after session will eventually "dam up the flow of the group" (Corey et al., 1988, p. 48).

Be an Active Participant

"You will help yourself most if you take an active role in the group. Silent observers are not as likely to get as much from their participation in the group, and others may believe their silence means they are being judgmental" (Corey et al., 1988, p. 48).

Give Feedback

Whether positive or negative, your honest and direct response to others will move the group toward a deeper level of trust. Occupational therapists look forward to a long career of giving constructive feedback to patients. It is essential for occupational therapy students to develop the skill of giving honest feedback in ways that are empathetic and respectful of the other member.

Be Open to Feedback

Others in the group may not have perfected the art of giving constructive feedback. When someone responds honestly but bluntly, it is natural to get defensive in justifying your own standard and therefore to reject their feedback. Instead of letting defenses sabotage your work in the group, use the group as an opportunity to discover your defenses, which might include "rationalizing, withdrawing, denying, or turning a specific criticism into a global 'I'm no good'"(Corey et al., 1988, p. 51). Try to get beyond your defenses and learn to use feedback constructively.

Take Responsibility for What You Accomplish

It is easy to blame others when you are bored, annoyed, or unable to self-disclose in the group. Take a look at your own contribution to this state of affairs, and instead of blaming the group, think about what you could do to make things better. You have a great deal of control and choice about how you interact with others in the group, and in the final analysis, what you accomplish is up to you. Corey's suggestions are some individual behaviors and beliefs that can help groups move toward cohesiveness. We as occupational therapists have many activities at our disposal that encourage the group to move in the direction of cohesiveness. An example is the structured group activity called "Giving and Receiving Feedback" (Session 3 in Chapter 11).

Secondly, because the stages are predictable, knowledge of group development prepares us for what is coming next. It makes us better able to plan occupational therapy activities that are appropriate at each stage of development. For example, a "Trust Circle" exercise, requiring members to intentionally fall into the arms of other group members and trust that they will be protected, may not be a good activity to introduce in the control stage of a group. Even the best laid plans might have to be changed because of changes in the stage of the group's development. For example, in a student training group, I had planned a structured exercise in setting priorities for the sixth session of the group. The group had developed beyond the control stage to a level of intimacy that made them almost cohesive. Sharing their priorities seemed too superficial so they rejected it and modified the activity to a discussion of how to rescue their troubled relationships. The group let me know very quickly that they needed to deal with something on a deeper level.

Another reason for studying group development is that the role of the leader changes with each stage. As occupational therapy leaders, we need to know what to expect. Imagine if you were a student leading a group and one week the patients all decided to rebel against you. Suppose you did not know that this is a normal process for groups? How would you feel? One student leading a time management

group for substance abusers was faced with a patient uprising. Quite unexpectedly, several members of the group refused to do the prescribed activity. Rather than forcing them to do it, she changed the agenda to a discussion of what they did and did not like about the group. This student did not get defensive (fortunately) but listened intently to the patients' complaints and wrote down their suggestions. Group development theory had given this student some guidelines about how to handle the conflict. She knew she could not give up her leadership role, but neither was there any way she was going to force six grown men to do an activity they did not want to do. By listening to them and taking them seriously, she allowed them to challenge her in a way that did not threaten her and did not threaten the integrity of the group either. The following week they were able to approach the activity (one they themselves had suggested) with renewed interest and enthusiasm.

Identifying Group Stages

A good way to learn about the stages of group development is to reflect on a group one has participated in for several sessions. If the group meets for 10 weeks, the self-reflection about the stage of development should not start until at least the fifth session. If the stages are discussed too soon, before the conflicts begin, the discussion will not be meaningful. Furthermore, too close a scrutiny will make the group self-conscious and therefore, inhibit its flow. The leader takes her cue from the group itself in the timing of a discussion of developmental stages.

As a self-learning tool, the student group member might look at the characteristics of each stage and see if these behaviors can be found in her group. Table 2-2 may be useful in assisting with this process. As behaviors are recognized,

Table 2-2.
Schutz's Stages of Development of Groups

I. Inclusion - behaviors
  1) Depend on leader to structure
  2) Look to leader for answers
  3) Rational approach dominates
       discuss topics/opinions/thoughts
       avoid feelings
       look for purpose/goals for group
  4) Individual behaviors predominate
       attention-getting or withdrawal
       humor/laughter
       territoriality/pairing
       talking but not listening
       referring back to prior experiences
  5) Search for similiarities
       energy is in keeping harmony
       find "what we agree on"
       avoid conflicts
  6) Concern over belonging/approval
       only say what will be accepted
       eye contact, verbalize mostly with leader
       seating changes frequently

II. Control - behaviors
  1) Ambivalence toward leader
       challenge structure/purpose
       challenge leader style
       challenge authority of leader
       test limits/rules
       need for leader protection/approval
  2) Disenchantment with group
       subgroups struggle among selves
       leader viewed with distrust
       members critical and discounting of group
  3) Sharing group responsibility
       dependence-independence struggle
       members share leadership functions
       suggestions for change in structure and task emerge
       member-leaders emerge
       competition, not cooperation, predominates
       leader bends will of group

III. Affection - behaviors
  1) Focus on feeling
       express feelings about each other
       express feelings about the leader
       consensual validation occurs
       direct hostility expressed constructively
  2) Delight in company of others
       identity with group
       feel one is lovable and loved
       concern that one is not lovable and not loved
       altruistic desire to help others
       separation anxiety
       new behaviors are explored

examples of these in one's own group may be cited. Generally, if three or four of the behaviors are present for a given stage, that one is likely to be correct. As an example, my student group lab was scheduled to do the "Giving and Receiving Feedback" exercise. Some of them questioned if they were ready for it. They claimed they did not know each other well enough to say anything critical. They asked me to allow them to modify the activity so they would not have to say anything negative. A few said, with hostility, they would just have to "make something up." A few others counterattacked with the rationale that they would soon have to give constructive feedback to patients and this would give them some practice. I did not allow them to modify the activity but did allow them to vent their frustrations and fears and make their suggestions. Clarification and examples were given on how to give constructive feedback. The activity was carried out with a great deal of anxiety, but ending in relief when it was "not as hard as we thought." Considering this example, try the Group Development Evaluation (Worksheet 2-2)

Group Norms and Roles

Norms

Norms are present in every group; they incorporate certain attitudes and standards of behavior that are acceptable to the group. Norms may be specified and verbalized by the leader, or they may not be verbalized but only implied by the behavior and interactions of members. The norms of a group may change as it develops or as members come and go. The therapist's awareness of the norms and their acceptance by the group helps him understand better the behaviors observed in the members.

The leader is responsible for establishing explicit ground rules for the group, like being on time and respecting the opinions of others. These are expectations the leader will announce at the outset and enforce as the group continues. Confidentiality has been mentioned earlier as a common explicit norm of groups. This means that what members say and do during group sessions should not be revealed or discussed with non-members. The agreement to keep group work confidential is an extension of the patient-therapist relationship: what patients say and do is considered privileged information. Knowing this, the patients can trust one another and are more likely to open up to the group.

Non-explicit norms are more elusive because they are seldom verbalized. These may even be beyond the group's awareness. They may be understood in terms of behaviors that are acceptable or non-acceptable in the group. For example, the avoidance of conflict may be a norm in the beginning stages of groups. Certain topics may be considered taboo, to be discouraged or avoided. Norms develop in all groups, therapeutic or otherwise. Yalom points out that the norms of a therapy group are radically different from the rules of etiquette in social groups. In therapy, not only must members interact freely, they must also feel free to comment spontaneously on their immediate feelings about each other and the leader. Yalom describes the desirable norms of a therapy group as "active involvement in the group, non-judgmental acceptance of others, extensive self-disclosure, desire for self-understanding, dissatisfaction with present modes of behavior, and eagerness for change" (Yalom, 1985, p. 117). These norms do not develop automatically. The leader uses considerable influence to shape the norms of a therapy group, with necessary help from its members.

Furthermore, the leader should closely

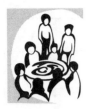

Worksheet 2-2
Group Development Evaluation

Directions: List six different behaviors or events in the group in the first column. Then in the second column, identify the stage of development in which this behavior would best be categorized using Schutz's stages (1—inclusion, 2—control, 3—affection).

Group Behaviors	Stage 1, 2, or 3
1.	
2.	
3.	
4.	
5.	
6.	

Stage of development for this group is _____.

From Cole, M. B. *Group Dynamics in Occupational Therapy, Second Edition.* © 1998 SLACK Incorporated.

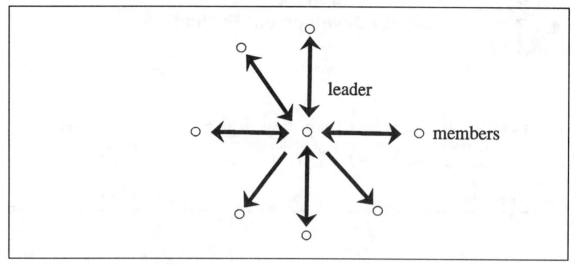

Figure 2-2. Leader-centered interaction.

monitor the non-explicit norms of the group. The adoption of non-therapeutic norms must be avoided at all costs, because once norms are established, they are very difficult to change. The therapist is the key influence in shaping norms. Yalom suggests that therapists do this in two ways: as a technical expert and as the model-setting participant.

As technical expert, the therapist relies on her experience and knowledge to introduce therapeutic norms and the reasons for them. Then, as the group goes on, the therapist may use social reinforcers to encourage the enactment of therapeutic norms, while discouraging anti-therapeutic norms. For example, one pattern that should be discouraged is the group members speaking only to the leader. We have already learned that dependence on the leader is a characteristic of the early stages of groups. A typical picture of this interaction is shown in Figure 2-2.

In the earliest stages, the leader establishes a norm of group interaction in several ways. She can refuse to answer the questions of members and reflect these to other members. For example, Mary asks the leader, "What are we supposed to talk

about?" The leader does not answer, but responds with a question, "What might be some meaningful issues to talk about today?" As members begin to give their ideas, the therapist might ask, "Mary, what do you think about Sally's idea?" or "Sally, why don't you give Bill some feedback about his suggestion?" In this way, the leader tactfully establishes a communication pattern that looks more like Figure 2-3.

Members are speaking not only to the leader, but addressing each other as well. This is an important norm to set in an interactive occupational therapy group, where members are expected to give each other feedback and learn from each other. This norm also helps the group to progress beyond the initial stage of development.

In this example, the therapist has used her role as both technical expert and model-setting participant. The therapist has guided the group by telling members that they should interact with one another, and demonstrated the behaviors by asking specific group members to respond to one another.

Self-disclosure might be another way to

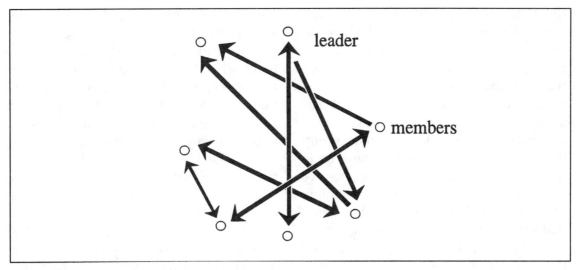

Figure 2-3. Group-centered interaction.

model expected behaviors. When asking members to share their feelings, the leader may begin by sharing her own. Referring to the situation described earlier, the therapist might say: "When Maureen criticized the student for not knowing what to do with a patient who cried, I felt very concerned about how that student was feeling. Yet I was frustrated, because the situation was presented anonymously and I didn't know who wrote it. I didn't want to force this student to reveal herself, but I was afraid she would really be hurt and I wanted to protect her from the attack. I wonder if other members had some of these feelings also." This example demonstrates several expectations. The norm of free expression of emotion in the group is demonstrated by the leader's expression of both concern (fear) and frustration. The focus on the here-and-now is demonstrated in the leader's encouragement of responses to one another within the group about what just occurred. The therapist's encouragement of concern for one another and not allowing members to criticize one another in a hurtful way helps establish a norm of safety and trust. Finally, this self-disclosing comment invites the group to

reflect on its own process, encouraging a norm of self-reflection in the group.

The norms in this example are some of what Yalom considers to be therapeutic norms. Some therapeutic norms Yalom refers to are: self-reflection of the group, encouraging self-disclosure, encouraging free interaction among members, reinforcing the importance of the group, regarding members as agents of change, and setting an atmosphere of safety and support.

Norms will necessarily change in different groups. In occupational therapy groups, norms will vary with the patient populations we deal with and our frame of reference. Norms also change as the group moves through the stages of development. A comment that is unacceptable in Stage 1 may be right on target in Stage 2 or 3. For example, the avoidance of conflict may be normal in Stage 1, but gives way to open criticism of the leader and the group structure in Stage 2. The norm of open conflict in turn gives way to a norm of acceptance of constructive feedback in Stage 3.

If a group is to progress in its development, norms must, from time to time, be challenged. Members who do so are considered to be taking a risk. Risks involve revealing yourself to the group in a way that makes you vulnerable, and taking the chance that you will be accepted and supported. In risks, there is always the chance that you may not get the response you are looking for. For example, after a very tense session in "Giving and Receiving Feedback," Roberta shared with the group that she was rather hurt that someone in the group considered her to be aggressive and intimidating. Another member, Jennifer, took Roberta's cue and shared that she was confused by someone's comment that she was a snob and "looked down her nose" at peers who were not as smart as she was. The comments of Roberta and Jennifer were met with silence. Shortly afterward, the group ended.

What risks did Jennifer and Roberta take? How did the group respond? How do you think the group changed (or should change) as a result of their risk-taking behaviors? What norms did these two students challenge? Use Worksheet 2-3 to evaluate a group experience.

In considering the example of Roberta and Jennifer, it is clear that neither left the group happy. They were both angry and silent during the next group session. The group, left on its own, perhaps would have continued to ignore the behavior, which in some ways threatened the group's status quo. In this case, the therapist has to make some judgment calls. Are Jennifer and Roberta mature and stable enough to handle the group's response or do they need support in continuing to take risks? Is the group ready to change its norms and open up to challenge and conflict? In the group exercise "Giving and Receiving Feedback" (Chapter 11, Session 3), the members' feedback to one another is anonymous. At what point are members ready to accept responsibility for their comments and give up the safety of

anonymity? The leader's intervention should be protective of Roberta and Jennifer and supportive of their vulnerability, while being sensitive to the level of trust within the group. The best intervention, considering these factors, would be to use these members' risk-taking behaviors as a way of encouraging the silent members to take risks also. Only when the writers of the seemingly hurtful comments take the risk of revealing themselves can the issues be discussed and resolved. Members can learn a great deal from this process, not the least of which is learning to give critical feedback in a caring and helpful way, and learning to accept critical feedback as an opportunity to grow and make therapeutic change.

Roles

Roles are the result of the members dividing the work of the group among themselves. Members play roles (e.g., follower, initiator, energizer, and blocker) spontaneously as the group progresses, or roles may be assigned by the leader. Researchers have identified the more frequent roles played in groups and have organized these according to their functions. Some roles tend to help the group accomplish a task, while others help maintain the group's lines of communication. Still other roles tend to interfere with group function, such as an attention seeker or a monopolist. The therapist not only needs to recognize these roles, she should help members take on a variety of roles, and to change those roles that are detrimental to the group. It is often through taking on different roles that much of the therapeutic learning takes place in the group setting.

The concept of group roles was introduced in 1948 by two researchers, Kenneth Benne and Paul Sheats. Their idea was to look at leadership of the group not as sole-

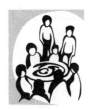

Worksheet 2-3
Monitoring Norms

Directions: As a learning exercise, complete the following after each group experience. Your comments can address many individual and group behaviors, but here are some suggestions: seating pattern, structure and format of the group, timing, silence, topics discussed, communication pattern, expression of emotion, discussion of process, and leader intervention.

List three behaviors that were accepted by the group.
1.

2.

3.

List three behaviors that were not (or would not be) accepted in this group.
1.

2.

3.

List three expectations established by the leader.
1.

2.

3.

List three of your own expectations for this group.
1.

2.

3.

What norms have changed from the last group? Which norms would you like to see changed?
1.

2.

3.

From Cole, M. B. *Group Dynamics in Occupational Therapy, Second Edition.* © 1998 SLACK Incorporated.

ly present in the identified leader or therapist, but as a shared responsibility of all the
members. These writers suggest that "the
quality and amount of group production is
the 'responsibility' of the group...(and) the
setting of goals and the marshaling of
resources to move toward these goals is a
group responsibility in which all members
of a mature group come variously to
share" (Cathcart & Samovar, 1974, p. 180).
Benne and Sheats developed from their
research at the National Training Lab in
Group Development in 1947 their now
classic breakdown of member roles into:

1. Group task roles
2. Group building and maintenance
   roles
3. Individual roles

A group role is a behavior pattern or
structured way of behaving within the
group. Group roles tend to remain stable
regardless of who is in them. Thus, a single group member can take on a variety of
roles within the group, and members can
change their roles as often as they wish.
Since there is a relationship between personality and the roles one typically plays
with others, the roles members find themselves taking on can, themselves, be
revealing. However, the roles are inter-
changeable. Group maturity of the members has been measured by the ability to
take on a variety of group roles.

Group Task Roles

These are the 12 roles that help the
group to get its work done.

1. Initiator-contributor—Suggests new
   ideas, innovative solutions to problems, unique procedures, and new
   ways to organize
2. Information seeker—Asks for clarification of suggestions, focusing on
   facts
3. Opinion seeker—Seeks clarification
   of values and attitudes presented

4. Information giver—Offers facts or
   generalizations "automatically"
5. Opinion giver—States beliefs or opinions
6. Elaborator—Spells out suggestions
   and gives examples
7. Coordinator—Clarifies relationships
   among various ideas
8. Orienter—Defines position of group
   with respect to its goals
9. Evaluator-critic—Subjects accomplishments of group to some standard of group functioning
10. Energizer—Prods the group into
    action or decision
11. Procedural technician—Expedites
    group's movement by doing things
    for the group, such as distributing
    materials, arranging seating
12. Recorder—Writes down suggestions
    and group decisions, acts as the
    "group memory"

Group Building and Maintenance Roles

These are the seven supportive roles
that keep the group functioning together.

1. Encourager—Praises, agrees with,
   and accepts the contributions of others
2. Harmonizer—Mediates the differences between other members
3. Compromiser—Modifies his own
   position in the interest of group harmony
4. Gatekeeper and expediter—Keeps
   communication channels open by
   regulating flow and facilitating participation of others
5. Standard setter—Expresses ideal
   standards for the group to aspire to
6. Group observer and commentator—
   Comments on and interprets the
   process of the group
7. Follower—Passively accepts ideas of
   others and goes along with the movement of the group

Individual Roles

These are opposed to group roles and indicate the use of the group to serve one's individual needs. These roles tend to interfere with group functioning. Benne and Sheats suggest that a high incidence of individual behaviors is symptomatic of various group malfunctions such as: inadequate group skills of members (including the leader); low level of group maturity, discipline, and morale; or an inappropriately chosen and inadequately defined group task. There are eight individual roles defined by these authors.

1. Aggressor—Deflates the status of others; expresses disapproval of the values, acts, or feelings of others; attacks the group or group task, etc.
2. Blocker—Tends to be negativistic or stubbornly resistant, opposing beyond reason or maintaining issues the group has rejected
3. Recognition seeker—Calls attention to self through boasting, acting in unusual ways, or struggling to remain in the limelight.
4. Self-confessor—Uses group as an audience for expressing non-group oriented feelings, insights, or ideologies
5. Playboy—Displays lack of involvement through joking, cynicism, or nonchalance
6. Dominator—Monopolizes group through manipulation, flattery, giving directions authoritatively, or interrupting the contributions of others
7. Help-seeker—Looks for sympathy from the group through unreasonable insecurity, personal confusion, or self-depreciation
8. Special interest pleader—Cloaks her own biases in the stereotypes of social causes, such as the laborer, the housewife, the homeless, or the small businessperson

Admittedly, the group roles are, in part, a function of the group's stage of development. More of the task and maintenance roles can be observed in a mature group than one that is less mature. No statements are made as to the relative value of the various roles. It can be assumed that all roles are equally valuable and necessary to the group's positive outcome. Too many opinion givers and not enough compromisers are likely to create chaos rather than productivity. A well-functioning group needs a balance of roles, and this requires members to take on a mixture of roles that are compatible.

As a learning experience, it is helpful to analyze member roles. This gives members some feedback about what roles they tend to take on in groups and how they are contributing to the group outcome. It is easiest to see roles in groups that require extensive interaction, problem-solving, and decision-making (Worksheet 2-4).

Remember, a single member can take on several roles. After everyone has written down their ideas, group members should compare notes and discuss their answers and the reasons for them. See if the group can reach a consensus about who played which roles.

For further self-awareness, the questions in the Self Role Analysis worksheet (Worksheet 2-5) can be answered concerning your own role in the group. Since flexibility in roles is considered a sign of maturity, it may be set as a goal in groups to have each member try a few new roles over the course of group meetings.

Special Patient Problems

It is evident from our discussion of individual roles that certain member behaviors can interfere with or severely constrict the functioning of groups. Knowledge of group dynamics also helps the leader know how to deal with special problems.

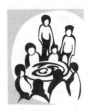

Worksheet 2-4
Role Analysis Exercise

Directions: After your group ends, take a few minutes to identify which members played the various identified roles. Give an example of the behavior that supports your choices.

Group Task Roles

Role	Member Name	Sample Comment or Behavior
1. Initiator-contributor		
2. Information seeker		
3. Opinion seeker		
4. Information giver		
5. Opinion giver		
6. Elaborator		
7. Coordinator		
8. Orienter		
9. Evaluator-critic		
10. Energizer		
11. Procedural technician		
12. Recorder		

Role Analysis Exercise (continued)

Group Building and Maintenance Roles

Role	Member Name	Sample Comment or Behavior
1. Encourager		
2. Harmonizer		
3. Compromiser		
4. Gatekeeper		
5. Standard setter		
6. Group observer		
7. Follower		

Individual Roles

Role	Member Name	Sample Comment or Behavior
1. Aggressor		
2. Blocker		
3. Recognition seeker		
4. Self-confessor		
5. Playboy		
6. Dominator		
7. Help-seeker		
8. Special interest pleader		

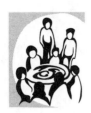

Worksheet 2-5
Self Role Analysis

1. What role(s) did you see yourself playing in the group?

2. Were these the same or different from the role(s) others saw you playing?

3. How does your role in this group compare with the one you usually play in groups?

4. What other roles would you like to try?

5. What comments or behaviors can you use to help you take on a new role?

For example, if the leader understands why the monopolist needs to monopolize and how his behavior affects the other group members, then the type of therapeutic intervention needed can be determined. Sometimes the problems that arise are best dealt with by the leader, while others are handled more effectively by the group itself.

Yalom (1985) points out that all patients are problems. Indeed, patients are often assigned to therapy groups for the purpose of attempting to change problem behaviors. The behaviors to be reviewed here are monopolizing, silence, attention-getting, and psychosis. It is very important for the occupational therapist leading groups to gain an understanding of each member's needs and develop skills in handling problem behaviors.

Members who display these problem behaviors are those who play the individual roles in groups, often blocking the group's progress and frustrating its members. Dealing effectively with these patients in the group involves several challenges for the therapist. First, the therapist should develop an understanding of the individual dynamics of the patient: What does this patient really need? Second, the therapist needs to develop strategies for preserving the integrity and cohesiveness of the group: What does the group need? How can the leader handle this patient so that the group can continue to function therapeutically? Ideally, both the patient need and the group need can be satisfied. Realistically, it is not always possible for the leader to do both. If a choice is to be made, the group should be preserved first, even if that means an individual member must leave it. A good group therapist will never sacrifice the whole group for the sake of an individual member.

The Monopolist

Harry came into the group angry. He refused to listen to the purpose of the group or to participate in the activity. "I'm not going to draw like I'm in kindergarten. Excuse me, but you girls (occupational therapy student leaders) don't know anything about alcohol abuse. When I was in County Hospital, they had me doing paintings and sculptures, and what-all, and it never did anything for me..." Five other members listened to this outburst in silence. They had heard Harry's routine before.

How should the leaders handle Harry? First, let us ask the two key questions. What does Harry need? Perhaps he needs to control the group, to attain the group's (or leader's) attention, or perhaps he needs to avoid his own hurtful issues. What do the members of the group need? Probably, they need to get Harry to "shut up." However, when a silent group allows a monopolist to control things, there is always an element of ambivalence. In some ways, Harry may be serving their needs as well, particularly if they, too, wish to avoid revealing hurtful issues or feelings.

In this example, Harry is playing the role of the aggressor, by devaluing both the task and the leaders of the group. The leaders, in this case, are more likely to stop Harry's tirade by appealing to the other group members. Ask them, "Why do you allow Harry to monopolize your group? Why are you silent?" The group might be encouraged to give Harry feedback by completing the sentence, "When you speak like that it makes me feel _____." If the group is able to express its frustration with Harry, then Harry might be helped by learning to control the behaviors that elicit negative feelings from others.

The Silent Member

Silent patients occur frequently in occupational therapy groups. In active groups, silent members may go unnoticed for a session or two, but will eventually block the group's progress. Why? Because as the group becomes aware of a member's silence, members begin to imagine what the silent member must be thinking. Soon resentment develops over the silent, passive member's "not pulling his weight" in the group. In truth, a silent member might feel inadequate, out of tune with the others, and fearful of self-disclosure. What the group wants most is for the silent member to talk, and to allay its fears about what he may be thinking. For example, in a group of students, Patty usually made two or three non-committal comments in each session, just enough to keep her from being noticed. Patty's greatest fear was becoming the center of attention. But as members got to know one another through mutual participation in group activities, it soon became clear that no one was getting to know Patty. Two group members finally confronted her angrily at the beginning of a group. Once begun, she continued speaking in a very pressured way, hard to interrupt: "I've been listening to you all discussing your life in the dorms and your problems with your boyfriends. But I'm a commuter. I leave right after class and go to my evening job and I don't get home until midnight. On weekends I help my handicapped mother with the housework and help her shop and pay her bills. I don't have time for a boyfriend and homework, too. I can't think about having fun when I'm wondering how I'll manage paying next semester's tuition or how I'll get the money to fix my car. I have nothing in common with this group. I'm not resentful or angry and I learn a lot from listening. But don't ask me to join in when I have nothing say." After allowing the group to respond, the occupational therapist suggested that the group try to find things Patty and they had in common, rather than things that singled her out as being different. Patty was still quiet, and had a hard time feeling like part of the group. But after this "event," the group no longer regarded her as an impediment. They empathized with her and collaborated to help involve her as much as she could tolerate.

Attention-Getting Behaviors

There are various forms of attention-getting behavior. Most represent self-centered patterns of interaction which reflect low self-esteem and the need for external evidence of one's worth. The three types we will discuss are self-depreciation, complaining, and narcissism or self-love.

The Self-Deprecator

The self-deprecator is the patient whose stories you hear over and over. She's always putting herself down, and seems unresponsive to overtures of acceptance from others. Janice loved to do activities, so she participated willingly in the occupational therapy group. But whenever she finished a project, she talked on and on about all of its flaws and imperfections. The group used to argue with her and tell her how nice her project looked. But the routine was repeated too often, so they stopped responding to Janice at all. This "fed up" group behavior made Janice feel all the more rejected. Getting the group to help Janice to see her self-defeating behavior was a key intervention here. Through group feedback, Janice learned how she made her expectation of rejection a self-fulfilling prophecy. The leader encouraged Janice to accept the group's support and stop devaluing herself before the group gave up on her.

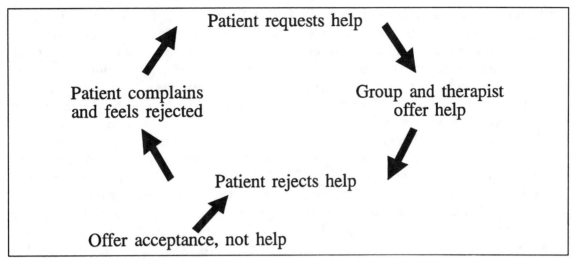

Figure 2-4. Self-defeating cycle of the HRC.

The Complainer

The help-rejecting complainer, referred to by Yalom as the "HRC" (1985, p. 389), chronically rejects the very help he asks for from the group. Yalom explains this behavior as unresolved dependency: the HRC is dependent on authoritative others, but at the same time is unable to trust others. After the fifth or sixth "yes, but..." response, the group usually becomes frustrated and angry at having all its advice rejected. The HRC is seen as using up a lot of time and energy and getting nowhere. Marge, for example, had chronic headaches and was addicted to several medications, which in turn, caused a barrage of other symptoms from constipation to irrational anger. An unknowing doctor tried to help Marge by lowering her pain medication prescription. Predictably, the doctor's well-meaning action not only did not help Marge, but it made him the target of all her irrational anger. She complained incessantly in group and would not be consoled. Marge had once again painted herself into a corner. Not only had the group rejected her, but she had rejected the only one (the doctor) who had the credentials to help her with her addiction prob-

lem. Why does this happen? Because the patient is stuck in a self-defeating cycle (Figure 2-4).

What to do? Do not give the patient the help requested. Why? Because she will reject the help and therefore reinforce the self-defeating cycle. The only hope for the HRC is to break the cycle. The therapist can help the group to empathize with Marge, to understand and acknowledge her feelings of defeat and frustration. As a bond with the group forms, the patient might be helped to see how her own behavior invites rejection.

The Narcissistic Member

These attention-seekers seem to demand the constant and undivided attention of the group. Narcissistic patients have an exaggerated self-love; they feel they deserve concern, compliments, gifts, and surprises, although they give none of these to others. For example, Franklin, a small, clever, attractive man, seemed to have a natural talent for comedy. He held the group's attention with his humor, but rarely listened to the other members. Franklin did a lot of talking about the women he had affairs with; he could not understand why these relationships never lasted. The group's need was to have Franklin contribute to the group by listening to and empathizing with others.

Groups can be very useful to patients like this, who need to alter their perception of themselves and others. It is important, however, for the therapist to protect them because of their high degree of vulnerability. The group's feedback can be accepted if it is presented in a gentle and caring way. Franklin, for all his humorous overconfidence about his sex appeal to women, had a very fragile sense of self-worth. He was highly dependent on the acceptance or rejection of others. The group, in its anger, could easily burst his bubble and its rejection would sink him to the depths of depression. Franklin needed the members' high regard to sustain him through their feedback about how his lack of caring makes them feel. The therapist might look for an opportunity to ask the group to comment about Franklin's rejection in ways that are not likely to evoke defensiveness.

Psychotic Patient Behavior

The patient who becomes psychotic and is out of touch with reality does not benefit from group treatment, according to Yalom. Irrational and illogical patients take up vast amounts of group energy and may bring the group process to a halt. Such patients should be removed from the group until their psychosis comes under control through medical treatment. Posthuma, however, suggests that psychotic patients may benefit from occupational therapy group treatment in which the activity is the focus, rather than discussion and social interaction (Posthuma, 1989).

Additionally, psychosis may not always be easy to identify. Some patients continue to interact in a seemingly rational manner, and may deceive the group by creating distractions or personal crises to cover their breaks with reality. Patients with borderline personality disorder provide good examples of this problem behavior. Borderline patients have been identified as exceedingly difficult to treat. Yalom describes them as having an "outward veneer of integration" which "conceals a chaotic, primitive personality structure" (Yalom, 1985, p. 407). Borderline patients often thrive in occupational therapy groups because they have developed a great deal of skill. Often they are excellent artists, craftspeople, and writers, as well as convincing talkers. In groups (as in life), they seem to go from crisis to crisis. Self-destructive acts can be an everyday occurrence, although often unpredictable. Group members and therapists alike are taken in by the borderline patient's great potential to achieve, and are disappointed again and again by his impulsive self-destructiveness.

Group treatment can be valuable to the borderline patient because of the many opportunities to test reality. Feedback from the group can keep his numerous perceptual distortions and primitive needs and fears in check. However, the therapist needs to be constantly in touch with the amount of the group's time and energy taken in meeting the needs of the borderline patient. Sometimes these patients leave little time for the other group members.

Termination of Groups

Finally, as the time for ending a group approaches, the leader will need to help the group through the process of termination. Some groups prepare for termination from the day they begin, while others avoid dealing with issues of termination altogether. The therapeutic learning that takes place in the group can be greatly enhanced by a good termination, or it can be destroyed by an inadequate termination. The leader should be keenly aware of the issues groups need to deal with in terminating so that she can help the group face them in a healthy and effective way.

This rather gruesome word "termination" is used here simply to mean the end of something. In the case of groups, it refers to the point at which groups cease to meet together as a group. Whether or not members expect to encounter one another as individuals in another context, termination of a group usually means the end of relationships as they exist within the group. The end of a group is a real loss and involves some of the same feelings associated with other losses.

Termination, when faced directly, usually involves pain and anxiety. Group members tend to avoid these feelings in a number of ways: withdrawal, devaluing the importance of the group, anger toward the leader or other members, silence and inactivity, or leaving the group prematurely. It was mentioned in the section on group development that some research shows group regression as the end approaches. A group that has reached maturity may go backward and re-enter a state of conflict prior to termination. Some groups just ignore the impending termination by bringing up new issues as if the group would continue as usual.

A healthy termination is never easy. However, leaders can help group members to go through the process, which involves several steps.

1. Review the group experience, the goals, and the learning that took place over the life of the group. Even though members may wish to devalue the group, the leader can encourage members to verbalize the goals they have accomplished or can help them recall positive learning experiences.

2. Review concerns and feelings regarding separation and loss. A good therapist will encourage the expression of painful, sad, angry, or anxious feelings to prepare the members for separation. Often the leader will experience these feelings and can share them with the group as an example.

3. Use counseling skills. Empathy and confrontation (detailed in Chapter 3) are often useful in this process to help members acknowledge their feelings instead of avoiding them.

4. Finish unfinished business. This seems obvious, but there may be various reasons why members wish to avoid doing it. A therapist should encourage members to bring up issues that are pending, and follow up on past conflicts to bring closure.

5. Give feedback on skills learned. Group members may be engaged in giving one another feedback about changes they have made, or learning what has been gained from the group's activities.

6. Help generalize learning. As a way to help members accept separation, an emphasis can be placed on how what was learned in the group can be practiced and applied elsewhere. When members understand how they can apply their skills to their lives outside of the group, they can move on without diminishing the importance of their group experience.

Summary
Students learn best about group dynamics through experience. So it is recommended that students meet in a series of six to 10 group sessions. These can be led by peers or can follow the format of Chapter 11, led by an instructor.

As a way to enhance an awareness of group dynamics, it is suggested that Worksheet 2-6 be used to record student reactions after each group session.

Bibliography

Benne, K., & Sheats, P. (1978). Functional roles of group members. In L. Bradford (Ed.), *Group Development* (2nd ed.). La Jolla, CA: University Associates.

Bion W. (1961). *Experiences in groups and other papers.* New York: Basic Books.

Cathcart, R., & Samovar, L. (1974). *Small group communication, a reader* (2nd ed.). Dubuque, IA: W. C. Brown Co.

Corey, G., Corey, M. S., Callanan, P., & Russel, J. (1988). *Group techniques* (Rev. ed.). Pacific Grove, CA: Brooks/Cole.

Posthuma, B. (1989). *Small groups in therapy settings: Process and leadership.* Boston: Little, Brown and Co.

Schutz, W. (1958). The interpersonal underworld. *Harvard Business Review* 36(4), 123-135.

Tuckman, B. (1965). Developmental sequence in small groups. *Psychological Bulletin, 63*(6), 384-399.

Yalom, I. (1985). *The theory and practice of group psychotherapy* (3rd ed.). New York: Basic Books.

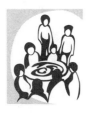

Worksheet 2-6
Personal Group Reaction Outline

Title/Theme:_____ Date of Session:_____

Seating Pattern Diagram:
1. Draw a diagram of the seating arrangement, listing names of each member present and his or her position within the group.
2. Discuss significance of seating pattern, positions near leader, opposite leader, pairing, subgroups.
3. Note absences and impact of these.

Norms: Identify "rules" of the group (confidentiality, respect, etc.). What behaviors are acceptable to the group? Not acceptable? Each week note any changes in group norms from previous weeks.

Content: Identify the major discussion topics of the group.

Process:
1. Theme—Based on the topics discussed, identify the predominant theme of the session in a few words or a phrase (this becomes the "title" of your paper). The theme should have both a content and a process (or feeling) component. Then explain how you arrived at this theme. How do the topics reflect the theme and why were they verbalized (or not verbalized) in this manner?
2. Stage—Identify the stage of development you think your group is in and why.
3. Verbal communication—What significant interpersonal interactions took place between group members? Be sure to name names. Vagueness is not helpful to the understanding of process. Interpret what was implied or hidden in the group discussion. What subjects were avoided and why?
4. Nonverbal communication—What was the general mood of the group? What was communicated by nonverbal behaviors of members, especially feelings of members? Interpret significance. How did nonverbal behaviors affect group functioning?

Personal Reaction: Identify your role and the impact you had on the group. Describe your personal feelings.
1. How did you respond to this group?
2. How do you feel about your relationship to the group?
3. How did you react to the leadership style?

Self-Evaluation: What did you learn about yourself today in group (e.g., strengths, weaknesses, values, interactive style)?

Goal: What are your personal goals for the next session?

SECTION TWO
Group Guidelines From Seven Frames of Reference

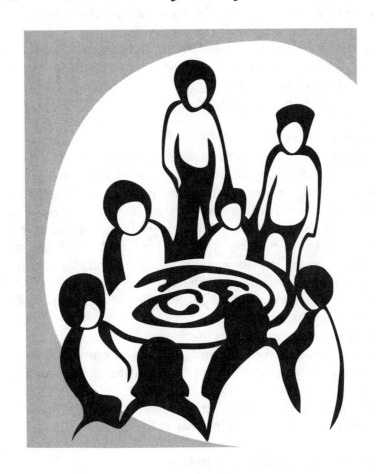

Chapter 3: A Humanistic Approach

Chapter 4: A Psychoanalytic Approach

Chapter 5: The Behavioral Cognitive Continuum

Chapter 6: Allen's Cognitive Disabilities Groups

Chapter 7: A Developmental Approach

Chapter 8: Sensory Motor Approaches

Chapter 9: A Model of Human Occupation Approach

Introduction to Section Two

Yalom (1995) writes that although there are presently many diverse "group therapies," there is a body of research that has been derived from a common ancestor. The oldest and most researched group is the long-term outpatient therapy group. This group consists of the most highly motivated patients and the most ambitious goals: to offer symptomatic relief and also to change character structure.

Once the basic dynamics and principles of this higher level group are mastered (as in Chapters 1 and 2), the student can then modify these to fit many specific clinical situations. Yalom suggests three steps for doing this:

1. Assessment of the clinical situation
2. Formulation of goals
3. Modification of technique

I have adopted Yalom's sound judgment in using these steps to plan occupational therapy groups, but have added an additional important step to the clinical reasoning process: identification and application of a frame of reference. Regarding the position of frames of reference in practice, Mosey writes that "many authors...[have] recognize[d] that no theory can be directly applied. A theory must first be transformed through a linking structure into usable information" (Mosey, 1989, p. 195). Mosey suggests that our research should focus on the development, refinement, and evaluation of the effectiveness of frames of reference. Occupational therapy uses a method called "extrapolation" (Mosey, 1989, p. 197) to make theory usable, involving several steps as follows:

1. Identification of appropriate theories
2. Selection of useful concepts from theory
3. Combining compatible concepts and postulates from various theories
4. Reformulating of the selected concepts and postulates to provide guidelines for treatment

In addressing the problem of planning and leading occupational therapy groups, I have used a similar technique in applying theory.

Identification of Appropriate Theories

First, I have identified seven appropriate practice theories:

1. Humanistic
2. Psychoanalytic
3. Behavioral cognitive
4. Cognitive disabilities
5. Developmental
6. Sensory motor
7. Model of human occupation

Some leaders in our profession would take exception to my choice of frames of reference. The psychoanalytic, humanistic, and developmental chapters draw widely upon psychological theory. The behavioral cognitive and sensory motor chapters draw mainly from the fields of neurology, anatomy, and physiology (and related medical fields). The model of human occupation, while identified by most as original to occupational therapy, draws upon systems theory, which is used widely in business and was originally derived from physics. My point is, most of the theoretical concepts that make up occupational therapy frames of reference have also been researched and applied in other disciplines. What makes these frames of reference different from similar theories in psychology and medicine is that the concepts were reorganized in a way that can guide us in planning and leading occupational therapy groups.

Selecting and Combining Useful Concepts

In describing each frame of reference, compatible concepts which are applicable to occupational therapy group treatment are selected from various theories. First, each concept or basic assumption is described according to the source or author where it originated. Then the relationship of the concepts to occupational therapy groups is facilitated through examples and learning exercises.

Combining Compatible Concepts

Compatible concepts are combined from various theories to formulate a point of view on function, dysfunction, change, and motivation. A frame of reference should guide our understanding of illness and disability in our patients. Before jumping into group treatment, occupational therapists should have some understanding of the state of health of the group members, and this understanding is different in each frame of reference. The definition of dysfunction can range from neurological malfunctioning in the sensory motor frame of reference, to the presence of unconscious conflicts in the psychoanalytic frame, to the lack of adaptive skill development in the developmental frame. Principles or postulates regarding change (Mosey, 1981) are the assumptions derived from theory that help us formulate how treatment will work. These are the "principles by which prevention of dysfunction occurs, function is maintained, interfering behavior is managed, and an individual is assisted in moving from a state of dysfunction to a state of function" (Mosey, 1981, p. 141).

Mosey further suggests that principles of intervention begin with the function to be developed (e.g., trunk balance, self-esteem), and end with the nature of the external environment that is likely to enact this therapeutic change. In other words, these principles help us predict how change will occur, and guide our designing of occupational therapy activities that will facilitate the development of function. For example, in using a developmental frame of reference for a group of elderly patients with Parkinson's, the postulate regarding intervention may be as follows: a sense of integrity and acceptance of one's life and death may be facilitated by participation in group activities where past accomplishments are the focus. In a behavioral cognitive frame of reference for the same patients, the postulate regarding change might be: socially acceptable eating habits that may be learned through the use of weighted utensils combined with peer examples. Each of these frames of reference suggests a different definition of function and dysfunction, different goals to be addressed, and a different kind of activity. Thus, the important parts of occupational therapy group treatment are addressed in the different frames. Within each chapter on a frame of reference, concepts are applied to group structure, limitations, role of the leader, appropriate goals, and suggested activity examples.

Reformulating Concepts to Provide Guidelines for Treatment

To provide the student with a concrete idea of how groups should be run in each of the frames of reference, the seven-step format for group leadership described in Chapter 1 is modified for each frame of reference covered. Suggested modifications to the introduction, use of activity, sharing, generalizing, application, and summary are described at the end of each chapter in this section. A chart reflecting these differences in the structure of groups may be found in Appendix E. It is hoped that with this breakdown, the application of theory will be, at least partly, demystified.

Bibliography

Llorens, L., & Gillette, N. (1985). Nationally speaking—The challenge for research in a practice profession. *American Journal of Occupational Therapy, 39*, 143-145.

Mosey, A. (1981). *Occupational therapy: Configuration of a profession*. New York: Raven.

Mosey, A. (1989). The proper focus of scientific inquiry in occupational therapy: Frames of reference. *Occupational Therapy Journal of Research, 9*(4), 195-201.

Yalom, I. (1995). *The theory and practice of group psychotherapy* (4th ed.). New York: Basic Books.

Chapter 3

A Humanistic Approach

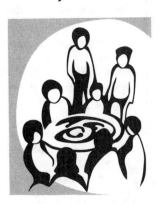

The humanistic frame of reference seems to correspond closely to what we have come to know as group dynamics theory. Many of the general concepts reviewed in Chapter 2 rely on the basic assumptions from existential and humanistic psychotherapy. The humanistic approach is also a major contributor to the core philosophy of occupational therapy. As the basic assumptions of humanistic and existential theory are reviewed, this connection will become evident.

Focus

This frame of reference, more than any other, helps us develop skills for forming and maintaining therapeutic relationships. Its philosophical roots encourage an accepting attitude toward mankind, and the writings of Carl Rogers, Abraham Maslow, Irvin Yalom, Rollo May, and others help us to develop an appreciation for what is special about being human. The counseling skills contributed by Gerard Egan (1986) are useful for students in the

helping professions when learning to communicate our understanding, concern, and guidance to patients, both as individuals and in groups.

The humanistic philosophy focuses on mankind as separate from animals and attempts to define those characteristics that are uniquely human. The value of human beings is paramount in the humanistic view. People are seen as equally valuable, regardless of their race, religion, sex, level of intellectual ability, socioeconomic position, and state of health. The very roots of occupational therapy, in the early 1900s, reflect these humanistic beliefs. The "Philosophical Base of Occupational Therapy," reprinted on page 62, emphasizes "intrinsic motivation," "self-actualization," and the ability to shape one's own state of health. These are statements that acknowledge the power of the human spirit within us all. The current interest in "spirituality" among occupational therapists indicates a renewed interest in the humanistic approach. The Principles of Occupational Therapy Ethics of the Amer-

---

The Philosophical Base of Occupational Therapy

Man is an active being whose development is influenced by the use of purposeful activity. Using their capacity for intrinsic motivation, human beings are able to influence their physical and mental health and their social and physical environment through purposeful activity. Human life includes a process of continuous adaptation. Adaptation is a change in function that promotes survival and self-actualization. Biological, psychological, and environmental factors may interrupt the adaptation process at any time throughout the life cycle. Dysfunction may occur when adaptation is impaired. Purposeful activity facilitates the adaptive process.

Occupational therapy is based on the belief that purposeful activity (occupation), including its inter-personal and environmental components, may be used to prevent and mediate dysfunction, and to elicit maximum adaptation. Activity as used by the occupational therapist includes both an intrinsic and a therapeutic purpose.

This statement was adopted by the April 1979 Representative Assembly of The American Occupational Therapy Association, Inc. as Resolution C #53-79. The text can be found as noted below:

American Occupational Therapy Association. (1979). The philosophical base of occupational therapy. *American Journal of Occupational Therapy, 33,* 785.

American Occupational Therapy Association. (1979). Policy 1.11. The philosophical base of occupational therapy. In *Policy manual of The American Occupational Therapy Association, Inc.* Bethesda, MD: Author.

Copyright American Occupational Therapy Association. Reprinted with permission.

---

ican Occupational Therapy Association continue to emphasize the rights of all human beings to equal treatment and to advocate the rights of the handicapped (AOTA, 1996).

However, as Mosey (1981) reminds us, a philosophy (fundamental belief) or a theory (concepts and postulates) cannot be directly applied. So, after reviewing the basic assumptions of existentialist and humanistic theory, the applications (plans of action) described by Carl Rogers and Gerard Egan will be discussed. These authors/therapists present applications of humanistic theory which are particularly useful to occupational therapists. Their techniques help guide our interventions in occupational therapy groups, as well as our choice of activities.

Basic Assumptions

Existential Concepts

Existential philosophy can be seen as the forerunner of humanism. The major contributions of the existentialists lie in two key concepts: freedom and anxiety.

Freedom

Freedom implies that an individual has a capacity for self-awareness and aware-ness of his environment that allows him to make choices. An individual who is aware need not allow his present behavior to be determined by others, his situation, or his past experiences. He alone is responsible for his own life dilemmas. Therapy that utilizes this approach is aimed at getting patients to see that they have choices, have always had choices, and helps them take responsibility for the choices that have made them who they are now. Adults can stop blaming their parents for their short-comings, and instead, take on the respon-sibility of correcting them. The concept of freedom to choose is what allows patients to take charge of their own lives, to leave the past behind, and to make positive changes for the future.

Anxiety

Anxiety, in the existentialist view, is a necessary condition of living. Rollo May defines anxiety as "the threat to our existence or to values we identify with our existence" (1977, p. 205). The concept is based on the idea that our existence or "being" (May & Yalom, 1989) has no intrinsic predetermined meaning. The meaning of life is developed by each individual for himself. Thus, in therapy, there is an emphasis on one's individual values, and in finding or defining what activities are meaningful to the individual. It is the existentialist view that while too much anxiety can immobilize a person, a certain amount of anxiety is normal and positive. It is anxiety that alerts one that all is not well, and that a change is needed. In this case, anxiety is seen as a motivator to make necessary changes in behavior, values, or life structure in order to maintain or promote healthy functioning.

Humanistic Concepts

The humanistic approach is overwhelmingly positive and is appealing to most therapists. Carl Rogers was perhaps its major spokesman. Rogers developed what is known as nondirective counseling, based on the assumption that the patient really knows what is best for him. Rogers viewed his patients with "unconditional positive regard" and allowed them to choose the direction of therapy, to set their own goals, and to provide their own solutions to problems (Rogers, 1967). Abraham Maslow added significantly to humanistic thinking, also. The key concepts of his humanistic approach are: respect, genuineness, non-judgmental acceptance, deep understanding, and self-actualization.

Respect

Respect in therapy is not a technique, but an attitude toward the patient. In the humanistic approach, the therapist sees the patient as the only real expert on his own life. Therefore, the therapist makes no predetermined assumptions about the patient, but seeks to learn all about him by asking open-ended questions and getting him to talk about himself as much as possible. Yalom translates this idea in his approach to group treatment by encouraging group members to respect each other and to talk to each other as much as possible. Respect also includes a belief that when people are realistically aware of their problems, they are capable of creating their own solutions. Therefore, suggestions and advice giving are discouraged and replaced by responses that show empathy. Empathy is expressed by both therapist and group members by statements that not only reflect what the patient has said, but also acknowledge how the patient is feeling. For example, a patient presents the problem that his wife does not understand his need to grieve the death of his mother. The therapist would encourage the group to ask for appropriate details in order to gain a thorough understanding of how this patient feels. Then empathy would be expressed with a statement like "You must be feeling abandoned when your wife cannot share your grief about the loss of your mother." Statements such as this encourage the patient to trust the therapist and/or group members and to move ahead to even greater self-disclosure.

Genuineness

Genuineness is also an attitude rather than a technique. It means that the therapist expresses real emotional responses to the patient. Patients are keen observers and are quick to sense any dishonesty on the part of therapists. When the therapist tries to cover up anger or frustration, the patient usually senses something wrong and the effect is often silence and with-drawal of trust. It is only by expressing negative feelings that honest communica-tion with the patient is facilitated. This is not to suggest that the therapist's anger (or other feelings) should be expressed indis-criminately. On the contrary, it takes con-siderable skill and self-understanding for a therapist to express feelings in a way that is therapeutic (Egan, 1986).

The value of genuineness has a pro-found effect upon groups. When the ther-apist encourages the members to be gen-uine, the responses they give to one anoth-er are much more meaningful and helpful. In the initial stages of groups, it is a natur-al tendency for members to hold back in their responses to one another. Patients are often reluctant to express negative feelings toward other members. Reasons for this have been discussed in Chapter 2. After members have established a certain degree of trust in one another, they feel much more inclined to share their real feel-ings. It is one of the therapist's roles to establish an atmosphere of safety and trust which allows group members to be gen-uine in their responses to one another.

Non-Judgmental Acceptance

Non-judgmental acceptance refers to the therapist's relationship with the patient as one of caring. In the humanistic approach, the patient is accepted for the human being that he is, regardless of his feelings or his behavior. This "uncondi-tional positive regard" allows the patient to reveal all his inner feelings and secrets without fearing the therapist's rejection. According to Rogers, research indicates that "the greater the degree of caring, priz-ing, accepting, and valuing the client in a non-possessive way, the greater the chance that therapy will be successful" (Corey, 1991, p. 214). The humanistic therapist needs to be very careful not to allow his

own values to enter into the therapeutic relationship. Judgments of bad and good feelings or bad and good behavior have no place in the humanistic approach.

Being judged by others is one of the greatest fears patients have in the group setting. For example, when a patient speaks in the group, he is often uncom-fortable with the silence of others. Patients often imagine that silent members are secretly disapproving of what is being said. It is most important for the therapist to establish the norm or expectation early in the group that members not judge one another in this way. All members have a right to have feelings and feelings are nei-ther good nor bad. Likewise, behavior should not be judged for itself, but looked upon in the context of the individual's per-ceptions of self and environment. If a patient got drunk on a weekend pass, this behavior can be seen as one of several responses the patient could have to a stressful situation. The object is not to con-demn the behavior, but to understand it and examine its effect on the patient.

Deep Understanding

In the humanistic approach, behavior change is considered to be the by-product of a deep self-understanding. For this rea-son, considerable time and energy in ther-apy is devoted to uncovering hidden aspects of the self. In occupational therapy groups, structured activities are often helpful in fostering self-understanding among group members. The therapist should continue to gather information from the patients until she can almost see the world through the patient's eyes. Only then is the therapist able to assist the patient in changing his behavior. New therapists have a tendency to push for behavior change too quickly. In their desire to be helpful, new therapists might even make a suggestion in the form of a

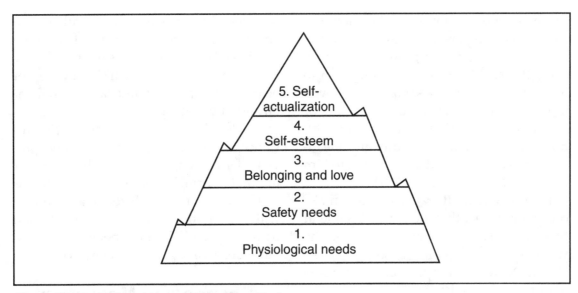

Figure 3-1. Maslow's mountain. Adapted from Maslow.

question, such as, "Have you tried talking to your wife instead of just getting drunk?" Such a question reveals a lack of respect as well as understanding. Questions should focus on further defining the problem until it is thoroughly explored. When it is revealed that the patient depends on his wife so much that he cannot risk disagreeing with her, then getting drunk to numb the pain is less contemptible. Furthermore, the problem is redefined not as one of drunkenness, but one of dependency. That dependency may be further explained by a lack of trust in oneself. Problems are seldom as simple as they may seem. Rogers believes that "when therapists can grasp the present experience of the client's private world as the client sees and feels it without losing the separateness of their own identity, then constructive change is likely to occur" (Corey, 1991, p. 214).

Self-Actualization

Self-actualization is the innate tendency of all human beings to achieve their potential. This concept assumes that each of us has within us an inherent potential that we

can actualize and through which we can find meaning. Maslow, the chief proponent of this concept, places self-actualization at the top of a continuum called the hierarchy of needs. Maslow sees at the core of human nature a push to satisfy the needs which ensure physical and psychological survival. The satisfaction of each need is a necessary prerequisite to the search for satisfaction of the next. Thus, in Maslow's hierarchy, 1) physiological needs, 2) safety needs, 3) needs for belonging and love, and 4) esteem needs are all prerequisites to the need for self-actualization. Maslow's hierarchy is often referred to as a pyramid or mountain with five successive levels (Figure 3-1). In his book *Toward a Psychology of Being*, Maslow elaborates the idea of self-actualization in his discussion of "peak experiences." These experiences are difficult to describe, but widely documented, according to Maslow. They are moments of ecstasy, self-discovery, and brilliant creativity or vision; moments when suddenly one's views of himself and the world change permanently. Peak experiences are said to cause symptoms to disappear; they can change self-perception in a healthy direction and can release the person for greater creativity, expressiveness, and growth. "The person (after such experiences) is more apt to feel that life in general is worthwhile, even if it is usually drab, pedestrian, painful, or ungratifying, since beauty, excitement, honesty, play, goodness, truth, and meaningfulness have been demonstrated to him to exist" (Maslow, 1968, p. 101).

If only we, as therapists, could make our patients feel that life is worthwhile in this way! The humanistic view of the world seems so optimistic, so holistic, so simple. Now let us apply some of its ideas to our view of patients.

Function and Dysfunction

In the humanistic view, a healthy functioning individual is one who is self-actualized, who is functioning close to his potential. Such a person is aware of the freedom to make choices, and takes responsibility for the decisions of the past. He is not inhibited by guilt over lost opportunities, and does not blame others for his dilemmas. A healthy person works toward satisfying his own physiological and psychological needs, and chooses an environment and life structure that allows growth and expression. Anxiety is replaced by meaningfulness and purpose; the individual feels good about himself.

Dysfunction would be the opposite of all these. But there is the difficulty. We as therapists need to find out where the dysfunction lies when our patient is stuck, and to help him identify the obstacles preventing him from pursuing self-actualization. Perhaps the patient is not aware of the freedom to make choices. Many patients I have worked with have felt so defeated by the "system," the bureaucracy of governments and organizations, or the prejudices of society that they no longer exercise their ability to choose. Many have

had negative life experiences rather than "peak" experiences. Perhaps their more basic needs are not being satisfied or they feel unsafe, unloved, or like they do not belong. People with handicaps, both mental and physical, often feel they are misfits, controlled by others, victims of circumstance, incapacitated by anxiety, and prevented from enjoying the fulfillments of life that "normal" people enjoy. As therapists, we may need to listen to and endure with our patients a great deal of pain before we can help them begin to find the more positive aspects of themselves.

Change and Motivation

Humanists often address motivation in their writings. Maslow views need satisfaction as a kind of thrust for survival, but this changes from physiological survival to psychological survival as it approaches the top of the needs hierarchy. Self-actualization is seen not as a search for what is missing, but an innate drive toward self-fulfillment. This differs somewhat from the existentialist view that anxiety is the major motivator, that the search for structure and meaning is largely motivated by the desire to escape the anxiety of meaninglessness and nothingness. In humanistic theory, there is an assumption that people have a natural tendency to improve the quality of their lives. This idea is certainly compatible with the basic tenets of occupational therapy. Perhaps we would add that our plan of action to improve the quality of life is the engagement in meaningful occupation.

Of central concern in the health professions is the knowledge of how change occurs, since it is upon this knowledge that we base our treatment. Here again, psychological theorists give us many clues. The humanists say that we cannot change our patients, that they must desire to change themselves. The function of the therapist is to create an atmosphere of safety and to help the patient build the kind of self-image and self-understanding that increases the likelihood of positive change. The humanistic therapist does this through the *therapeutic relationship* and through the facilitation of therapeutic groups. Rogers said that behavior change is really a by-product of a deep self-understanding. To change their lives in a positive way, patients must first feel and believe that they have the ability and power to make changes. This requires a feeling of self-worth and self-esteem as well as a belief that one has the needed skills and capacities required. A prerequisite for change is the belief that change is possible. All of these are appropriate issues to be addressed in occupational therapy groups.

Group Treatment

Yalom in his book *The Theory and Practice of Group Psychotherapy* (1995) describes a basically existential humanistic approach. Patients are treated in groups not only because it is practical, but because of the many unique advantages that only a group can offer in treatment. The goals for an individual in this frame of reference have mostly to do with increasing self-understanding, self-worth, and self-actualization. In the group setting, members are expected to discuss their own lives, their problems, and their successes. Through their self-disclosure, members develop relationships with one another and learn to trust each other. The feedback and support they give one another is of far greater value than what they can get from any individual.

Furthermore, many of the therapeutic factors described by Yalom (instillation of hope, universality, altruism, group cohesiveness, and interpersonal learning) will help the members achieve their goals. The therapeutic factors are those aspects of groups which make them therapeutic. Instillation of hope conveys the positive expectation members have at the outset of groups that the group experience will help them. Patients in group treatment often feel great relief when they discover that their problems are not unique, that others share their misery (universality). Altruism implies that patients benefit not only by receiving from others, but also from giving. Learning to give to others in the group may in fact be the most important lesson of all. Group cohesiveness has been described as the final and most desirable stage of group development. It is an attraction for each other that is shared by all its members. Cohesiveness makes possible all the positive, productive work that can be accomplished by the mature group described in Chapter 2. Interpersonal learning incorporates a broad range of factors about the give and take of emotional and social relationships. The reader is referred to Chapters 1 and 2 of Yalom (1995) for further discussion of the therapeutic factors of groups.

A humanistic group is best suited to a higher functioning clientele. It is the approach suggested for personal/professional growth of student or staff groups. A certain level of self-awareness is expected, and members should be able to communicate their self-perceptions to the group reasonably well. In short, members must be capable of insight. Insight means not only acknowledging one's own problematic behavior, but having some understanding of the reasons behind it.

For example, I have treated groups of substance abuse patients using this approach. Most of these patients have been employed, have developed intimate relationships with others, and have in times past functioned in the world with relative success. Self-awareness activities and discussion of values are helpful in defining problems. These patients understood all too well how abusing substances interfered with functioning, since many had endured severe losses (e.g., spouses, jobs, financial losses) due to their drug/alcohol habits. They were able to discuss the dilemmas and the pain openly and to help each other learn alternative strategies. Often their problems seemed to be related to an inability to assert themselves emotionally or to cope with stress. There are other problems, of course, but occupational therapy groups in this example tended to focus on expression of emotion and managing stress.

Irving Yalom (1995) acknowledges the reality of acute inpatient psychiatry (short hospitalizations, rapid turnover, dual diagnosis) by suggesting some modified goals for groups in acute settings. He suggests that groups should occur daily, use a more directive leadership, and create a supportive atmosphere through structured interaction. Each group should be designed as if it were the only one, since repeat attendance is not guaranteed. The goals in a single session, using the humanistic approach, should be as follows:

- Engage the patients in the therapeutic process. The group activity should demonstrate how therapeutic interaction can be helpful to each member.
- Problem spotting. The activity should give members an opportunity to present their problems to the group for discussion and feedback. Solving the problem is not as important as defining it, using skills in concreteness and primary accurate empathy (PAE), and directing patients to the appropriate resources for addressing problems fully on their own.
- Decreasing isolation. Group activities in the acute hospital setting should encourage sharing of common concerns and focus on communication with others and improving interpersonal relationships.

Role of the Leader

The occupational therapist who follows a humanistic frame of reference focuses on skills that help develop the therapeutic relationship. These skills will be used extensively in planning and leading occupational therapy groups. A thorough knowledge of group dynamics is extremely important in helping him to select members, set goals, and plan appropriate activities.

The facilitative and advisory leadership styles are the most appropriate for humanistic groups. Both give group members an active part in the direction and process of therapy, while allowing the leader to guide them through the establishment of therapeutic norms.

Knowledge of the stages of groups is important, as well as what skills are appropriate for each stage. The reader is referred to Gerard Egan's *The Skilled Helper* (1986) for a more thorough discussion of these skills. Egan's text is intended for teaching basic counseling skills for those who will be doing individual psychotherapy. However, the stages of counseling which parallel the development of groups and the use of specific skills in group intervention will be the emphasis here.

Egan describes three stages of counseling:

I. Problem definition
II. Self-understanding
III. Behavior change

Stage I is concerned with problem definition. This stage is parallel to the beginning stage of a group, in which members get to know one another and begin to lay the ground rules for how they will interact. The skills Egan suggests for this stage are attending, concreteness, and PAE.

Attending

Attending is something most of us do without even thinking about it. The leader of the group needs to be especially alert and observant since she is attending to not one, but several people at one time. Attending refers to the attentive physical presence the therapist focuses on the patient; it is evident even before anyone begins to speak. Taking note of appearance, body language, posture, seating position, eye contact, and facial expression are all part of attending. The therapist gets from these factors important clues as to how members are feeling and how the group is likely to respond to various activities or interventions.

Skill Practice in Attending
Completing Worksheet 3-1, First Impressions, will make you aware of how powerful these first impressions really are. Read the example of a completed First Impressions worksheet below.

1. Draw a diagram of where people are seated in the room.
2. Write a one- or two-word phrase describing the appearance of each member. For example:
   Glenn—Sloppy, poor hygiene
   Mary—Dressed up, neat
   Sue—Provocative, overly made up
   Joe—Preppy, well-groomed
3. Write one or two adjectives to describe the posture of each member. For example:
   Glenn—Relaxed, slouching
   Mary—Watchful, tense
   Sue—Uncomfortable, fidgety
   Joe—Alert, open
4. Note with whom each member has eye contact. For example:
   Glenn—Looks at no one, looks down
   Mary—Looks at everyone
   Sue—Looks only at Joe
   Joe—Looks at leader primarily

5. Write a feeling word(s) describing the emotional message given by the facial expression of each. For example:
   Glenn—Defiant
   Mary—Anxious, fearful
   Sue—Distracted, blunted
   Joe—Eager, anticipating

It is most helpful to put the descriptions of each individual together so you can begin to get a more complete picture of each.

Knowing these impressions before starting the group, the leader can predict some responses that can be expected from the four patients. Even if the therapist does not know anything about the patients except their names and ages, an observant leader will begin to adapt his approach to the group to accommodate the different expectations.

Which of these patients is most likely to be cooperative? Uncooperative? Which patient is most likely to disrupt the group? Which member might be expected to leave prematurely? Attending and forming impressions of members becomes second nature to the skilled therapist, but the beginning therapist perhaps needs some practice. Worksheet 3-1 may be used to practice these observations on your own group.

Concreteness

Concreteness refers to the ability to elicit specific information about a patient or problem. If the humanistic therapist's goal is to obtain a thorough understanding of the patient, many clarifying questions must ultimately be asked. The most basic skill in concreteness is to ask open-ended questions. These are questions that cannot be answered with a simple "yes" or "no." Open-ended questions encourage the patient to clarify his perceptions, elaborate on important points, and give specific per-

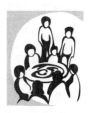

Worksheet 3-1
First Impressions

Directions: First, draw a diagram of where people are seated in the room. List names of group members in first column. Then use one or two descriptive words to denote appearance, posture, and facial expression. Before beginning to speak, note the persons each member makes eye contact with. This information will make up your first impressions of group members.

Member Name	Appearance	Posture	Eye Contact	Facial Expression
1.				
2.				
3.				
4.				
5.				
6.				
7.				
8.				

sonal examples. A therapist may use open questions to get the patient to discover concrete solutions to problems, but that often happens in a later stage of treatment.

Constructing open-ended questions is not always as easy as it seems. Some beginning therapists are in the bad habit of asking closed questions one after the other, and this kind of habit is hard to break. Consider the following opening of an occupational therapy session:

OT: Would you like to do some drawing today?

Joe: No.

OT: Are you too tired?

Joe: Yes.

OT: Can you just talk to me for a while?

Joe: I'd rather not.

OT: Do you find it hard to talk?

Joe: Yes.

OT: Why?

Joe: I don't know.

Now consider the following alternative opening:

OT: To begin our session, I'd like to learn how well you express your feelings. What can you tell me about how you're feeling right now?

Joe: Nothing.

OT: What makes it difficult to talk about feelings with me?

Joe: It's nothing against you, I'm just in a bad mood.

OT: What put you in a bad mood?

Joe: My doctor just told me I can't go home this weekend.

In leading occupational therapy groups, open questions are more effective because they encourage communication and interaction among members. Closed questions tend to cut off communication. This is an important point to remember when planning questions for discussion when processing an activity group. In asking open questions, it seems most useful to begin with the words "what" or "how." Using the word "why" is not advisable because it tends to elicit vague answers, and because it may sound judgmental, reminding some patients of their angry parents' interrogations. Also, avoid beginning a question with "do you," "can you," "would you," "are you," or "have you," because these can easily be answered with "yes" or "no," as observed in the preceding example. Now try Worksheet 3-2.

Primary Accurate Empathy

PAE is discussed by several humanistic theorists, particularly Carl Rogers. The importance of its use early in therapy cannot be overemphasized. PAE is the reflection of the feeling and content expressed by the patient. If composed and delivered effectively, an empathetic comment from either the therapist or another group member will convince the patient that he is being listened to and understood. The effect of empathy is to encourage this patient to open up even more. PAE, used often in groups, will help build an atmosphere of safety and trust, and will help the group progress toward a state of cohesiveness.

PAE is considered "primary" because it does not reach far below the surface. It reflects, but does not repeat, what the patient has actually said. Empathy requires that the feeling of the patient be recognized, and that may require careful observation of nonverbal cues as well as what the patient actually says. (In the practice exercise, you will just have to read between the lines.) The "accurate" part of empathy requires that the emotion be identified accurately. Emotions vary in both kind and intensity. Some psychologists have divided feelings into the categories of mad, sad, bad, and glad. It is not enough to just say "you feel angry." Anger varies from low intensity, like annoyed or

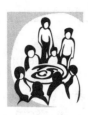

Worksheet 3-2
Open-Ended Questions

Directions: In each of the following examples, respond to the patient with an open question that can:
- Elicit more specific information
- Focus the discussion on a specific problem
- Help define the problem

1. "I'm always so unlucky!"
Therapist response:

2. "No matter what I do, I can't win."
Therapist response:

3. "I'm not thinking right today."
Therapist response:

4. "Boy, did I have a boring weekend!"
Therapist response:

5. "My doctor gave me new medication, and I'm just not myself."
Therapist response:

6. "Life is so unfair. Do you think there's any justice in the world?"
Therapist response:

7. "What good does it do to write down a schedule? When I go home, it's all for nothing."
Therapist response:

8. "I'm really afraid to talk about how I feel."
Therapist response:

9. "Just let well enough alone. I feel great today."
Therapist response:

10. "Why should I care what my mother thinks?"
Therapist response:

perturbed, to very high intensity, like rage. Patients often do not have a very wide "feeling" vocabulary; many are not used to expressing their feelings in words. Often patients need the help of the therapist to find the right words to describe their feelings accurately. Worksheets 3-3 and 3-4 will help you to develop a better "feeling" vocabulary.

After expanding our knowledge of "feeling" words, we will apply them to the skill of PAE. When practicing PAE, we will use sentence completion to facilitate finding the right feeling words. We will complete the sentence "You feel _____because _____." "You feel" refers to the feeling word that best reflects how the patient is feeling. "Because" refers to the thoughts or behaviors that are seen to have caused the feeling. When leading a group, you will learn to use your own words to show empathy. Now try Worksheet 3-5.

According to Egan (1986), the goal of Stage II in counseling is self-understanding. The middle stage of group development is more complex than this, with its subgroups, leadership struggles, and questioning of purpose/value, but the outcome is still a greater self-understanding. It is helpful to groups if the leader uses and teaches the skills of Stage II to get through this vital phase of group development. The skills of Stage II are immediacy, advanced accurate empathy, and confrontation.

Immediacy

Immediacy is the direct mutual communication between therapist and patient. It enables the therapist to discuss openly and directly what is happening in the here-and-now of their interpersonal relationship. It is an invitation to process the relationship, and this is how it is best used in groups. When a group bogs down, and nothing seems to be happening, a question like: "What is happening right now?" or "What do you think the silence means?" will serve to refocus the group on its own process. The group's relationship to its leader is commonly a troubled one in Stage II, with which immediacy can help. For example, the leader can often sense anger, resentment, or rebellion in the members and invite the group to discuss it. She could ask, "Are you angry with me for insisting that you give each other constructive feedback?" This direct question encourages the members to examine their own feelings about the leader, an essential task in the "control" stage of groups. Trust is another important issue to help therapist immediacy. A comment like, "I can see that you're having a hard time trusting one another in this group today," will invite the group members to examine their relationships with one another. Now try Worksheet 3-6.

Advanced Accurate Empathy

Advanced accurate empathy (AAE) goes a step further than PAE. This skill enables the therapist to bring feelings and thoughts that the patient may only be implying to the forefront. Therapists find AAE difficult because it involves forming a hypothesis about the underlying or hidden feelings/topics the patient just hints at with her statements. Egan says that PAE means "sharing hunches about clients and their overt and covert experiences, behaviors, and feelings which the therapist thinks will help patients see their problems and concerns more clearly, and in a context that will enable them to move to goal setting and action" (Egan, 1982, p. 79).

AAE helps the patient in several specific ways. First, it can help the patient become aware of hidden or forbidden feelings. Male patients, for example, often try to hide their sad or hurt feelings because they

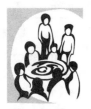

Worksheet 3-3
Feeling Words

Directions: This exercise may be done as a group or individually. Take 10 or 15 minutes to list as many feeling words you can think of in each category listed at the top of the first four columns. A fifth column is provided for those words that seem to defy categorization, but are nevertheless expressive of feelings. You may use a thesaurus to form a more complete list (at least 20 words per column). When you are finished, go to Worksheet 3-4.

Mad	Sad	Bad (fearful)	Glad	Other Emotions

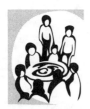

Worksheet 3-4
Developing Your Empathy Vocabulary

Directions: From the list you made in Worksheet 3-3, sort the words in each column into the three levels of intensity described to the left: mild, moderate, or severe. For example, in the "Bad" column, a mild emotion might be "worried," a moderate emotion might be "fearful," and a severe one might be "petrified." Refer to your completed list when completing the Primary Accurate Empathy worksheet (Worksheet 3-5).

	Mad	Sad	Bad (fearful)	Glad	Other Emotions
Mild					
Moderate					
Severe					

From Cole, M. B. *Group Dynamics in Occupational Therapy, Second Edition.* © 1998 SLACK Incorporated.

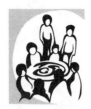

Worksheet 3-5
Primary Accurate Empathy

Directions: After reading each patient's comment in group, write a response which completes the sentence: "You feel _____ because _____" and communicates:

- What emotion that patient is feeling (as accurately as possible)
- A summary of the thoughts or behaviors that are seen to have caused the feeling

1. "I can't draw very well (shows a very faintly drawn picture to the group). This is supposed to be my sofa and my dog."
   "You feel _____ because _____."

2. "He just accused me of being prejudiced! I say he's a moron!"
   "You feel _____ because _____."

3. "Brian is doing so well. He's leaving tomorrow to start a new life, and here I am, still in the hospital."
   "You feel _____ because _____."

4. "Can I leave now? This group is making me very upset, especially when Mark sounds so angry."
   "You feel _____ because _____."

5. "This group just isn't helping me. None of you understand what I'm going through!"
   "You feel _____ because _____."

6. "I didn't want to come to occupational therapy group today. Setting goals is too much work."
   "You feel _____ because _____."

7. "When Laurie tells me I'm being insensitive, I don't know what she means."
   "You feel _____ because _____."

8. "All I know is that I'm restricted to the ward again. They seem to like punishing me."
   "You feel _____ because _____."

9. "My boyfriend always picks on me when he's had a bad day. Now I am too upset to participate in this group."
   "You feel _____ because _____."

10. (Tara crying) "I don't know why I'm so upset. Just hearing Roy talk about being old and alone. He reminds me of my grandfather who died 2 months ago."
    "You feel _____ because _____."

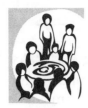

Directions: In the following examples, respond with a direct question or statement that encourages the group to examine its here-and-now relationships.

1. Group of adolescents hospitalized for drug abuse.
    Tina: "If we discuss our problems in group, you'll just tell our parents. They're the ones who sent us here in the first place."

    Bob: "Yeah, how do we know you won't rat on us?"

    Mikki: "I'm not telling you nothin'. I may have to come to this group, but I don't have to talk."

    Therapist response:

2. Group of eating disorder patients working on vocational readiness. This group has chosen to do one small craft project after another. None of the members have opted to take on anything more challenging, yet three of the members face discharge with only three or four more occupational therapy sessions.

    Therapist response:

3. Group of arthritis patients attending the third session of a leisure planning group.

    Morgan: "What are we in this group for anyway? All I want to do is go back to work. Then I won't have any leisure time."

    Jackie: "I stopped participating in sports back in high school. Sure, it would be good for me, but it's just too much effort."

    Ellie: "Sure, my doctor told me I need to plan time for relaxation and enjoyment, but I'm not sure I need someone telling me how or when to do it."

    Therapist response:

From Cole, M. B. *Group Dynamics in Occupational Therapy, Second Edition.* © 1998 SLACK Incorporated.
(Adapted from Egan, 1982)

consider them to be a sign of weakness. Second, the therapist can use AAE to help the patient see patterns of behavior or general trends. A bad experience with one doctor, for example, may lead a patient to mistrust all doctors. A third way that AAE can help a patient is to help her draw logical conclusions to her behaviors or comments. An older teen who feels trapped by her parents' rules and says she's tired of her parents treating her like a child may be expressing a desire to leave home and become more independent. Actually moving out may be very scary to an adolescent who has never been on her own, but that is where her comments seem to be leading.

Since AAE is really the therapist's hypothesis or educated guess about the patient's implications, it is best to present these ideas tentatively. Always leave yourself a way out, by using phrases like "could it be that...," "it seems likely that...," or "I could be wrong, but...." The fact is, you could be wrong, and it should always be acceptable for the patient to correct you if you are. Even if you are not wrong, if the patient really is hiding a seething rage at his spouse, he may not be ready to face or accept such intense feeling. Tentativeness also leaves the patient a way out, without damaging the therapeutic relationship.

The easiest way to learn AAE is to begin with PAE. Practice both PAE and AAE by doing Worksheet 3-7.

Confrontation

Confrontation involves the resolution of possible discrepancies, distortions, games, and smokescreens patients use to avoid self-understanding and/or behavior change. It includes challenging the undeveloped, unused, or misused potentialities, skills, and resources patients may have as well. Confrontation as a technique is actually an extension of AAE or inter-

pretation. However, whereas interpretation involves the therapist's understanding of a patient's behavior, confrontation permits the patient himself to put his own meaning to the behavior. In confrontation, the therapist points out maladaptive behaviors or inconsistent actions and comments, and invites the patient to explain or make sense of them.

Confrontation has a reputation for being harsh and accusing. However, the skilled confrontation is not harsh, but an act of caring. It should offer genuine feedback to the patient about his comments or behavior, while leaving the judgment of the behavior up to him. The tone of voice used by the therapist is very important here. The correct words, conveyed in an angry or accusing tone, will not achieve the desired result. What is hoped for is self-discovery on the part of the patient, using the confrontation as a guide.

For example, when Ben expresses that he's "happy-go-lucky and able to cope with almost anything," the therapist might ask, "If this is true, what are you doing on an inpatient ward of a psychiatric hospital?" In this confrontation, it is Ben who has to explain the discrepancy between his healthy self-presentation and his psychiatric inpatient status. The therapist might say, "One doesn't get admitted to a psychiatric ward by being healthy and able to cope. How did a healthy person like you end up on a psychiatric ward?" There must be problems Ben is not talking about. However, the point of the confrontation is not to accuse Ben of having problems; the point is to get Ben himself to stop denying or hiding his problems, and instead try to solve them.

Use Worksheet 3-8 to practice your skills in confrontation as an act of caring and promoting self-understanding. (Note: The lectures of C. Huber, University of

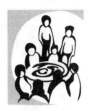

Worksheet 3-7
Advanced Accurate Empathy

Directions: First, respond with a primary accurate empathy statement to the patient. Then, respond with some statement of advanced accurate empathy. Freely interpret so as to assist the client in taking a larger view of his situation, see the implications or examine the logical conclusions of what is said or done.

1. Sam, age 54
   Situation: This man has a variety of problems. This time he has just undergone surgery to repair a back injury. His tendency is to ruminate constantly on his defects.
   "To feel bad, all I have to do is review what has happened in my life. This past year I let my drinking get the best of me for 4 months. Over the years, I've messed up my marriage. Now my wife and I are separated. I don't have the kind of income that can support two households, and the job market is really tight. I'm not so sure what skills I have to market anyhow."

Therapist PAE response:

Therapist AAE response:

2. Adele, age 44
   Situation: This woman has been admitted for the third time with a bleeding ulcer.
   "I'm completely depressed. I don't feel like working anymore. Actually, I work all the time. I can't think of any day I get up and don't intend to work. I think I begrudge myself the time I take for relaxation. There's been no day for the past 2 years when I said, 'Today's a day off.' I always feel so good about myself after I've worked hard, and after all, it's my choice to spend the time the way I want, isn't it?"

Therapist PAE response:

Therapist AAE response:

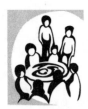

Worksheet 3-8
Practice in Confrontation

Directions: Respond to each of the following clients first with primary accurate empathy, then with confrontation.

Example: Sheila says "Everything is fine" as she stares at the floor and looks sad.

Therapist confrontation: You must feel sad, judging from the downcast look on your face. Yet you're telling me everything is fine. How do you see that?"

1. Mike, a spinal cord injured patient, age 25, comments after a visit from his wife. "It really hurts me when I think about what she said to me." He smiles and shrugs his shoulders.

   Therapist confrontation:

2. Anne, age 35, is an arthritic patient who has become socially isolated except for a few friends. She is seeking ways of getting along better with others interpersonally. "I give a lot to my friends, but I expect a lot in return. Unfortunately, it seems like many of them don't recognize my caring and I react by getting angry with them."

   Therapist confrontation:

3. Robert, age 54, a cardiac patient, is recently divorced, has lost his job, and is broke. He keeps joking about it.

   Therapist confrontation:

From Cole, M. B. *Group Dynamics in Occupational Therapy, Second Edition.* © 1998 SLACK Incorporated.
(Adapted from Egan, 1982)

Bridgeport, Dept. of Psychology, are acknowledged as the inspiration for learning exercises in counseling skills.)

Goals

The goals of groups using the humanistic frame of reference, as mentioned earlier, are self-awareness, self-understanding, and self-actualization. These give the occupational therapist very clear guidelines about what types of issues need attention. Many aspects of the self can be explored, such as feelings and their expression, self-identity and characteristics of the self, style of interaction with others and with groups, body image and feelings about the body, values and attitudes of individuals, and an exploration of the barriers which prevent people from achieving their potential.

Whatever the goal, it is important that it be relevant to the here-and-now, and applicable to the person's present life situation. Historical causes of difficulty are only a focus in humanistic therapy if they affect present behavior.

Structure

Since the humanistic approach is person-centered, it is best to give minimal structure in occupational therapy groups using this frame of reference. This allows the individual members to have more say about the direction of therapy. Order can be maintained and direction kept clear by providing appropriate activities and limiting the range of choices in the group sessions. As the group is introduced, it is important for the therapist to set ground rules and communicate norms that reflect the basic assumptions of humanistic theory. Respect for one another, non-judgmental acceptance, and genuineness are important basic values for the occupational therapist to explain and to model.

Examples of Activities

Occupational therapy modalities that are appropriate for this frame of reference are those which promote the goals of humanistic therapy. Creative activities are well suited to these purposes, as well as the practice of specific skills. Self-awareness and self-understanding are addressed by all of the Activity Examples given at the end of the chapter. Group activities dealing with values and meaning in daily activities are "Leisure Collage," "My Ideal Job," "Activities Wheel," and the "Purpose in Life Chart." Emotional issues are discussed in the following group activities: "Positive Attitudes," "Saying Goodbye," "Draw Your Wall," and "Primary Concerns." The "Primary Concerns" activity is designed specifically for acute hospital settings, and emphasizes the value of follow-up therapy. "My House" asks members to get in touch with their dreams and to think about ways to achieve those dreams.

Humanistic groups should place an emphasis on human spirituality. Personal choices, ideals, and dreams and the quality of relationships are examined through structured activity and discussion. As such, these Activity Examples are not limited to positive and supportive issues. Separation, loneliness, solitude, and loss are all too real to our patients, and should not be avoided in group activities. It is only through open discussion of the full range of human emotion that persons begin to feel supported by each other. It is often through the human connections that begin in group treatment that members find the strength to seek out other helping relationships in their lives. The humanistic approach uses creative media (e.g., drawing, collage, storytelling) to help patients get back in touch with their intrinsic motivation and to develop a philosophy to live by. Activity Examples 3-1 through 3-10 are appropriate for humanistic groups.

Group Leadership

The general group format presented in Chapter 1 is based on a humanistic approach. Therefore, the seven steps remain basically the same.

Introduction

The therapist gives her name and the title of the group followed by the acknowledgment and introduction of each member. The environment should facilitate group confidentiality, trust, and safety (i.e., a private, soundproof room with a door that closes, free of interruptions for the time allotted).

The warm-up should be carefully selected to reflect therapeutic norms, such as respect and caring for one another, a focus on feelings, and open self-disclosure.

Expectations for a group in the humanistic frame of reference will be high, since it assumes that members have the capacity to understand and resolve their own problems without directive intervention from the therapist. This approach is generally not appropriate for patients who are cognitively impaired.

In humanistic groups, the purpose should be thoroughly explained, since member self-understanding and insight is assumed to be possible. Care in this initial explanation will make it possible for the members themselves to strive to accomplish the purpose as they do the activity.

The timeframe for the group should allow for longer, more complex, and thought-provoking activities. A greater portion of time in these groups should be set aside for discussion and group interaction. Perhaps 90 minutes or even 2 hours would not be too long for groups in a humanistic frame of reference.

Activity

Selecting activities is guided by the therapeutic goals of the humanistic frame of reference. The goals are self-awareness, self-understanding, and self-actualization. Thus, exploring interests, making choices, and developing new skills are also fair game, as long as these activities are patient directed. Creative activities like drawing, painting, sculpting, and storytelling or drama often encourage the expression of hidden aspects of the self, and are helpful in the goals of self-awareness and insight. The therapist selects and structures the activity to maximize goal achievement.

For example, she might choose to have the group draw a "Circle of Feelings." This requires each member to draw a circle in the center of a piece of 9- x 12-inch white drawing paper. Then the members use colored markers to indicate layers of feelings. The outer edge of the circle represents the outer self, the feelings they show to others, while the center of the circle represents the inner core, those feelings kept well-hidden and seldom shown to others. Such an activity serves to focus and guide the group toward a frank discussion of their inner feelings, promoting the goal of greater self-understanding among members.

The timeframe for such an activity should adhere to the rule of no more than one third of the entire group time. Emphasis in this frame of reference should always be on discussion and processing.

Sharing

Considerable time should be taken with this stage to be sure each member's work is correctly understood and explored by the group. The therapist might ask questions of each member to help clarify and focus their issues. Leader skills in concreteness, PAE, immediacy, confrontation, and AAE can be used effectively in all of the discussion stages of humanistic groups. The occupational therapist can use patient issues as examples to demonstrate the techniques of reality testing and consensual validation for the group. In the humanistic frame of reference, feedback is the most vital therapeutic tool available, and should be encouraged early in groups, beginning in the sharing stage. The purpose of feedback goes beyond the acknowledgment of member contributions. It is a skill to be taught to all the group members if they are to help one another.

In our example of the "Circle of Feelings" exercise, members may question one another about the meaning of color and about reported feelings. They may agree or disagree about the outer circle a patient describes. If Ben draws an outer circle of yellow, and reports feeling that others see him as cheerful and carefree, the statement invites other group members to comment. Some may agree with Ben, that he presents a jovial exterior. Others may see beyond this, to his inner pain and suffering. Ben and the group both benefit from a discussion of how he really comes across to others.

Processing

The potential of members sharing the leadership of groups is maximized in the humanistic frame of reference. Thus, the skill of giving and receiving feedback is further defined in the processing stage. As members discuss their feelings about the activity, the leader encourages them to also express feelings about one another. The best that we hope for is a genuine curiosity about one another, leading to concern and caring in the later stages of group development. The focus on feelings in the processing stage is consistent with the humanistic frame of reference. The therapist can further apply this frame by getting members to use their own experiences and capabilities to help one another.

Generalizing

In humanistic theory, the meaning of life is a central concern. The generalizing stage of the group is devoted to deriving the meaning of a small slice of life, the group experience. The therapist should encourage the members to verbalize the meaning of the experience for them. Looking at similarities and differences in what is meaningful will help reinforce the values of each member. Using our "Circle of Feelings" example again, some members might find meaning in becoming more aware of their own inner feelings, while others might value the opportunity to learn how others really see them. It may surprise some members to find themselves able to express feelings verbally, while others may be more guarded and unwilling to trust their inner feelings to others. Some people seek the understanding of others through self-disclosure and these people find meaning in close relationships with others. For other people, the impression they leave with others might be more important, the "never let them see you sweat" approach. Therapists need to be careful not to judge any value as right or wrong. Accepting differences among members is an important norm to promote in this stage.

Application

In this phase, meaning is expanded and personalized. In humanistic groups, action is not the emphasis. Thus, the group experience will more likely be applied to the enhancement of self-concept or deeper insight rather than the changing of behavior. The meaningfulness of activity encourages members to take steps toward further development and ultimately self-actualization.

Summary

The summary, as with every phase, should involve the group members whenever possible. They are presumed capable of analyzing the entire group experience and judging which parts are most significant. The therapist's role is to encourage them to do this, and not to do it for them. When the therapist asks for a summary of the group, about 5 minutes before it is time to end, members will quickly learn that this is what is expected, and may eventually do it spontaneously.

Bibliography

American Occupational Therapy Association. (1996). *Reference manual of official documents of the AOTA.* Bethesda, MD: Author.

Corey, G. (1986). *I never knew I had a choice* (3rd ed.). Monterey, CA: Brooks/Cole.

Corey, G. (1991). *The theory and practice of counseling and psychotherapy* (4th ed.). Monterey, CA: Brooks/Cole.

Egan, G. (1982). *Exercises in helping skills.* Monterey, CA: Brooks/Cole.

Egan, G. (1986). *The skilled helper* (3rd ed.). Monterey, CA: Brooks/Cole.

Huber, C. (1981). *Counseling techniques.* Presentation at University of Bridgeport Department of Graduate Psychology.

Maddi, S. R. (1980). *Personality theories: A comparative analysis* (4th ed.). Homewood, IL: The Dorsey Press.

Maslow, A. H. (1968). *Toward a psychology of being* (Rev. ed.). New York: Van Nostrand Reinhold.

May, R. (1977). *The meaning of anxiety* (Rev. ed.). New York: Norton.

May, R., & Yalom, I. (1989). Existential psychotherapy. In R. J. Corsini & D. Wedding (Eds.), *Current Psychotherapies* (4th ed.) (pp. 363-402). Itasca, IL: F. E. Peacock.

Mosey, A. C. (1981). *Occupational therapy: Configuration of a profession.* New York: Raven Press.

Mosey, A. C. (1989). The proper focus of scientific inquiry in occupational therapy: Frames of reference. *Occupational Therapy Journal of Research, 9*(4), 195-201.

Rogers, C. (1967). The conditions of change from a client-centered viewpoint. In B. Berenson & R. Carkhuff (Ed.), *Sources of Gain in Counseling and Psychotherapy.* New York: Holt, Rinehart, and Winston.

Rosenfeld, M. (1993). *Wellness and lifestyle renewal.* Bethesda, MD: American Occupational Therapy Association.

Simon, S. (1972). *Values clarification.* New York: Hart Publishers.

Yalom, I. (1995). *The theory and practice of group psychotherapy* (4th ed.). New York: Basic Books, Inc.

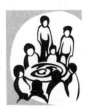

Humanistic
Activity Example 3-1
Self-Awareness

Directions: Fill out all the information listed on the worksheet. Then select what parts you would like to share with the group.

I am (name you prefer):

Some of my needs are:

Some of my hopes are:

I would describe myself as:

Some things that are important in my life now are:

Some things that may become important to me are:

Three things I am trying to achieve are:

I am good at:

Some things I would like to improve about myself are:

I run away from:

I feel confident when:

I am proud of:

My most striking quality is:

From Cole, M. B. *Group Dynamics in Occupational Therapy, Second Edition.* © 1998 SLACK Incorporated.
(Adapted from Simon, 1972)

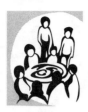

Materials: Magazines (at least two per patient) with pictures on a variety of subjects.

Directions: Select from these magazines pictures of negative scenes, problems, or situations. There is no required number, so find as many as you like. You have 15 minutes for this task.

Procedure: Each member presents his or her pictures and describes the negative situation. Then the group is asked to point out all the positive aspects of the pictures. For example, appearance or personal hygiene of the people, weather conditions, communication and support available, etc. Then the group can choose a few situations to problem solve. Answer the question: "What can be done to give this situation a happy ending?"

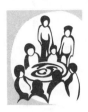

Humanistic
Activity Example 3-3
Leisure Collage

Materials: Magazines on varied topics, scissors, glue, white paper, and markers.

Directions: Cut pictures of things you like to do from these magazines and then arrange and paste them on the paper. You have 20 minutes to do this task. After you have finished pasting, use a marker to label each picture with a word ending in "ing" (e.g., eating, talking, playing volleyball, singing).

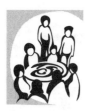

Materials: Writing paper and pens.

Directions: At some point in our lives, we have all had to leave someone we love. Either we left, or we got left behind (i.e., a best friend moving away, a lover finding a new love, a relative's death, a child going away to school). Often we do not have the chance to say the things we want to say before the separation. So here is another chance. Take the next 15 minutes to write a letter to a loved one, telling him or her the things you would like the person to know. Begin with "Dear _____" and end with some form of goodbye.

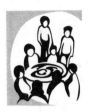

Humanistic
Activity Example 3-5
My House

Materials: Worksheets, rulers, colored markers, and pencils with erasers.

Directions: Imagine you are going on a 1-month vacation, and will live in a small house on the beach by yourself. The beach has a path that leads to town where you can buy food or other supplies. Visualize what the house would look like. You arrive in a taxi with your bags. You step onto the deck, unlock the front door, and walk in. What would you like to see? Now fill in the floor plan on the worksheet with whatever you would like in your house. Some suggestions are: sofa, bed, dresser, rug, television set, bookshelf with books, refrigerator, stove, washer, dryer, bicycle, sailboat, etc. (Figure 3-2).

While doing this activity, think about what necessities you will need and also what items you would like to help you enjoy your vacation. You may assume there are other people to socialize with at the beach, but they will not be staying with you. You are the only one living in your house.

From Cole, M. B. *Group Dynamics in Occupational Therapy, Second Edition.* © 1998 SLACK Incorporated.

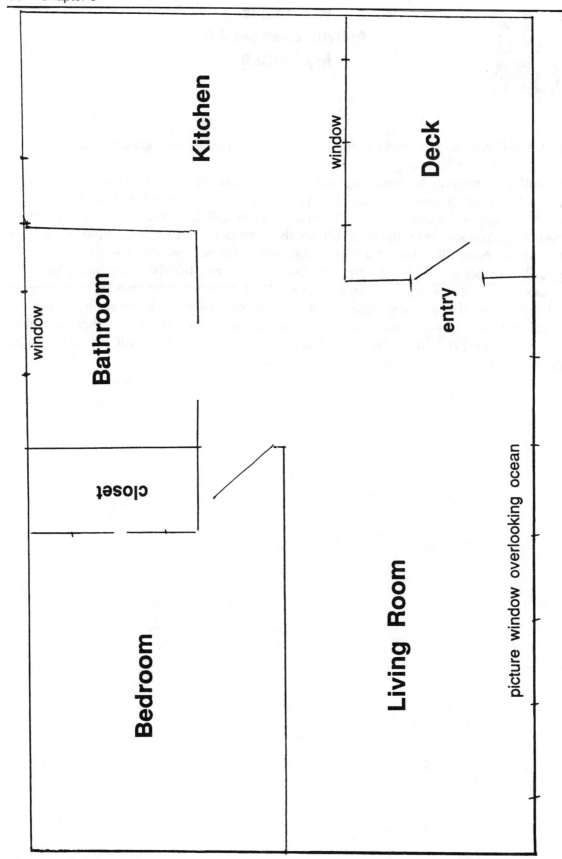

Figure 3-2. "My House" design (for use with Activity Example 3-5).

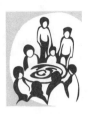

Humanistic
Activity Example 3-6
My Ideal Job

Materials: Worksheets and pencils.

Directions: Suppose you had the opportunity to be trained to do whatever job you want. What would be your ideal job? To help you define your ideal job, first circle your answers to the following questions. If you circle more than one, write "first choice" or "second choice" next to the answer.

1. What work setting do you prefer?
   Contemporary office
   Well-equipped workshop
   Home-like setting
   Outdoors
   Other

2. What other people would you prefer to work with?
   Work by yourself
   Be part of a working team
   Be the expert who gives help and advice to others
   Be your boss' right-hand man/woman

3. What skills do you prefer to use while working?
   Manual skills, work with hands or tools
   Artistic or creative skills
   Intellectual skills, knowledge, and ideas
   Political skills, strategies, or persuasion
   Technical problem-solving skills

4. What rewards would you seek from your job?
   Lots of money
   Satisfaction from helping others
   Having others recognize your skills
   Achieving your own potential

5. How much risk are you willing to take in your job?
   Prefer doing something familiar with regular pay
   Do not mind being paid on commission
   Willing to try new ideas, even if they are not a sure thing
   An element of danger might make work more exciting

Now consider your answers to those questions and circle the jobs that might fit your critera from the list below.

Salesperson in a small clothing store

Licensed electrician

Mechanic

Nursery school teacher

Medical technician

Nurse in a large hospital

Medical receptionist in a doctor's office

Advertising artist

Newspaper reporter

High school coach

Hairdresser

Interior decorator

Telephone lineman

Insurance claims adjuster

Traveling salesperson for a large company

Chef in an expensive restaurant

Hostess in an expensive restaurant

Manager of a small delicatessen

Manager of an expensive antique shop

Home health nurse

Musician in a band

Public relations representative for a hotel

Counselor in a drug rehabilitation center

Landscape designer

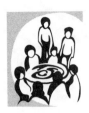

Humanistic
Activity Example 3-7
Draw Your Wall

Anne Golensky, MS, OTR, is acknowledged for creating this activity for use with recovering alcoholics.

Materials: White drawing paper and sets of colored markers.

Directions: The purpose of this activity is to discover the barriers we face that prevent us from moving toward self-actualization. Members introduce themselves and each completes the sentence "Something I've always wanted to do is _____." Then, with paper and markers, members draw their "wall," which symbolizes the things that hold them back from achieving their dreams.

From Cole, M. B. *Group Dynamics in Occupational Therapy, Second Edition.* © 1998 SLACK Incorporated.

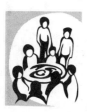

Humanistic
Activity Example 3-8
Primary Concerns

Materials: Three 3- x 5-inch index cards for each member, pens, and area telephone directories.

Directions: This activity is for acute inpatient groups. Members introduce themselves giving names and stating one reason they are in the hospital. They may briefly discuss where they intend to go when they leave, if known.

Write on each of three index cards the following information:

Card 1—What are you most concerned about at this moment?

Card 2—What are you most worried about after you leave the hospital?

Card 3—Who can you count on to help you with your concerns after you leave this group? List names and phone numbers of your doctor, a pharmacy near your residence, your closest family members and friends, and any other resources available to you. (Phone numbers may need to be filled in afterwards.)

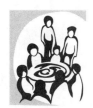

Humanistic
Activity Example 3-9
Activities Wheel

Materials: Worksheet with two circles representing 24-hour days. A calculator on hand would be helpful.

Directions: For each hour, fill in the name of the activity you are typically doing at that time of day. Then, total the hours for each general category at the bottom of the circle. Finally, approximate the percentage of the total for each category.

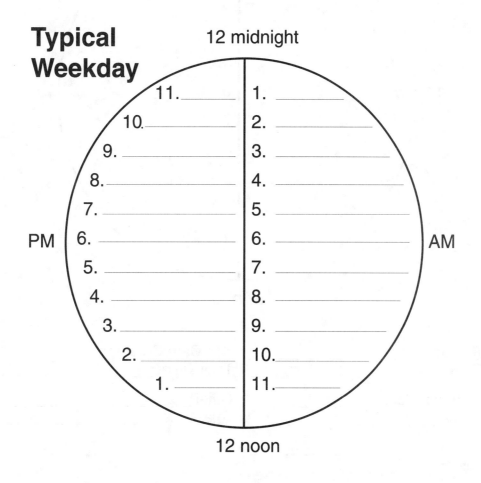

Work/Obligations:_____
Time: _____

Leisure/Relaxation: _____
Total Time: _____

Sleep/Rest: _____
Total Time: _____

Self-Care/Caregiving: _____
Total Time:_____

Other:_____
Total Time: _____

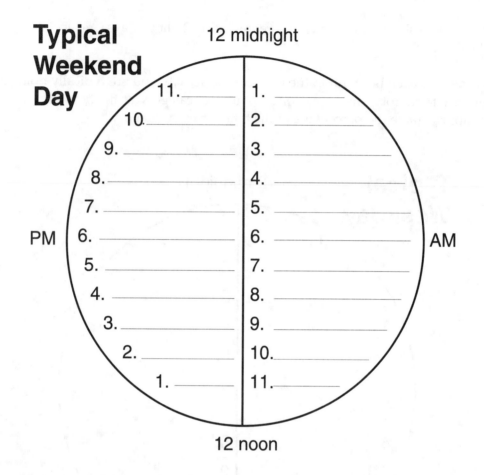

Typical Weekend Day

12 midnight

11._____ 1._____
10._____ 2._____
9._____ 3._____
8._____ 4._____
7._____ 5._____

PM 6._____ 6._____ AM

5._____ 7._____
4._____ 8._____
3._____ 9._____
2._____ 10._____
1._____ 11._____

12 noon

Work/Obligations:_____   Self-Care/Caregiving: _____
Total Time: _____   Total Time: _____

Leisure/Relaxation: _____   Other:_____
Total Time: _____   Total Time:_____

Sleep/Rest: _____
Total Time: _____

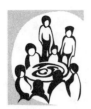

Humanistic
Activity Example 3-10
Purpose in Life Chart

Things I love:
1.

2.

3.

4.

5.

Things I am proud of:
1.

2.

3.

4.

5.

Things I want to strive for:
1.

2.

3.

4.

5.

Things I hate:
1.

2.

3.

4.

5.

Things I am ashamed of:
1.

2.

3.

4.

5.

Things I never want to become:
1.

2.

3.

4.

5.

Things I can do today to feel better about myself:
1.

2.

3.

From Cole, M. B. *Group Dynamics in Occupational Therapy, Second Edition*. © 1998 SLACK Incorporated.
(Adapted from Rosenfeld, 1993)

Chapter *4*

A Psychoanalytic Approach

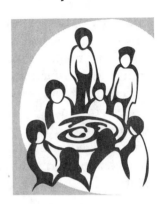

Historically, occupational therapy theorists have been acknowledging the usefulness of various forms of psychoanalytic theory in guiding our treatment of patients with mental illness. Diasio (1968) explores the psychoanalytic view of motivation and the environment. The Fidlers (1963) point out the importance of the unconscious and view activities as part of a communication process with human and non-human objects to effectively gratify instinctual needs. Mosey (1986), in considering analytical frames of reference, emphasizes the "structure for linking psychoanalytic theories, the symbolic potential and reality aspects of activities, and the process of altering intrapsychic content in the direction of providing a more adaptive basis for interaction with the environment." Llorens (1966) refers to "socially acceptable, ego-adaptive functioning" in describing the effect of patient involvement in activity groups, thus focusing on occupational therapy techniques that help develop and strengthen the functions of the ego.

Focus

Psychoanalytic theory has been out of favor, even in the field of mental health from which it originated. This fact is generally attributed to the lack of efficacy research, and the slowness and abstractness of the therapeutic process itself. As an occupational therapy approach, it is probably due for a comeback, perhaps in a redefined form. There are two reasons for this. First, there is no more effective framework for dealing with human emotion. When our patients refuse treatment, fail to follow through, or lack motivation to improve their state of health, emotional issues are usually to blame. We need psychoanalytic principles to identify conflicts and break through defenses and resistances that interfere with functional outcome. Second, the complexity of the psychoanalytic theory provides an explanation for many of the irrational, even bizarre behaviors we observe in persons with a variety of illnesses, for example, suicide attempts, risk-taking behaviors, paranoia, self-starvation, or obsessive compulsive behaviors, that are otherwise unexplainable.

Following the early theorists, two general goals of occupational therapy groups will be considered: alteration of personality and development of ego skills. This chapter will first review the basic assumptions of psychoanalytic theory which are useful in planning occupational therapy groups. Ego functions and their relevance to occupational therapy will then be reviewed. Finally, contributions from the occupational therapy literature will be summarized, and group leadership guidelines will be derived from these psychoanalytic theoretical concepts.

Psychoanalytic Theory

Psychoanalytic theory, based on the work of Sigmund Freud in the late 19th and early 20th centuries, has had a profound influence on all theories of group treatment. Corey (1991) describes Freud as an "intellectual giant" whose work represents "the most comprehensive theory of personality and psychotherapy ever developed." In the 1990s, there is a tendency to underestimate the influence of psychoanalytic theory because many subsequent theorists have either developed it further or reacted against it. The current emphasis on brain biochemistry as a determinant of human behavior has overshadowed the importance of personality dynamics in our understanding of mental illness. New technology has enabled researchers to observe the physiological and biochemical functioning of the brain in ways never before possible, and thus new genetic links have been discovered.

However, for occupational therapists, these new scientific discoveries do not alter the fact that there are many mental illnesses currently being diagnosed for which psychoanalytic theory offers the only plausible explanation. For example, there is a growing interest in borderline personality disorder, which is thought to originate from a failure to separate from parents and achieve an autonomous sense of self at around age 2. If the parent does not allow the child to explore his environment and do activities of his own choosing in a safe environment, then as an adult, he is unable to derive any satisfaction from activities. Knowing this, the occupational therapist can offer patients with borderline personality disorder an opportunity to explore activities according to their own interests. Recent research shows that for some borderline patients, it is possible to strengthen autonomous functioning through participation in task-oriented occupational therapy groups (Greene & Cole, 1991).

For occupational therapists, psychoanalytic theory is also useful in the physical disability areas of practice. The concept of self-worth and the many defenses of the ego can help us understand why some of our patients use denial of their illness or resist our suggestions for treatment. It is important for occupational therapists to determine the symbolic meaning of illness or trauma in the structure of personality, and how symptoms are incorporated into the patient's perception of self. For example, Julia, an 83-year-old woman with osteoporosis and chronic arthritis, was in and out of doctors' offices all her life, with many failed attempts to increase her independent functioning in occupational therapy. Only at age 79, after her husband died, did she learn to perform self-care independently. In her earlier years, Julia's many illnesses symbolized her helplessness. Her dependency on her husband for personal self-care fulfilled her need for attention and love. The patient's sense of self is vital to her acceptance or rejection of occupational therapy treatment, whether the illness is mental or physical.

The original form of psychoanalytic theory, sometimes called "id psychology" (Fine, 1979, p. 319), has been widely criticized by psychologists, social scientists, and occupational therapists during the past 20 years for its vagueness and its unsuitability for research. The link with psychoanalysis and its questionable appropriateness for treating many types of mental illness has added fuel to the fires of discontent. Psychoanalysis is a therapeutic approach developed by Freud, in which individual patients are assisted in uncovering their unconscious conflicts by conversing with a therapist, a process which could take many years. Critics feel that one cannot research the unconscious, since it is not observable or measurable.

A more current emphasis on ego psychology focuses on the conscious rather than the unconscious aspects of the personality and is therefore, by definition, more observable and measurable. The ego is best understood as the "self." A patient's sense of self, his self-concept, can determine his degree of involvement in occupational therapy treatment. If a patient sees himself as a capable and worthwhile individual, he will be motivated to overcome disability. If Dean defines himself as an accountant, he will make the effort to overcome his depression and to return to that occupation. In this frame of reference, the ego is seen as a powerful motivating force which can either resist or facilitate therapeutic change.

Bellak and colleagues (1973) operationalized the functions of the ego, making them more amenable for research purposes. They define 12 ego functions:

1. Reality testing
2. Judgment
3. Sense of self and the world
4. Control of drive, affect, and impulse
5. Object relationships
6. Thought processes
7. Adaptive regression in service of the ego
8. Defensive functioning
9. Stimulus barrier
10. Autonomous functioning
11. Synthetic integrative functions
12. Mastery/competence

The functions most applicable to occupational therapy will be further defined later in this chapter.

Basic Assumptions

The following is intended as a brief review of the original concepts of Freudian psychoanalytic theory. A more thorough understanding may be obtained by referring to other basic psychology texts. Psychoanalytic theory is exceedingly complex, and there are many variations currently in use. It must be remembered that Freud's theory provides an intellectual understanding of the personality and its development. The parts described as id, ego, and superego do not parallel structures or functions of the brain, nor do they represent distinct developmental stages. The purpose for which psychoanalytic theory will be used in this text is to define those concepts that help us understand the dynamics of illness, both mental and physical, and to develop treatment techniques to address these dynamics. Because of the focus on group treatment, many important aspects of Freudian theory will be left out.

Personality Structure

Freud organized personality into three parts: the id, the ego, and the superego. This structure is still accepted by many psychotherapists regardless of their discipline or theoretical preferences. While a balance of these components is considered ideal, the functions of the ego in this text will be emphasized because of their direct relevance to occupational therapy groups.

The Id

The id is seen as largely unconscious. It is the part of the personality which houses primitive drives and instincts, needs, and conflicts that the ego is unable to integrate. The id is the biological component of the personality, and is thought to operate through primary process thinking. Primary process thinking is the earliest to develop in the infant. It is illogical and undisciplined and operates on the pleasure principle, demanding immediate gratification of needs and drives.

The Ego

The ego is the psychological component and has contact with the external world. It functions logically and works to achieve a balance between internal drives and external expectations. The ego operates through a secondary process, one that is learned through experience in reaching compromises and applying logic and discipline in an attempt to adapt to the environment.

The Superego

The superego is the social component of the personality which serves as an individual's moral code, his sense of good and bad, right and wrong. The superego is often illogical and unrealistic in its quest for idealism and perfection. The superego is the last part to appear in the developmental process and its beliefs are learned from parents and from society.

Psychosexual Stages

Freud believed that personality is largely determined by one's early childhood experiences. Psychosexual stages of development, spanning a range of 18 years from birth to maturity, are differentiated by changes in the objects which potentially provide need satisfaction. An object is someone or something that gratifies or frustrates a need; objects can be human or non-human. The classic example of an object in the oral stage is a mother's breast. A non-human substitute for a mother's breast is the bottle. When a child's needs are gratified, he thrives and is able to develop and move on to the next stage. However, when the child's needs are continually frustrated, he develops a fixation which can remain in the unconscious and cause many of the problems in adulthood which we know as symptoms of illness. Freud's psychosexual stages of development are outlined in Table 4-1.

The psychosexual stages are critical to our understanding of mental illness. In spite of current discoveries of the genetic and biochemical origins of some illnesses, most psychopathology is still explained in terms of Freud's levels of personality organization. In general, the earlier the conflict occurs, the more severe the illness. While there are not rigid parallels between the stages and the development of certain illnesses, fixations in the early stages are likely to result in faulty or incomplete development in later ones. For example, failure to develop self-control in the anal stage may result in the overdevelopment or misuse of defense mechanisms as the ego attempts to compensate for lack of self-control in later stages.

When we, as occupational therapists, observe patients in our therapeutic groups who are unable to work together and get along with one another, a knowledge of how the patients have progressed through the psychosexual stages may help us understand the reasons why. In addition, the stages may offer guidelines as to what type of therapeutic intervention is needed. For example, trust is an issue dealt with in the oral stage. Groups in which members seem to lack a basic trust of one another might benefit from activities which assist patients in feeling more comfortable with self-disclosure. This self-disclosure can

Table 4-1.
Freud's Psychosexual Stages

Age (years)	Stage (source of gratification)	Fixation Characteristics (potential problem areas)
Birth-1 year	*Oral Stage* early - sucking late - biting	Theme: trust, dependency Regression: psychosis
1-3 years	*Anal Stage* early - excreting late - retaining	Theme: control, autonomy Regression: neurosis, character disorders
3-5 years	*Phallic Stage* genital interest penis envy	Theme: Oedipal/Electra complex
5-12 years	*Latency Stage* sublimation of sexual drive superego develops	Theme: Skill development social role development emergence of guilt
11-adulthood	*Genital Stage* puberty capacity for intimacy	Theme: Sexual identity adult responsibility for love and work

form the basis of establishing trusting relationships with the therapist and with one another.

Psychic Energy, Libido, Aggression, and Anxiety

In Freud's view, the amount of psychic energy is limited and must be shared by all three parts of the personality. This explains why people cease to function when too much energy is being used up in trying to deal with unresolved conflicts from the past. A healthy individual is able to resolve conflicts as they arise and therefore keep psychic energy available for the ego to grow, develop, and interact effectively with the environment. In mental illness, psychic energy may be trapped in the id and may produce non-adaptive behaviors which we call symptoms.

Two specific forms of psychic energy are described by Freud: the libidinal and the aggressive drives. Libido is the sexual energy which represents the urge to perpetuate life, to be intimate, to love, and to reproduce. This is also called the life-force, and is demonstrated by a person's tendency to form relationships with other people. The aggressive drive is equated with the death-force, and is associated with hostility, hatred, and the urge to destroy. It is expressed in the tendency to be self-sufficient and to keep others at a distance. Both the libidinal and the aggressive drives are part of the id, and both seek expression through objects. It is a function of the ego to control these drives and to allow their expression in ways that are socially acceptable. It is a function of the superego to guide an individual's libidinal and aggressive drives toward constructive and morally acceptable expression.

Anxiety, in Freud's view, is defined in relation to both drives and the ego's control function. Anxiety is an alerting response which lets us know that something is wrong and needs to be changed, and that some action needs to be taken to get us out of danger. However, unlike the existentialists who view anxiety as a normal condition of life, Freud views anxiety as pathological. Freudian anxiety develops out of the conflicts over control of the available psychic energy within the personality itself. This anxiety goes beyond fear of realistic danger from the external world. It is the fear that the id may take over, forcing the individual to act irrationally or in ways that are morally wrong, or that the superego may take over, causing a pervasive sense of guilt and self-punishment. As long as the ego maintains control, anxiety can be safely held in check and dealt with realistically. High levels of neurotic anxiety, however, may necessitate the unconscious use of ego defense mechanisms to help reduce the tension and protect the survival of the ego. These mechanisms will be reviewed later in this chapter.

Occupational therapists may facilitate the expression of psychic energy through activities. This helps the patient in a variety of ways. Through activities, the aggressive drive can be directed toward productive work, constructive homemaking, or competition in sports. The libidinal drive can energize the patient to development of social skills, nurturing skills, and cooperation with others. Various ego functions might be encouraged in occupational therapy groups, such as appropriate expression of feelings, both loving and aggressive, or the sharing of perceptions to help members develop a realistic sense of self.

Symbols, Projections, and Communication with the Unconscious

Rarely, except in episodes of psychosis, does the content of the unconscious become known. Psychoanalytic therapy's main thrust is to help an individual become aware of his unconscious conflicts and fixations, so that the mature ego can deal with them effectively and resolve them. However, the nature of primary process makes awareness of unconscious material very complex. Primary process is not organized or logical, and is not remembered in words or complete thoughts. Highly emotional material may take the form of symbols that represent experiences which originally produced them. For example, a child who experienced the violent death of a parent in an automobile accident may have repressed the original memory. If as an adult, she draws a car as part of an occupational therapy activity, she may suddenly reexperience an overwhelming feeling of grief and loss without knowing why. It is the therapist's role to help the adult patient to interpret the meaning of the symbols she produces, and with the help of a psychiatrist, remember and work through the original traumatic experience.

Object Relationships

Object relationships were previously mentioned as the organizing principles of the psychosexual stages. Freud viewed object relations as the foundation of an individual's capacity to love and to work. The Fidlers (1963) define occupational therapy in terms of the development of relationships with human (therapist) and non-human (environment) objects. In human relationships, the patient develops the ability to satisfy some of his basic needs, such as recognition, self-esteem, and belonging, through a therapeutic relationship with the occupational therapist. In the safety of a therapeutic environment, the patient uses realistic feedback from the therapist or other patients to correct his unrealistic concepts and expectations of self and others.

Non-human objects are related to the patient's ability to work. The patient can learn, in occupational therapy, to use the symbolic as well as actual properties of objects to help satisfy instinctual drives and needs. For example, Bob can satisfy his need to express hostility by flattening a ball of clay or sawing a piece of wood. Mary can express her compulsive needs by maintaining a perfectly clean and organized kitchen. Using this principle, occupational therapy activities can be selected according to the instinctual needs of group members.

Assumptions of Ego Psychology

Alfred Adler (Fine, 1979) is credited with making the first significant break with Freud over the nature and importance of the ego. He believed that the ego is responsible for shaping the personality, rather than the person being shaped by biological forces and early childhood experiences. Another theorist who recognized the importance of the ego was Heinz Hartmann. Hartmann (1939) looked at the process of psychoanalysis and suggested that it was not a reconstruction of what once existed buried in the unconscious (the Freudian view). He saw that psychotherapy requires that the mature ego establish correct causal relationships and judgments of the emerging memories. The significance of Hartmann's work is in establishing the autonomy of the ego as separate from the id in psychoanalytic theory. Ego psychology has been developing since 1923, and has had many spokespersons, including Adler, Sullivan, Hartmann, Erikson, Lewin, and Rapaport (Fine, 1979). The common element is an emphasis on the ego. For the sake of brevity, not all the functions of the ego can be reviewed. Those selected for emphasis are reality testing, sense of self, thought processes, self-control, defense mechanisms, and mastery/competence.

Reality Testing

Reality testing is perhaps the most important function of the ego in therapy. It is the ego's ability to use perception and judgment to differentiate between internal needs and external demands. This process involves the use of interaction with the environment and with others in shaping and reshaping one's views of self and the world. It is precisely this process which is responsible for adaptation to the environment. The ego becomes aware of needs and drives from the id, but delays their gratification until they can be satisfied in ways that are socially acceptable.

Consensual Validation

Reality testing is an integral part of the therapeutic use of groups. As members share their perceptions of themselves and the world with others in the group, they have the advantage of hearing the responses of others. It is through this feedback that group members gather evidence to support their self-other perceptions. When perceptions of others are clearly different from one's own, then one needs to question whether her own perceptions are realistic. The process of integrating one's own perceptions, views, or beliefs with those of others is called consensual validation.

For example, Lisa shared with the group a painful experience involving her father's rejection of her. Lisa believed she had to live with this rejection and was powerless to change it. Several other members recounted similar feelings about their own fathers, based on similar experiences. This feedback helped validate Lisa's feelings of rejection; based on clear evidence, she had a right to feel rejected—in her situation, anyone would. However, another member of the group, Roberta, also told Lisa how she had begun speaking to her father after a 7-year period of silence. Roberta was able to significantly improve her father-daughter relationship through some more adult conversations and sharing of feelings. This feedback made Lisa reconsider her position; perhaps she was not as powerless as she believed herself to be. The group helped Lisa to see which parts of her self-perception were real (being rejected) and which were not real (being powerless).

Exploring Outer Reality

Occupational therapy groups involving the use of concrete tasks provide another kind of reality testing, one on a sensory level. Manipulation of objects and materials provides sensory input: taste, touch, smell, vision, hearing, and proprioception (position, pressure, balance, etc.), which can lead on to challenge internal perceptions. Robert felt he had no energy and therefore could not complete a woodworking project. When the group members persuaded him to try it, however, the sensory stimulation provided by sawing and hammering the wood (proprioceptive and auditory) helped release the needed energy. Robert learned through experience that by engaging in appropriate motor activities, he was able to direct his energy to produce a positive effect on the environment (a completed project). If the group then also provides positive feedback on his wood project, Robert is further inclined to change his view of himself from ineffectual, "I can't," to effective, "I can!" It is important here for the occupational therapist to be aware of Robert's abilities in choosing a task, ensuring that his experience is likely to be a successful one.

Sense of Self

Many aspects of sense of self appear in the literature, and their meanings can be somewhat confusing. Three discrete aspects will be defined here: self-concept, body image, and self-esteem.

Self-Concept

Self-concept and self-identity are sometimes used interchangeably with the word ego. Developmentally, the idea of self originates when the infant begins to differentiate self from mother, and then from the environment in general. Psychotic individuals are understood by ego psychologists to have regressed beyond the point where they are able to differentiate self from others. These psychotic individuals are said to have "poor" or "loose" ego boundaries. This factor makes psychotic patients particularly sensitive to their environment. When someone in the group is angry, for example, it is often the psychotic patient who is first to notice it, although he may not express his awareness realistically or appropriately.

Following Freud's original formulations, the attempt was made to correlate the various clinical entities with the points of fixation in psychosexual development. Primarily, the oral stage is associated with psychosis, the anal stage with neuroses, and the phallic stage with hysteria. Ego psychologists have elaborated and changed this original oversimplified concept of mental illness, but have retained the idea that the ego or self-concept is fundamentally different in these three levels of psychiatric diagnosis. Psychological testing such as word association (Jung, 1910), interpretation of inkblots (Rorschach, 1921), and association with photographs (Murray's Thematic Apperception Test, 1938) are a few of the earliest attempts to measure ego functions with particular regard to self-concept.

The idea that concept of the self is a common problem area for mentally ill individuals has led occupational therapists to make self-concept and its related ideas—body image, self-esteem, and self-perception—the focus of occupational therapy treatment. Groups using movement, dance, physical sports, or exercise may be helpful to patients in developing a realistic body image. Drawing and word association activities, often taking their cue from the various psychological tests, have been useful in promoting knowledge of the self. Self-esteem is better approached in occupational therapy through successful experiences and feedback from others. Person drawings in particular are a useful therapeutic tool, for both evaluation and treatment in occupational therapy.

Body Image

Body image is the perception of one's physical self that forms the basis of self-awareness. According to theories of child development, the earliest learning involves the association and differentiation of somatosensory sensations. These provide a kind of geographical knowledge of the body and how it works that defines "me." Body sense, according to Allport (1958), allows a child to develop a sense of personhood. It is the sensory motor exploration of early play that helps the child define the boundaries of his body and distinguish "me" from "not me." In adulthood, body sense continues to provide a basic reference point from which environmental interactions take place. The sensory systems, for example, help people know how they feel. Influences from the body guide day-to-day behavior. For example, you may stay home from work because you feel fatigued, or you may go for a walk because you feel restless. The child achieves a sense of control over his body by reaching out to the environment to satisfy body needs: a bottle satisfies hunger, a toy satisfies need for pleasure, mother satisfies the need for comfort. As adults, we continue to reach out to the environment and to others based on our perceptions of our bodies and what we need.

Illness tends to produce distortions in body image, and this may be the source of problem behaviors. As occupational therapists, one of our goals is to determine whether our patient's body image is realistic. Using activities that encourage patients to become aware of their feelings and sensations can help to correct body image distortions. Movement activities and person drawings are two examples of this.

Self-Esteem

Self-esteem describes the subjective feelings of one's own ability. As with sensory motor, perceptual, and cognitive processes, feelings are innate and develop as the child matures. However, feelings or affects are intricately tied to objects, and their expression determines how people relate to one another and to their world. The idea that affects are ego states comes from Freud's 1926 work *Inhibitions, Symptoms, and Anxiety*. Rapaport (1953) attempted to articulate a theory of affect, suggesting that affect originates as psychic energy and is seen as a signal emitted by the ego to indicate an internal feeling state needing to be noticed. Spitz (1959) offered a theory of affect development in the infant as crying, smiling, and stranger distress or fearfulness. Language development then allows the child to express a multiplicity of feeling states of increasing complexity.

The expression of affect or emotion is an important function of the ego. As suggested by Rapaport, it is one of the ways the ego has to control and direct energy from the id. Acting out has been described earlier as a more primitive, less socialized form of expression of affect through action. Those with special talents are able to express affect through artistic media, such as painting, music, poetry, or drama. While these ways are socially acceptable, the most commonly acceptable way to express affect is by describing it verbally with words.

As occupational therapists, we often observe in our patients (and sometimes in ourselves) a lack of ability to communicate emotions to others. In the ego adaptive frame of reference, a common goal of occupational therapy groups is the appropriate expression of emotions.

Thought Processes

Thought processes are the cognitive functions of the ego having to do with attention, memory, learning and logical thought, compromise, problem-solving, and judgment.

Attention

Attention is the ability of the ego to focus on something for a period of time. It requires not only alertness of the mind, but a readiness to take in new information. Information coming in through the sensory systems is screened for relevance and the brain focuses on aspects of the environment to which a response is appropriate. Sustained attention, or concentration, is needed for the individual to participate in occupational therapy groups.

Memory

Memory is central to psychoanalytic theory, as seen in Freud's persistent efforts to recapture early childhood events. Rapaport (1942) recognized the relationship between memory and emotional factors. The ego was thought to censor memory in accordance with the intensity of associated emotional factors. In other words, events that were extremely painful are repressed; the ego stores them below the level of consciousness and they cannot be remembered at all. Or, the ego can alter the perception of a traumatic event, so that the senses are numbed and the brain will not receive more stimuli than it can handle. In this case, the memory of the event would be inaccurate or unrealistic. The current metaphor most closely associated with memory is that of the computer, with information storage and retrieval as the primary activities. It is believed that one's memory process reflects individual styles of secondary process functioning. In other words, what someone remembers is dependent upon how she perceives and understands an event in the first place.

When an occupational therapist hears a patient report a remembered event in a group, it becomes the task of the therapist to listen not only for the facts, but also for the emotional bias the patient expresses. This is particularly important if the patient's emotional response is problematic. For example, Shelley reported at the beginning of the group that something about the last group had been bothering her all week. Last week, during a serious discussion among several group members, Shelley had gotten up from her chair and stepped into the center of the group to kill a spider that was crawling on the floor. She felt "terrible" that her action would be viewed as a violation or mocking of the members whose discussion she had disrupted. The group's response to this confession was surprising. Two or three members remembered the incident in passing, but said it was "no big deal." The three members who were involved in the discussion had no recall of the event at all, just as though it never happened. The facts of the spider killing event were the same for everyone, but Shelley remembered them in the context to a strong emotional bias which put herself in a negative light. It was only with the feedback of the other group members that she was able to shed the bias and put the event in a more realistic perspective.

With most significant events in our lives, we do not have the advantage of the feedback of the others to help us correct our emotional bias. Hence, when past events not witnessed by the group are reported to the group, it is difficult for members or the therapist to separate the facts from the emotions involved. It is only in the context of here-and-now events that groups can be helpful in this way. This is one reason that it is suggested that our occupational therapy groups have a here-and-now focus.

Learning and Logical Thought

Learning is a skill of the ego which has been given little attention by followers of psychoanalysis, yet it is central to the notion of making therapeutic change. It has been noted by ego psychologists that intellectual development (learning) occurs most favorably in a warm, secure environment. This observation is helpful to occupational therapy so we can recognize the importance of creating and maintaining this kind of safe environment in our groups. Physical safety should be a given; this means that the occupational therapist removes any dangerous objects or factors from the environment (i.e., sharp objects, loose wires, wet or slippery floors). Psychological safety is provided when the occupational therapist maintains control through the establishment of group norms, such as mutual respect and prevention of verbal attacks on one another.

The kind of thinking attributed to the ego is secondary process thinking. This is also called reasoning or logical thought. It is the ability of the ego to consider facts in the light of reality and put them to use in guiding behavior. Problem-solving is a cognitive skill which requires the use of logical thought. In fact, all of the functions of the ego contribute to problem-solving: accurate perception and reality testing, memory and control of impulses, as well as appropriate use of defenses. The process of solving problems is quite complex, but the ability to do so is often a deciding factor in whether our patients are considered to be competent in activities of daily living. Occupational therapists are often asked to evaluate a patient's problem-solving ability. Observation of the patient in a group activity is one way to determine this skill. For example, Rich, a patient in a cooking group, was unfamiliar with the process of peeling and slicing carrots for a salad. However, since he had arrived late, that was the only job available. Rich picked up the knife and proceeded to chop the carrot, leaving the skin on and cutting only part way through with each chop. When another patient handed Rich a vegetable peeler, Rich turned on the would-be helper and waved the knife at him in a somewhat threatening way. After a few more attempts to cut the skin off the carrot with the knife, Rich put down the carrot and abandoned the task. After observing Rich's behavior, the occupational therapist discussed the situation with Rich and determined that Rich's ability to solve problems was poor.

How can occupational therapy groups be helpful to Rich in learning to solve problems? Clearly, teaching him to use a vegetable peeler will only help temporarily in the specific situation. In general, Rich's tendency to act alone and reject help are the real issues that need to be dealt with. Group discussion following the cooking task helped Rich to understand what his options were in solving the carrot problem. Asking for help and being able to accept it in a non-threatening way were agreed upon as goals for Rich in future group tasks.

Judgment

Judgment is another function of the ego which is often the focus in occupational therapy groups. Good judgment requires the following cognitive processes: accurate and realistic perception of the situation, identification of intended behaviors and likely consequences, prediction of the behaviors' effect on others, control of response until options are considered, and an appreciation of what it takes to accomplish something. On a well-known psychological test, the patient is asked the question, "What is the thing to do if you find an envelope in the street that is sealed, addressed, and has a new stamp?" The most acceptable answer is "mail it" (Wechsler, 1981, p. 126). How one arrives at this response requires a complex process of perception, reasoning, and anticipation of consequences. Judgment is a cognitive skill of the highest order, and one of the most difficult to learn or teach.

Self-Control

Control was the earliest of the ego functions to be recognized, when Freud conceptualized the ego's main function to control the instinctual drives from the id. Impulse control may be seen as a derivative of this earlier conceptualization.

In occupational therapy groups, we often encourage impulse control in a number of ways. We expect group members to arrive on time and to remain attentive for the length of the group, usually 50 to 60 minutes. We expect members to consider others in the group, listen to them, wait their turn to speak, share tools and materials, and pass the glue or the scissors. In a cooking group, we would ask members not to taste the food with their fingers, and to wait to begin eating until the whole group is seated. On a shopping trip, we ask our patients not to taste items in the store, not to buy items impulsively, and to wait to light their cigarettes until they have finished shopping. Following social norms and interacting effectively in groups requires good control of impulses.

Defense Mechanisms

Defenses are broadly understood as a way of warding off anxiety and ensuring the safety and preservation of an intact

ego. The strengthening of healthy defenses is a common goal in occupational therapy groups. In addition, the concept of defenses helps us as occupational therapists to understand better our patients' responses to activities. Through our recognition of defenses in our patients, we as occupational therapists are better able to plan activities and make therapeutic interventions in our groups to help patients achieve a healthy balance in their lives.

Defense mechanisms are an important part of the structure of the ego. Early psychologists focused on this aspect when developing the techniques of psychoanalysis. The goal of psychoanalysis was to break through a person's defenses so as to uncover the memory of critical childhood events.

Kaplan and Sadock (1998) have classified defense mechanisms into four categories:

1. Narcissistic defenses—Projection, denial, and distortion
2. Immature defenses—Acting out, blocking, hypochondriasis, introjection, passive aggressive behavior, projection, regression, schizoid fantasy, somatization, and turning against the self
3. Neurotic defenses—Controlling, displacement, dissociation, externalization, inhibition, intellectualization, isolation, rationalization, reaction formation, repression, sexualization, and undoing
4. Mature defenses—Altruism, anticipation, asceticism, humor, sublimation, and suppression

The contemporary ego psychologists view mature defenses as performing a healthy adaptive function, and these will be most relevant to our work in occupational therapy. Those defenses that are dealt with most often in occupational therapy are reviewed here. The reader is referred to Kaplan and Sadock (1998) for a more thorough description of the above defenses.

Sublimation

Sublimation was identified by Anna Freud in 1936 as a healthy and acceptable rechanneling of libidinal and aggressive drives into constructive activity. While sublimation is no longer a focus in psychological literature, the concept remains central to occupational therapy because of its implications regarding activity, creativity, and tasks or work. As occupational therapists using a psychoanalytic frame of reference, we continue to see clear evidence of this rechanneling of energy. The concept allows us to understand why work is such a central part of living, and why the loss of the work role produces both aggressiveness and anxiety and a sharp decline in one's self-worth. Neutralization (Hartmann's updated substitute for sublimation) refers to the de-energizing of the libidinal and aggressive drives. It is the "successful defense" by which the mature ego masters reality.

Projection

Projection is another defense, originating with Freud (1914), which continues to hold value in occupational therapy. The modern day variation was described by Melanie Klein (1948) as projective identification. In this mechanism, parts of the self are split off and projected onto an external object or person. Projection provides the ego with a means of getting rid of bad parts of the self. Sam is angry with his boss, but he believes the anger is bad, so he projects the anger onto his boss. Now Sam can like himself and feel justified in believing his boss is the bad guy who gets angry. Good parts of the self may be projected also, to avoid separation or keep them safe from the bad parts. Projection at higher levels leads to misinterpreting the motives, feelings, attitudes, or intentions of others.

Projection as a concept is used extensively in occupational therapy in the form of projective techniques. Projective techniques are generally creative modalities, such as drawing, sculpture, poetry, creative writing, or drama, which allow or encourage a person to express the hidden parts of the self. A patient is said to project parts of himself, particularly affects such as anger or love, in the form of symbols or shapes in art or characters and situations in writing or drama. When done in adulthood, these images or fantasies are then open to interpretation by the mature ego. As therapists, we encourage our patients to apply logic and mature judgment to the products of their projective creations when we ask them to explain them to their fellow group members. One Vietnam veteran participating in an occupational therapy projective arts group was asked to explain his elaborate drawing of the atrocities of war. The guns, the dead body parts, and the destructive remains of buildings symbolized for him the bad parts of himself which he found so hard to accept.

Regression

Regression was also an emphasis of Freud's early work as it helped to explain "fixations" as a cause of mental illness. Regression is going backward from a later to an earlier stage of development. In 1964, Arlow and Brenner defined regression as "the re-emergence of modes of mental functioning characteristic of earlier phases of psychic development." They further state that regressions are usually transient and reversible. Pathology is not determined by the depth of the regression (oral, anal, etc.) but by its irreversible nature, by the conflicts which it engenders, and by its interference with the process of adaptation. The importance of regression has recently been enhanced by its relation to borderline and psychotic conditions.

Psychotic individuals are said to be regressed to the oral stage (birth to 1 year), the earliest stage in Freud's psychosexual stages of development. Persons with borderline personality disorder are thought to be regressed to the anal stage (1 to 3 years), and fixated there. This view of regression may help to explain the behavior of our patients with these diagnoses in terms of the functioning of the ego. To do so, however, would require a thorough understanding of Freud's psychosexual stages of development.

Regression has another implication that is important for the occupational therapist in planning treatment. This is the concept of "regression in the service of the ego." Ernst Kris (1936) first used this term to imply a purposeful regression to earlier modes of functioning without the loss of overriding ego control. The artist who smears paint on a canvas to express extreme affect but retains the control to return to the normal world (while the psychotic patient cannot) is a good example. The technique of "free association," or the uncensored, often illogical associations of words and images, has been cited as another example.

The therapeutic usefulness of regression to the ego lies in its contribution to a clearer self-understanding. When we ask our patients to wedge clay or use finger paints, these processes reflect the typical (sometimes forbidden) fascination of the anal stage (smearing feces). Our therapeutic purpose for doing this is not to encourage regression, but to free the individual to express affect in an uninhibited way, with the hope of recapturing the innate urge toward mastery which may be trapped there. The patient, after engaging in such a creative process, returns to a more mature level of functioning, but he retains an awareness of the affect discovered during the regression. This affect is essential if the

patient is to change the way he understands and uses activity as a part of his return to healthy functioning.

Acting Out

Acting out can best be defined as an action, usually repetitive and compulsive in nature, and often self-destructive, that serves the unconscious purpose of resolving a repressed internal conflict by external means. This is a popular way to explain self-destructive behavior in analytical terms. It reflects a primitive lack of control over actions that are typical of the infant, and regressively present in psychosis and character disorder.

In groups, we often see emotions being "acted out" instead of talked about. For example, anger at someone in the group is expressed by walking out of the room and slamming the door. An action is substituted for a mature verbal description of a feeling state. Occupational therapist group leaders should discourage acting out responses. These are inappropriate and unproductive for both the patient and other group members. The more mature ego skill of verbal expression of affect should be encouraged.

Identification

Identification, as a defense described by Freud, was meant quite literally as the taking onto oneself the characteristics of another. The concept originated as a logical outcome of the Oedipal conflict, in which sexual desire for the opposite sex parent is replaced by identification with the parent of like sex. Anna Freud (1936) described this phenomenon as "identification with the aggressor." The child's identification with the feared "aggressor" is used, in part, to explain the repetition of behavior patterns in families. Child abuse is an example when the abused child grows up to abuse his own children. Erikson (1950) contributed greatly to the popularity of this concept in his extensive discussion of the identity crisis occurring in late adolescence.

Mastery/Competence

Bellak and colleagues (1973) define this function of the ego as adaptive performance in work and relationships, and the subjective feelings of competence. R.H. White defines competence as "an organism's capacity to interact effectively with its environment..." (Bellak, Huruich, & Gediman, 1973, p. 260). "Fitness to interact with the environment," in White's view, includes language and motor skills, cognition, and higher thought processes. The affect or feeling of efficacy is what White called "effectance motivation" (Bellak et al., 1973, p. 260), referring to the individual's tendency to put more effort and energy into producing responses that will have a desirable effect on the environment. The feelings of competence are the result of a well-developed ego, and include a history of successful experiences in coping with the environment.

The ego's ability to cope is what rescues a person in times of illness or crisis. In an emotional crisis, many of the ego defenses described earlier may be viewed as coping mechanisms, protecting the ego from destruction by diverting psychic energy. In the case of physical trauma, the ego uses body sense and reality testing to determine what functions of the body remain intact. The ego's sense of self will often provide the motivation to find ways to compensate for lost functions. For example, a patient with right-sided hemiplegia will learn to write with her left hand. Compensation is a coping strategy.

Another example of a coping strategy is energy conservation. When physical and mental deterioration occur, energy for use in everyday activities is severely limited. Careful planning before embarking on a task can prevent the patient from wasting energy in needless movements. For example, after I had an operation, I was only able to stand up or walk for 15 minutes before stopping to take a rest. When preparing a meal, I had to learn to use the 15 minutes to gather absolutely everything I needed to make meatballs, then assemble them while sitting at the kitchen table. The cooking had to be done in an electric frying pan on the table, rather than at the stove. I had to learn to be satisfied with accumulating a mess around me, rather than cleaning as I went along, and to use a wet sponge to wipe my hands, rather than washing at the sink every few minutes. For patients with chronic disability, conserving energy is a coping skill that is absolutely essential for continued functioning at a level that is consistent with the patient's self-identity.

Function and Dysfunction

A functioning adult is free of conflicts and fixations, and is able to satisfy his needs and direct his drives in ways that fit in with the social environment and culture. A balance exists in the functioning individual that allows the psychic energy to flow freely between the id, ego, and superego. The ego is in control and defense mechanisms are not exaggerated, so that the individual with a healthy ego can use most of his energy to grow and develop and interact effectively with others. In Fidler's model, the healthy person is able to work productively with others to accomplish a task. As an adult, he has acquired all six of Mosey's adaptive skills (Mosey, 1981, see Appendix A). The defenses the individual uses are mature ones, like sublimation of aggression in work, identification with idealized others, and the suppression of immediate gratification. A healthy ego is synonymous with a strong sense of self; body image, self-identity, and self-esteem are realistic, and can serve as the basis of adaptive function.

Dysfunction in the psychoanalytic frame of reference is defined in terms of inadequate psychosexual development, the presence of conflicts and fixations, and the imbalance of psychic energy among the three parts of the personality. These abnormal states can produce symptoms of neurosis, psychosis, or character disorder, which imply a disturbance in the ability to carry out activities of daily living.

Dysfunction can be seen as a lack of ego skills. This can take the form of poor reality testing, poor or unrealistic body image, poor self-identity, poor self-esteem, impulsiveness or passivity, unbalanced use of defenses, and an inability to cope. Assessment of the ego functions will guide our setting of goals in occupational therapy. Patients with similar goals may be treated together in groups.

Change and Motivation

Change occurs through the learning and performance of adequate ego adaptive skills. These skills can be learned within the social context of therapeutic groups, where the consequences of problem behaviors can be readily seen and discussed. Foundation skills can be worked on through simple, well-structured, reality-oriented tasks that focus on the development to sensory motor, perceptual, and cognitive skills. Motivation can be enhanced through successful experiences in occupational therapy.

Motivation comes from the directing of psychic energy toward the mastery of ego skills. When energy is bound up in dealing with conflict, persons may not be motivated to develop ego skills. As the ego is available to help reduce tensions and to satisfy needs through mature relationships and meaningful work activities, persons will be motivated to increase ego skill

development. The occupational therapist can set up therapeutic groups that allow patients to practice adequate ego skills and experience successful and satisfying consequences for patients. A strong self-concept and high self-esteem are also motivating; these foster a sense of control and lead people to direct their energy toward even greater skill development.

Review of Occupational Therapy Perspective

The next portion of this chapter will review three authors from occupational therapy whose work has reflected the principles of the psychoanalytic frame of reference: Gail Fidler, Lela Llorens, and Anne Mosey. Occupational therapy groups using this frame of reference became popular during the 1960s and 1970s, and consequently many of the published works of these authors began about then.

An important influence in occupational therapy at the time of the early writings of Fidler, Llorens, and Mosey was a treatment approach begun in England by Maxwell Jones, known as the therapeutic community. The therapeutic community represented in the 1960s and 1970s a fundamental change in approach to the treatment of mental illness. Both psychodynamic theories of personality and theories of sociology contributed to this unique approach, which called for the patient role to change from a "sick role" to that of a responsible community member. Hospitals and institutions all over Europe and America began therapeutic communities on their psychiatric units and occupational therapists were an integral part of this new approach.

Prior to the 1960s, occupational therapy, although administered in groups, had a task skill focus with an emphasis on the use of crafts and productive work skills. The rise of therapeutic communities called for occupational therapists to incorporate milieu principles into their treatment approach. Examples of these principles are:

1. Those most affected by a decision should be involved in making, according to Jones.
2. "In the context of responsibility for self and others, patients will alter their self-perception from that of subordinate to that of peer group member" (Fairweather, 1964).
3. Patients learn best when they are allowed to experience the consequences of their own actions.

The Task-Oriented Group—Fidler

In keeping with her times, Gail Fidler published her classic article, "The Task-Oriented Group as a Context for Treatment" in 1969 (Appendix A). She mentions several spokespersons for ego psychology in her rationale, such as Sullivan and Lewin, and points to the "emerging focus on ego functions and adaptive skills" (Fidler, 1969, p. 43). Fidler also alludes to a focus on the use of groups in therapy as "a dynamic force in facilitating learning and behavior change" (Lewin, 1945).

Fidler, in incorporating occupational therapy principles with those of the therapeutic milieu, pointed out the value of observing patients doing tasks. She noted that "as patients engaged in activities or creating objects, they expressed characterological difficulties, and that attention to these problems as they emerged and were operant in the here-and-now seemed to be of benefit to the patient" (Fidler, 1969, p. 45). There appeared to her to be a relationship between problems encountered by a patient in his activity experiences and those difficulties he encountered in the outside world. The assumption here is not unlike one made by the ego psychologists. If the patient's difficulties

either interpersonally or in task performance are brought to his attention (whether by experience itself, group feedback, or feedback from the therapist), the patient can utilize ego skills to cope with the difficulties. The strengthening of ego skills, then, becomes the goal of the task-oriented group.

Although the task is defined as either an end product or a service that is done by the group as a whole, Fidler points out that task accomplishment is not really the purpose. Rather, the task is intended to "provide a shared working experience wherein the relationship between feeling, thinking, and behavior, their impact on others and on task accomplishment and productivity can be viewed and explored" (Fidler, 1969, p. 45). Through the task group experience, ego skills and deficits can be observed in the patient. Patients demonstrate, in the process of participating in the group, their problems in interaction and in doing, and these problems can then be the focus of group problem-solving. Through both therapist and group feedback, "alternate patterns of functioning can be considered and tested within the context of the here-and-now, to the end that such learning may induce ego growth and improve function" (Fidler, 1969, p. 45).

In other words, patients are expected to reflect on their behavior in the group and to come to some understanding of its consequence on other members and on task accomplishment. Behavior that is disturbing to others or counterproductive is identified as such, and presumably more adaptive modes of behavior are suggested and tried. The occupational therapist facilitates this process during the group; she intervenes as problems arise, points them out to the group, and helps the group problem solve. (See Appendix A for Fidler's article.)

Occupational Therapy in an Ego Adaptive Milieu—Llorens

Lela Llorens also wrote about occupational therapy programming using the psychoanalytic frame of reference. Her article "Occupational Therapy in an Ego Oriented Milieu" with P. Johnson (1966) and her book *Developing Ego Functions in Disturbed Children* with E. Rubin (1967) present useful occupational therapy assessment and treatment ideas using this practice model. Llorens writes that "a program of occupational therapy designed to enhance and support adaptive functioning must provide for the development of ego skills, opportunities for practice, and support for mastery" (1966, p. 179). She describes occupational therapy groups in three phases of treatment: evaluation, convalescence, and rehabilitation.

In the evaluation phase, observation is emphasized. The group meets for 3 consecutive days for 1 hour each day, and activities include orientation to occupational therapy, written completion of a background information sheet, and completion of a small mosaic tile tray. This small sample of behavior allows the occupational therapist to observe the patient's mood, relationships, motivation, performance, and skills. Results of the evaluation show how well the patient's ego is functioning in helping her adapt to the environment. Those whose egos are functioning less than normal are assigned to the convalescent phase of treatment.

The goals of the convalescent phase are to promote increased feelings of adequacy and to encourage independence in functioning. Modalities suggested to achieve these goals are sewing and needlework, art, leather and metal work, and woodwork. Convalescent groups consist of five to 15 patients with two therapists. Some ego skills worked on in this phase are:

- Expression or sublimation of needs in an acceptable manner
- Attention span and work tolerance
- Reality testing and orientation
- Verbal and nonverbal communication of feelings

The therapist takes responsibility for planning in these groups according to the patient's ability.

Patients whose egos are more highly functional are placed in the rehabilitation phase of occupational therapy treatment. Modalities for groups in this phase include more interaction: male and female interest groups, activities of daily living discussion groups, graceful living, typing, and cooking. A less authoritative leadership style is used in these groups. Mastery is both the motivation and the goal.

Adaptive Skills and Developmental Groups—Mosey

Mosey's concept of adaptive skills is also useful in the psychoanalytic frame of reference. While she frames the adaptive skills in a developmental context (recapitulation of ontogenesis), discussed in Chapter 7, the skills themselves closely resemble many of the functions of the ego described earlier. According to Mosey, "the term adaptive is used to indicate that these skills are acquired and utilized by the individual so that he may satisfy his inherent needs and the needs of others, interact with the environment in order to attain personal goals, and knowledgeably select those environmental demands he wishes to meet" (1970b, p. 134). Mosey acknowledges the influence of psychoanalytic theory on the adaptive skills by accepting the concepts of conscious, preconscious, unconscious, complex formation, and regression, but adds the need for mastery as an important component. She proposes that fixation may be the result of deficient adaptive skill learning. She identifies six adaptive skills, which are learned in sequence, with some overlap and interdependence as the child matures:

1. Perceptual-motor skill
2. Cognitive skill
3. Dyadic interaction skill
4. Group interaction skill
5. Self-identity skill
6. Sexual identity skill

The idea that group interaction skill precedes and therefore needs to be mastered before self-identity or gender identity are possible is significant. For an elaboration on these, the reader is referred to Mosey's book *Psychosocial Components of Occupational Therapy* (1986). (See Appendix C for a complete list of Mosey's adaptive skills and subskills.)

Summary of Mosey's Developmental Groups

Of particular interest to occupational therapists working with groups are the components of group interaction skill described by Mosey. She suggests five types of nonfamilial groups which simulate those which may be encountered in normal development. The intention of these groups is to provide opportunities to develop group interaction skills in the correct developmental sequence. Group interaction skill is "the ability to participate in a variety of groups in a manner that is satisfying for oneself and for one's fellow group members" (Mosey, 1970a, p. 273). The five types of groups are (Mosey, 1986):

1. Parallel
2. Project
3. Egocentric-cooperative
4. Cooperative
5. Mature

(See Appendix B for Mosey's article describing these groups.)

Parallel Groups
Parallel groups are the lowest level, made up of patients doing individual tasks side by side. Preschool children may be observed in a similar process on a playground, one swinging, another climbing, another digging in the sandbox. Little interaction is required, and the therapist defines the task and provides patients with the necessary assistance and emotional support.

Project Groups
Project groups emphasize task accomplishment. Some interaction may be built in, such as shared materials and tools and sharing the work. Social interaction outside of the task is not expected. The therapist structures the group with tasks that require interaction of two or more persons to complete.

Egocentric-Cooperative Groups
Egocentric-cooperative groups require the members to select and implement the task. Tasks are longer term and social interaction is expected. Although the task serves to organize this group, members are expected to respond to one another's social and emotional needs. The therapist facilitates this process.

Cooperative Groups
Cooperative groups require the therapist only as an adviser. Members are "encouraged to identify and gratify each other's social and emotional needs in conjunction with task accomplishment" (Mosey, 1970a, p. 273). The task in the cooperative group may be secondary to social aspects.

Mature Groups
In mature groups, the therapist is a co-equal member. The group members take on all the necessary leadership roles in order to balance task accomplishment with need satisfaction of the members.

Group Treatment
Two models are presented for occupa-

tional therapy groups in the psychoanalytic frame of reference: the projective arts group and the task-oriented, ego-building model.

The projective arts are aligned with the older, Freudian psychoanalysis. Theoretically, the creative process involves the production of drawings, paintings, sculptures, collages, poems, stories, dance, or music, which symbolizes unconscious drives or conflicts. The appearance of these symbols, however primitive, becomes open to interpretation within the therapy group. Patients do not need to be artistically talented to participate successfully in these groups. Patients often respond by feeling inadequate or child-like as they attempt to paint or write a poem because often they have not attempted to do these creative activities since they were in elementary school. Many of the so-called creative therapies, such as art therapy, music therapy, dance therapy, and psychodrama, as well as others, have been based on similar principles.

Activity Examples 4-1 through 4-6 are group activities that capitalize on projection of the unconscious. One caution must be heeded by group leaders when discussing patient creations in this context. Never attempt to interpret what the patient creates. Expressions of aggressive (e.g., desire for power, success, and victory) and libidinal (e.g., desire for love and intimacy) drives can be very powerful, and discussion of symbols and their meaning can lead to emotionally sensitive areas. The drawings and writings of patients must only be used as a context for discussion, and the patient's explanation of his own work will provide the basis for insight and learning.

The second approach described here is the ego building "task-oriented" group. Occupational therapy writers have implied that ego functions can be both evaluated and developed (learned) in the context of task-focused groups. The task, in groups using a psychoanalytic frame, takes on greater importance than in humanistic groups. Even when the task is not the focus, it is the context in which discussion, problem-solving, and therapeutic change take place. Therefore, the structure of the occupational therapy group in this frame is fundamentally different.

Structure and Limitations

After the introduction, the task predominates the group session providing both the structure and the timeframe for the group. Tasks can last for part of one session, or go on for several sessions. A task might take 3 hours at one time. Discussion depends on problems that arise and how the therapist chooses to intervene. Evaluative discussion is left for the last 15 minutes of each session, with a longer evaluation reserved following the end of the task. This alternative structure is primarily based on Fidler's "task-oriented group" but has been expanded and further defined. Mosey's concept of developmental groups is reflected in the changing role of the leader. The leader gives more help and structure to groups that are less capable, and less help to groups that have a higher level of ego functioning. The task group is not limited to high functioning patients. It can be adapted to fairly low levels of group interaction skill, with some changes in structure and the amount of help given by the leader.

Role of the Leader

Fidler defines the role of the occupational therapist as one of a facilitator. The leader's major goal is to make learning possible, and not to take over the group. Facilitation, then, requires that the therapist maintain and communicate a basic belief in the group's capacity to be "constructively self-determining" (Fidler, 1969,

p. 46). This means she does not make decisions for the group or rescue the group from its difficulties. Rather, she intervenes in the group's process in ways that encourage the group to make its own decisions and solve its own problems. The therapist decides how much freedom she will allow the group to be self-determining, based on her assessment of the level of ego functioning of group members. There is a delicate balance between success and failure, and she should not permit the group to become immobilized with frustration when it is truly incapable of doing a task or solving a problem without her help. This kind of leadership requires a thorough understanding of group dynamics.

Goals

The goals of groups in the psychoanalytic frame are for patients to develop and practice ego skills. These skills, reviewed from the beginning of the chapter, are reality testing, body image, self-identity, self-esteem, sense of control, and the use of healthy defenses and coping strategies. Providing the foundation for these skills are cognitive, perceptual, and sensory motor skills. Patients can be encouraged to develop and practice these skills within the group context through the shared working experience of tasks.

Examples of Activities

The group itself should decide on the task, using the resources of its members. Some of the successful task groups are reviewed here. Most tasks offer many opportunities to develop and reinforce ego skills. A few of these are highlighted for each group, but it is likely that many others are also possible.

A Group Newspaper

The group consisted of six Vietnam veterans who exhibited symptoms of substance abuse and post traumatic stress syndrome. This was significant in their choice of a task. They decided that what was most meaningful to them was to "tell the world the truth" about Vietnam veterans. The group took a trip to the library, where books and articles on the Vietnam war and on post traumatic stress syndrome were read and notes taken. From the notes, articles were written. Group members added their own stories, poems, and drawings, as well as old newspaper articles they had saved. The result was a 20-page booklet that was typed, copied, collated, and widely distributed to veterans hospital patients and staff by the group members.

In this group, members' common self-identity as "the unsung heroes" was reinforced. The task facilitated a sense of control by giving members a vehicle for expression of feelings and opinions that was acceptable in the social environment. Self-esteem was increased by the recognition of their work by others.

Easter Chocolates

The chocolates were really a combination of a product and service project. The group knew of a local residential school for handicapped children and wanted to do something for them. Since Easter was the next holiday, they decided to give them Easter candy. But they were on a limited budget, so they came up with the idea of making candy instead of buying it. Candy molds, baker's chocolate, sugar, and tinfoil were the only purchases. Members were able to collect enough old Easter baskets to hold the wrapped candy. The candy was made in the shapes of eggs, chicks, and small bunnies. Members wrapped each piece in foil and placed them in the baskets. Two of the group members delivered the baskets to the staff of the residential school the week before Easter. A week later they were very proud to receive a big thank you letter from the children.

Self-identity and self-esteem were reinforced in this group through doing for others. Members learned that they were capable of producing a product that brought pleasure to others, and were recognized for their altruism. Identification as a healthy defense was encouraged through nurturing the children (by giving candy) as perhaps they might have wished to be nurtured themselves.

A Walk to the Pet Store

The most important factor to this group was to get away from the hospital. They were psychiatric patients and not even allowed to walk around the grounds unescorted. In the task group, walking to the pet store gave them a way to go out as a group during scheduled group time, escorted by the occupational therapy staff. They decided on the destination because it was only a 15-minute walk, it was always interesting to see, and it would not cost any money. This task group gave them the opportunity to plan something together to meet their needs, restoring in them some sense of control. The sensory stimulation of walking and being in the outdoor environment also increased sensory motor skills.

Cooking a Spaghetti Dinner

Almost every group seems to enjoy a cooking task. It is relatively short term, provides enough work for all the members to participate, and satisfies a basic need for everyone—the need to eat. If possible, the group can do the menu planning and shopping, as well as the actual meal preparation. Since spaghetti and salad can feed the whole group for relatively little money, the group was able to afford soft drinks and dessert as well. This group made brownies from a mix before beginning the main course. Members were divided into salad makers, spaghetti mak-

ers, dessert makers, and table setters. The meal was enjoyed by the whole group and everyone was expected to help clean up.

This group requires many adaptive ego functions. Members identify with different roles to work on a realistic goal. They use their skills to cope with their part of the task, and receive feedback from others about their performance (reality testing). All of the senses are stimulated through the cooking task, and impulse control is necessary when using the tools and equipment (knives, stove).

Group Car Wash

This task required the cooperation of the hospital or sponsoring institution to provide permission, a space to work, and a source of water. At the VA hospital, the group took on the responsibility of writing letters to the various hospital administrators asking for permission. The letters were followed up with phone calls from the occupational therapist and other staff. Supplies included buckets, soap, rags, sponges, and a nozzle for the hose, most of which were borrowed from relatives and friends. Members prepared for the car wash 1 week ahead by making signs to post all over the hospital. On the day of the car wash, a few group members, accompanied by staff, went outside to post signs and arrows on the street and in the parking lot directing customers to the car wash location. Patients and staff took shifts of 2 hours each for 6 hours. At $3 a car, the group made almost $200, which they spent on a videotape player so the whole ward could watch movies on weekends.

Patience and perseverance were required in the planning of this extended task. There were many opportunities to reality test, reinforce body image (gross motor actions), self-identity (through working roles), and self-esteem (through the concrete result of their effort).

Group Leadership

In this frame of reference, as suggested earlier, the structure of the group is modified to include most of the discussion areas in the context of the activity or task. The activity, sharing, processing, generalizing, and application are not done as separate phases of the group, but are incorporated into the process of doing the task. Since the goal is to develop ego skills, the leader may stop the group whenever an opportunity for members to learn becomes evident. The evaluation portion should include all of the discussion phases of the group and should end with a summary.

Introduction

This part of the group can dispense with the warm-up and replace it with choosing a task. In beginning a task-oriented group, it is helpful for the leader to set forth some ground rules. Some of these will be specific, such as when and where the group will meet, for how long, and the practical limitations to their choice of task, such as availability of supplies. The leader also needs to set forth the expectation that the group will choose a task that they can all work on together, and that once decided, every member of the group is expected to contribute to task accomplishment. Three phases of a task group are introduced: planning, doing, and evaluating. The timeframe may vary according to the task, and a thorough discussion will be delayed until the task itself is finished.

Phase 1—Planning

After a brief introduction by the facilitator, the planning phase begins with brainstorming.

Brainstorming

Brainstorming involves the suggestion of possible tasks for the group by all members. Cooking a meal, planning a group walk, learning to do needlepoint, and making Easter baskets for the pediatrics ward are some examples of group tasks. It is often useful for a member of the group to record the ideas. The therapist should caution the group not to make judgments of the ideas suggested during brainstorming, but just to collect a list of ideas.

Persuasion

The next step in planning is persuasion. Members consider the pros and cons of each suggestion and attempt to persuade the group to do one of them. Here the therapist may need to introduce the idea of meaningfulness. A task which is likely to succeed is one that has meaning for its members. It is very tempting for some groups to plan something easy to accomplish, but often the easy tasks hold little value for the members. This results in member resistance in the doing phase. While the therapist should not under any circumstance influence the decision of the group, she should perhaps point out that a better decision will be made when the opinions of every member have been voiced and considered.

Interventions of the leader should be carefully thought out so as not to exert more authority than is necessary. Groups with poor ego skills will need more help than those with stronger ego skills. When in doubt, it is best to allow the group to experience the consequences of its actions, and then to find something to be learned from whatever happens. Occupational therapists often have difficulty with allowing groups to "fail" or to turn out badly. In the task-oriented group, however, it is often from the "failures" that patients can learn the most. Successful groups are of benefit in many ways also, but it is often the failures that promote real therapeutic change.

For example, I have sometimes observed in task-oriented groups with members of varied diagnoses, ages, and functioning levels an inability to make a group decision, even after 45 or 50 minutes of group discussion. Nothing is more frustrating to a group than sitting and doing nothing for an hour because nothing was planned. It is a mistake groups usually do not make twice. The planning session following such a group usually turns out to be quite productive.

Decision

After more or less persuasion, the group is expected to reach some kind of decision. Group decisions are made in several ways. Someone in the group can take a vote, with the majority ruling. Perhaps a consensus will be reached on the last suggestion discussed; if no one voices an objection, it may be assumed that everyone agrees. A patient leader might emerge in the group whose preference might be deferred to by the other members, or a decision can be made by a process of elimination. However the decision is made, it must be considered at some point during planning to be final. Often the group needs for the decision to be acknowledged and approved by the leader in order to proceed.

Specific Planning and Division of Labor

Once a decision is made, how the task will be accomplished should become the topic of discussion. Questions about what equipment and supplies are needed, how these will be obtained, where the group should be held, and how necessary procedures will be learned are addressed. The facilitator, in this phase, often needs to be a resource to the group, offering his knowledge of supply sources, procedures, and space availability. In lower functioning groups, this information should be offered more readily; in higher functioning groups, the therapist may offer information only if asked. The discussion of procedures naturally leads to the division of labor (who will do what). It is best when all the planning and preparation can be done by group members. Often each patient is charged with the responsibility of obtaining some item and bringing it to the group. Each member bringing one ingredient for a fruit salad or a pizza is an example of this. In this way it is easily seen that the success of the group task is dependent on each member of the group remembering and carrying out his or her responsibility.

Phase 2—Doing

It is usually most practical for the doing phase to be done at least 1 or 2 days later than the planning. This gives members a chance to prepare adequately. On the day of the activity, gathering and organizing are best left up to group members, although they may need some help. If moving right into activity is something that works for the group, then the leader should allow this. Generally, if careful planning has been done, then not a great deal of time is needed to organize the doing. As members proceed with doing the activity, the facilitator's role may expand to include consulting, advising, and providing information. The leader should be careful to offer these services only when asked, or when group disorganization is imminent. It is the role of the facilitator, however, to look for problems and to bring these to the attention of the group along the way. As problems arise, the leader may apprise the group: "Mary seems to be feeling left out" or "Sam seems to be doing all the work." Care should be taken not to suggest solutions until it is evident that the group cannot cope with the problem on its own.

Phase 3—Evaluation

Doing is not complete until the task is finished. However, evaluation of the group should be done before the end of every session. Sessions should be sufficiently long to allow for this process to occur. It is usually necessary for the leader to let the group know when it is time to stop doing and start talking. Discussion should focus on the process of the group and the role each member has chosen to play. The discussion phases of processing, generalizing, and application are incorporated into this evaluation phase of task groups.

Reflection of Behavior and Its Consequences

This should be verbalized if members are to learn from their experiences. Why was Mary feeling left out? Did she withdraw because she is shy? Was she seeking attention through non-participation? Was she uncertain about how to do her part of the task? Was she threatened by the perceived dominance of another member? How well did the group cope with Mary's problem? How did Mary feel? How did others feel about her? What other choices did the group have regarding Mary? These are the types of issues that should arise in evaluation of the group.

Feelings of Members About the Group

This "processing" aspect is an important part of evaluation. If Sam feels really good about the group, but Mary feels terrible, what are the reasons for this? Could Sam be feeling good because he is doing the whole thing himself and not allowing Mary an opportunity to contribute? How do other members see this? Suppose most of the members are bored with the task? What do they think makes it boring? How are they responsible for the boredom? What can they do about it? A leader should be very reluctant to allow a group to abandon a task part way through. Opportunities to learn should determine what is to be gained or lost from the abandonment.

Most of the time the group can learn more from following through on a task, even if to do so is frustrating and problematic. However, if the group is overwhelmed by frustration, the members' anxiety may interfere with their ability to learn. This is another judgment call which may be difficult for the leader to make.

Evaluation of Task Accomplishment

Finally, an overall evaluation of task accomplishment is in order. How does the group feel about the result? How does it compare with what they hoped for/expected? What did each member contribute to its accomplishment? To what extent did planning affect outcome? It is in this phase that the relationship among thinking, feeling, and behavior is most evident, and the therapist should never miss an opportunity to emphasize it. Good planning (thinking) generally produces successful action (behavior) and results in good feelings about oneself and the group. Concurrently, bad planning often produces an unsuccessful outcome and promotes bad feelings about self and the group. Individual examples of this process might also be pointed out. In all cases, learning from mistakes should be emphasized, so that members develop the strength and skill for making things turn out better next time.

Task-oriented groups are an excellent example of occupational therapy treatment using the psychoanalytic frame of reference. It is a context in which all of the ego skills discussed can be evaluated and worked on. However, it should be noted that it is not the only approach that works in this frame. Groups that use the symbolic meaning of activities or encourage self-expression through art, poetry, drama, dance, movement, or creative writing are alternative group goals. Occupational therapy groups that encourage exploring the unconscious and uncovering painful or conflictual memories to be resolved remain a less popular, but an equally legitimate, application of psychoanalytic theory.

Bibliography

Allport, G. (1958). *Becoming: Basic considerations for a psychology of personality.* New Haven, CT: Yale University Press.

Arlow, & Brenner. (1964). *Psychoanalytic concepts and the structural theory.* New York: International University Press.

Bellak, L., Huruich, M., & Gediman, H. (1973). *Ego functions in schizophrenics, neurotics and normals.* New York: Wiley & Sons.

Bergman, M., & Hartman, F. (1976). *The evolution of psychoanalytic technique.* New York: Basic Books.

Bruce, M., & Borg, B. (1987). *Frames of reference in psychosocial occupational therapy.* Thorofare, NJ: SLACK Incorporated.

Corey, G. (1991). *Theory and practice of counseling and psychotherapy* (4th ed.). Monterey, CA: Brooks/Cole.

Diasio, K. (1968). Psychiatric occupational therapy: Search for a conceptual framework in light of psychoanalytic ego psychology and learning theory. *American Journal of Occupational Therapy, XXII*(5), 50-57.

Erikson, E. (1950). *Childhood and society.* New York: Norton.

Fairweather, G. W. (1964). *Social psychology in treating mental illness.* New York: Wiley & Sons.

Fidler, G. (1969). The task-oriented group as a context for treatment. *American Journal of Occupational Therapy, XXIII*(1), 43-48.

Fidler, G. (1984). *Design of rehabilitation services in psychiatric hospital settings.* Laurel, MD: Ramsco.

Fidler, G., & Fidler, J. (1963). *Occupational therapy: A communication process in psychiatry.* New York: Macmillan Co.

Fine, R. (1979). *A history of psychoanalysis.* New York: Columbia University Press.

Freud, A. (1936). *The ego and the mechanisms of defense.* New York: International University Press.

Freud, S. (1914). History of the psychoanalytic movement. In J. Strachey (Ed.), *The Standard Edition of the Complete Psychological Works of Sigmund Freud.* London: Hogarth.

Greene, L., & Cole, M. (1991). Level and form of psychopathology and the structure of group therapy. *International Journal of Group Psychotherapy.*

Hartmann, H. (1939). *Ego psychology and the problem of adaptation.* New York: International University Press.

Jung, C. (1910). The association method. *American Journal of Psychology, 21,* 216-269.

Kaplan, H., & Sadock, B. (1998). *Synopsis of psychiatry* (8th ed.). Baltimore: Williams & Wilkins.

Kernberg, O. (1983). Psychoanalytic studies of group processes: Theory and applications. In L. Grinspoon (Ed.), *Psychiatry Update* (Vol. II) (pp. 21-35). Washington, DC: American Psychiatric Press.

Klein, M. (1948). *Contributions to psychoanalysis 1921-1945.* London: Hogarth Press.

Kris, E. (1936). The psychology of characterature. *IJP, 17,* 285-303.

Lewin, K. (1945). *Dynamic theory of personality.* New York: McGraw Hill.

Llorens, L. (1966). Occupational therapy in an ego-oriented milieu. *American Journal of Occupational Therapy, XX*(4), 178-181.

Llorens, L. (1976). *Application of a developmental theory for health and rehabilitation.* Rockville, MD: American Occupational Therapy Association.

Llorens, L., & Rubin, E. (1967). *Developing ego functions in disturbed children.* Detroit: Wayne State University Press.

Mosey, A. (1970a). The concept and use of developmental groups. *American Journal of Occupational Therapy, XXIV*(4), 272-275.

Mosey, A. (1970b). *Three frames of reference for mental health.* Thorofare, NJ: SLACK Incorporated.

Mosey, A. (1981). *Occupational therapy: Configuration of a profession.* New York: Raven Press.

Mosey, A. (1986). *Psychosocial components of occupational therapy.* New York: Raven Press.

Mosey, A. (1989). The proper focus of scientific inquiry in occupational therapy: Frames of reference. *Occupational Therapy Journal of Research, 9*(4), 195-201.

Murray, H. A., et al. (1938). *Explorations in personality.* New York: Oxford University Press.

Rapaport, D. (1942). *Emotions and memory.* New York: Harper.

Rapaport, D. (1953). On the psychoanalytic theory of affects. *IJP, 34,* 177-198.

Rorschach. (1921). *Psychodiagnostics: A diagnostic test based on perception.* New York: Grune & Stratton.

Spitz, R. (1959). *A genetic field theory ego formation: Its implications for pathology.* New York: International University Press.

Wechsler, D. (1981). *Wechsler Adult Intelligence Scale* (Rev. ed.). New York: The Psychological Corp.

Witkin, H., et al. (1954). *Personality through perception.* New York: Harper.

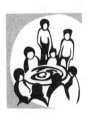

Psychoanalytic
Activity Example 4-1
Out on the Town

Materials: Colored crayons or pastels and 9- x 12-inch white drawing paper for each member.

Directions: Imagine that it is Saturday night and you have big plans. Choose anyone you like to be your companion, a significant other, a relative, a friend, even someone you have not yet met. Write the name of this person at the top of the paper.

Next think about where you would like to be going—a romantic dinner, a concert, a play or movie, a sports event, a social event—really anything you can imagine.

Now draw yourself, as you imagine, ready to go out for the evening. Pay attention to how you would look, what you would be wearing, and what would be your emotional state. Choose colors that represent your emotions as well as your outward appearance. You have 20 minutes to complete this drawing, so do not worry about artistic perfection.

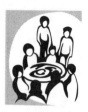

Psychoanalytic
Activity Example 4-2
My Room

Materials: 8 1/2- x 11-inch white paper, pencils with erasers, and rulers for each member. Colored pencils may also be used.

Directions: Introduce yourself by saying your name, and recalling a name your parents called you before you were 5 years old, or recalling a toy you remember playing with as a child.

Use the paper, pencil, and ruler to draw the floor plan of the room you slept in as a child. Try to remember as much about the room as you can.

- What was its size and shape?
- Whom did you share it with, if anyone?
- What color was it (paint, wallpaper)?
- Where was the bed? The window? Other furniture?
- Where did you keep your clothes and belongings?
- How old were you when you began sleeping there?
- What do you remember doing in this room besides sleeping?
- What else was in the room (carpets, curtains)?
- How did the bed look (bedspread, pillows, stuffed toys)?
- How did it feel to be in the room (sunny, dark)?
- What did it smell like?
- What was on the floor?

When you feel that you have a sense of this memory, begin drawing. You have 25 minutes to complete this floor plan.

From Cole, M. B. *Group Dynamics in Occupational Therapy, Second Edition.* © 1998 SLACK Incorporated.

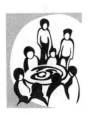

Psychoanalytic
Activity Example 4-3
Pass the Hat

Materials: A collection of various hats (sun visor, cowboy, baseball, ski hat, beret, etc.).

Directions: Choose a hat from the center of the circle and try it on. Think about who might wear this hat. As you introduce yourself, describe for what occasion you might wear a hat like this, if ever.

Put the hats back in the center of the circle. Now ask someone to volunteer to begin a story about a character wearing one of these hats. If no one volunteers, the leader may begin the story. After 1 minute, the first person stops and passes the hat to the next person in the circle. That person continues the story for 1 minute, and on around the circle. At any time during the storytelling, a member may choose to change the main character or add a new character by choosing a different hat. Ask members to describe interaction between the characters.

Discussion centers around the fantasized characters.
- Who did you like or dislike?
- Who do you know that any imagined characters reminded you of?
- Who are you vs. who might you rather be?
- How would you change if you could?
- Which hat fits most comfortably?
- What does your imagination say about yourself?

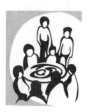

Psychoanalytic
Activity Example 4-4
A Poem for Myself

Materials: Pens and paper for each member and an assortment of used greeting cards (e.g., birthday, anniversary, wedding, sympathy, get well, friendship) that contain some form of a short poem.

Directions: Ask members to choose a greeting card and read the poem to the group. Collect the cards and put them away. Give out pens and paper. Ask members to think about how they are feeling right now, and what kind of card they might like to receive from someone. Ideas for this may be shared and discussed.

You have 15 minutes to write the first draft of a poem to yourself. This may be written as if it were from someone specific, or may be anonymous. The poem does not have to rhyme. It does not have to be in complete sentences. However, it should contain some words of inspiration relating to your current emotional state. Possible themes include:

- Needing a friend
- Sharing a joy
- Feeling alone
- Praying for guidance
- Missing someone
- Wishing to be healed
- Finding something (or someone) that was lost
- Discovering the truth about yourself

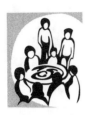

Psychoanalytic
Activity Example 4-5
Introducing the Empty Chair

Materials: 3- x 5-inch index cards and pens. Members sit in a circle with one extra chair in the center.

Directions: Everyone has troubled relationships in their lives. Is there someone you wish you could become emotionally closer to or have more supportive of you? As you introduce yourself, say a few words about someone in your life with whom you might like to have a better relationship.

Now, on the index card, write the name of one such individual. Then write the answers to the following questions.

- How is this person related to you (relative, spouse, friend, parent, neighbor)? Write a few sentences about the quality of this relationship.
- Where and when did the relationship begin?
- How many years have you known this person?
- What activities did you share with this person? Describe one such activity.
- When and where was your last meeting?
- Describe the nature of your most recent interaction.
- What about your relationship with this person do you wish to change?
- What would make the relationship better?

Sharing: When members have finished writing, ask them to focus on the empty chair in the center of the circle and imagine the person each member has chosen seated in it. Members then take turns standing behind the chair and introducing their significant person to the rest of the group, giving details from their writing.

Discussion: Focus on mutual support and give-and-take of relationships. Encourage feedback and suggestions.

From Cole, M. B. *Group Dynamics in Occupational Therapy, Second Edition.* © 1998 SLACK Incorporated.

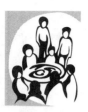

Psychoanalytic
Activity Example 4-6
Paint Your Day

Materials: Roll of bond paper large enough to cover the center of a 72-inch oblong table, 12 poster paints in a variety of colors, a paintbrush for each color, large jars of water, and sponges for cleaning up. No chairs are allowed.

Directions: Group members (no more than eight) introduce themselves and describe how they are feeling today. They are then instructed to do a group mural. The group members take a few minutes to organize how they will do the painting , such as if there will be a "top" and a "bottom" and how space will be divided. Members are encouraged to move around the table as they paint and to exchange colors as they wish. The subjects should relate to the feelings presented, and should **not** be reality-oriented (e.g., garden scene, ocean scene). Abstract shapes and symbols are best. About 20 minutes usually suffices to cover most of the surface of the paper.

Discussion: This centers around how members interacted with each other, as shown in the group mural. Sharing will reveal each member's painted creations, as well as what they might mean to that individual. Over-assertive or bold painting, color choices, and shapes and lines all reveal emotional states as well as personality traits. Group roles may also be identified this way (imitator, follower, orienter, elaborator, etc.). Refer to Chapter 2 for a review of potential group roles.

Chapter 5

The Behavioral Cognitive Continuum

From a historical perspective, most of the cognitive frames of reference in occupational therapy are derived from "learning theory," which grew from the roots of behaviorism in the 1950s and 1960s. The works of Skinner, Pavlov, and others revolutionized the field of psychology by applying the scientific method to human behavior. This idea was directly opposed to the concept of the unconscious in psychoanalytic theories, because behaviorists believed that only what was "observable and measurable" could legitimately be the subject of scientific study. Modern day thinking has mellowed the radical thinking of early behaviorism. Most current theories include cognition in the definition of observable behavior and acknowledge the internal control of the individual. However, some concepts from behaviorism remain useful, and may be recognized in the occupational therapy practice of today. Therefore, this chapter begins with an overview of those behavioral concepts which still apply to group leadership in occupational therapy: behavioral goals and objectives, conditioning and habits, shaping and chaining, rehearsal and practice, modeling, and reinforcement.

Next, the biomechanical approach is briefly reviewed. Therapy in the biomechanical frame of reference relies on behavioral concepts such as practice and repetition, behavioral objectives, and the formation of good habits of posture and body mechanics, and often requires external reinforcement. The biomechanical frame of reference also provides the background for certain behavioral cognitive techniques, such as biofeedback, progressive relaxation, and systematic desensitization, which are useful in groups when addressing issues like stress management, the management of pain, or the modulation of emotions. Frames previously described as "rehabilitative" or "acquisitional," including those of Denton, Mosey, and Trombly, are briefly included as their concepts contribute to group treatment.

Two different cognitive approaches are then described in this chapter. The first is cognitive rehabilitation, developed by

Abreu and Toglia (1983) and updated by Toglia as the "multicontext approach" (1991) and the "dynamic interactional approach" (1997) to cognitive rehabilitation. Previously, this model was included in the chapter on "Acquisitional Approaches," but the theory has developed beyond that category by moving away from separate and distinct cognitive subskills toward a more integrated approach. This model uses the works of Luria, a noted Russian brain physiologist, and other current brain research to develop a more holistic approach to cognitive rehabilitation. This theory, as updated, is particularly well suited to group treatment, especially as it impacts "metacognition," or the ability to monitor, regulate, and predict one's own functional performance.

The second set of concepts discussed in this chapter is cognitive behavioral therapy, recently dubbed CBT by Duncombe (1997). Duncombe has presented this approach as a legitimate occupational therapy frame of reference, which uses principles similar to those used in its psychological counterpart. Cognitive behaviorism is one of the most frequently used in mental health settings for several reasons. It sounds simple and logical, it easily lends itself to advances in technology, such as computer programming and biofeedback, and it is appropriate and useful in short-term treatment. Occupational therapists use the psychoeducational approach from cognitive behaviorism in treating patients on a verbal and symbolic level. To benefit from this approach, it is suggested that patients be capable of learning through logic and reasoning. The principal spokesmen for the cognitive behavioral therapies in psychology are Aaron Beck, Albert Ellis, and Albert Bandura. A more recent outgrowth of cognitive behaviorism used by occupational therapists, called dialectical behavior therapy (DBT) developed by Linehan (1993a), is described. This approach is widely used a basis of group treatment with psychiatric populations. Both Toglia and Linehan share the guiding principle that therapy should focus on the cognitive process, and that it is changes in thinking that will produce adaptive changes in patient behavior.

Focus

This group of approaches, some more behavioral, others more cognitive, were all developed through application of the scientific method to human behavior. They are expressed in a continuum, and their relationship to occupational therapy groups is described in Table 5-1.

Basic Assumptions

Behavioral Concepts

This section selects for review those behavioral concepts which still appear as an integral part of occupational therapy: behavioral goals and objectives, conditioning and habits, shaping and chaining, reinforcement, and rehearsal and practice.

Behavioral Goals and Objectives

One of the most fundamental contributions of behaviorism is the concept of behavioral goals. Only observable behavior was thought to be an appropriate focus for treatment. Therefore, behavioral goals and objectives should always be observable and measurable. The early behaviorists taught us to identify problems narrowly and specifically, so that focused treatment could be designed and its effects measured. The goals for our occupational therapy groups should be written in specific, measurable terms, so that necessary documentation of progress is possible. Often these goals are set by the patients and therapist together, and progress

Table 5-1.
Summary of Behavioral Cognitive Continuum

	Behavioral	Biomechanical, Rehabilitative	Cognitive-Perceptual Rehabilitation	Cognitive Behavioral, Dialectical Behavioral
Theorists	Skinner, Pavlov, Lazarus	Trombly, Denton, Mosey, Fidler	Toglia and Abreu	Bandura, Beck, Ellis, Linehan
Patient Applications	all populations	physically disabled	brain injury, stroke, mental illness	mental illness, emotional aspects, character disorder
Concepts and Techniques	goals and objectives, conditioning and habits, shaping and chaining, reinforcement, rehearsal and practice, role playing and role reversal, systematic desensitization, biofeedback	strength, ROM, endurance, positioning, prevention, restoration, compensation, adaptation, skill acquisition, lifestyle performance, biofeedback	orientation, attention, visual processing, motor planning, cognition, ADL, multicontextual treatment, metacognition, generalization, criteria for transfer of learning	social learning, modeling, self-regulation, cognitive distortions, automatic thoughts, disputing irrational beliefs, cognitive restructuring, dialectical strategies
OT Group Themes	graded tasks, social skills training, assertiveness, relaxation, stress, time or emotion management, coping skills training, conflict management	group exercise, group games involving movement, graded strength and endurance, prevention education, work readiness, work hardening	strategy themes (any of the six cognitive areas) in multiple contexts, group discussion of strategy generalizations, self skill assessment in group context	psychoeducational modules/groups, reading/films and discussion, role playing groups, worksheets and discussion in interpersonal effectiveness, emotion regulation, distress tolerance and mindfulness

toward the goals are openly discussed with the group. In behavioral cognitive groups, an evaluation of the group should be set up to see if goals are met. Worksheets 5-1 through 5-3 are designed to help students learn how to write behavioral goals.

Long-term goals are not always measurable. Sometimes when we set lifetime goals, such as "be successful at my job," it is not clear what it is that success really means. Even when these goals are measurable, such as "become a millionaire by age 40," how these goals will be accomplished remains unplanned. Until these goals are broken down into smaller, do-able steps, they will remain only dreams. Short-term, measurable goals are the actions and behaviors that help us and our patients make

dreams a reality. A measurable goal is one that describes behavior that can be observed. For example, your goal might be to improve self-esteem. How can you tell when self-esteem has improved? What behaviors would you look for? What actions could you take? Some possibilities might be standing taller, taking more care in dressing and hygiene to look your best, and verbalizing several positive aspects of yourself. The measurable goals in Worksheet 5-2 are 2, 4, 9, 10, 12, 14, 15, 17, and 18. One key to writing a measurable goal is the language used. Words like "learn," "understand," "encourage," "improve," "handle," and "manage" are vague because they do not specify how these things can be accomplished. Measurable goals are usually specific, and they incorporate behaviors that

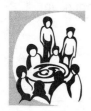

Worksheet 5-1
Writing Long-Term Goals

Directions: Begin by writing your lifetime goals for yourself. Write at least one goal from each of the following categories.

1. Professional

2. Educational

3. Monetary

4. Family

5. Health

6. Social

7. Spiritual

8. Emotional

9. Recreational

10. Creative

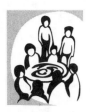

Worksheet 5-2
Recognizing Measurable Goals

Directions: From the list below, circle the goals that you think are measurable. Answers may be found on page 133.

1. Encourage decision-making

2. List one strength and one weakness

3. Develop a better self-concept

4. Discuss feelings about parents

5. Relate better to authority figures

6. Manage time better

7. Conserve energy in cooking a meal

8. Handle frustration

9. Demonstrate pride in personal accomplishment

10. Plan a weekend activity and carry it out

11. Define assertive behavior

12. Complete a task within time limit

13. Relieve stress

14. Eat a well-balanced diet

15. Plan time to study for a test

16. Take responsibility for behavior

17. Attend school regularly

18. Stay on a diet 80% of the time

19. Understand yourself better

20. Strengthen feminine/masculine identity

From Cole, M. B. *Group Dynamics in Occupational Therapy, Second Edition.* © 1998 SLACK Incorporated.

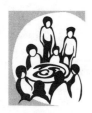

Worksheet 5-3
Making Our Lifetime Goals Measurable

Directions: In Worksheet 5-1, we wrote down some lifetime goals. First, go back to that list and check off which of those goals are measurable. Next, choose three goals from your list that are not measurable and write them down below. For each one, list several measurable short-term goals or steps to be completed.

Lifetime Goal 1
    1.

    2.

    3.

    4.

    5.

Lifetime Goal 2
    1.

    2.

    3.

    4.

    5.

Lifetime Goal 3
    1.

    2.

    3.

    4.

    5.

can be observed. Words like "define," "list," "discuss," and "complete" refer to either words or actions that can be readily observed, heard, or read. In the behavioral cognitive frame of reference, thoughts are also considered to be behavior. However, thoughts must be verbalized in order to be measurable.

Conditioning and Habits

Pavlov has been credited with identifying classical conditioning as a process through which much of human behavior is learned. When a piece of chocolate candy is placed in the mouth, the mouth waters and the person experiences a pleasant taste sensation. The autonomic response is soon associated with the visual stimuli, so that it only takes a glance at the candy bar in the store window to make the mouth water. Likewise, many associations in the brain are formed which attach meaning to incoming stimuli. Pavlov was able to recreate this phenomenon in the laboratory, and he called it "classical conditioning." Much of today's advertising uses this principle.

Skinner (1953) identified a more complex, but less controlled form of learning, which he called "operant conditioning." According to this principle, behavior that is reinforced by the environment tends to be repeated, while behavior that is discouraged or ignored tends to become extinct or disappear. Humans are continually subjected to random or chance reinforcement as they go through life, causing maladaptive as well as constructive learning. Therapy, therefore, must involve the identification and control of environmental factors that reinforce a behavior, so that the stage can be set for positive behavior change.

The development of habits is explained by the principle of operant conditioning. Persons repeat behaviors that are reinforced repeatedly until they become habit-

ual; however, once a habit is formed, reinforcement is no longer necessary. Habits are routine or customary ways of doing things. James (1985) explains that an "acquired habit, from a physiological point of view, is nothing but a new pathway of discharge formed in the brain, by which certain incoming currents ever after tend to escape"(1985, p. 55). This statement implies that certain stimuli, when encountered in the environment, evoke predictable responses which have been "conditioned" or learned. Waking up in a familiar environment, most people can wash, dress, eat breakfast, and otherwise get ready for the day without much conscious thought. James writes that "habit diminishes the conscious attention with which our acts are performed"(p. 59). In the above example, the familiar objects in the environment serve as stimuli for the habitual performance of these necessary tasks, so that brain energy is reserved for the more challenging tasks at work or school. Using this principle, cognitive rehabilitation seeks to re-establish habitual ways of performing functional tasks after brain trauma. When familiar ways of accomplishing a task are no longer possible, new pathways must be formed through the rehearsal and practice of the most efficient alternative strategies.

Shaping and Chaining

Skinner once demonstrated before a large audience teaching a live pigeon to turn around, using the technique of shaping. The pigeon's cage was set on the stage, where it could be readily seen. Using the principle of operant conditioning, he waited until the pigeon turned slightly in the desired direction, and reinforced this behavior with a pellet of food. Each time the pigeon turned a little farther in the desired direction, it was reinforced again with a pellet of food. Within 2 or 3 minutes, the pigeon had learned to turn a full 360 degrees before being reinforced. The technique of shaping requires that each step in a sequence be reinforced until the entire task is learned. When occupational therapists analyze activities, we break them down into component parts or steps. Instructing a patient in using a reacher, for example, we may begin with the correct grip, then practice the movements of the handle, and finally, practice picking up first lighter, then heavier objects. We may use approval or praise after each step is done correctly, without even realizing that we are using reinforcement to shape the patient's behavior.

Chaining refers to the learning of steps in a specific sequence, so that each action serves as the stimulus to provoke the next action (James, 1985). When a sequence follows along smoothly, without hesitation or making a decision among alternatives, then the sequence has become a habit. James suggests that it is the sensation of the movement just finished that provides reinforcement and signals readiness for what comes next.

Reinforcement

From the discussion of behavioral concepts so far, it is evident that reinforcement comes in many forms. Early behaviorists identified reinforcement as external to the individual. Positive reinforcement is a reward, something desirable to the individual—an edible treat, a gold star, a hug, words of praise, a paycheck. In negative reinforcement, something desirable is removed—privileges, freedom, participation in a social or recreational activity, a holiday. Later behaviorists believed that reinforcement can also be internal. Bandura, a cognitive behavioral theorist, identified two kinds of internal reinforcers: vicarious and self-produced. Vicarious reinforcers are symbolic, such as

a person's learned images of success and failure, or reflections of his values and ideals. Self-produced reinforcers come from the person's sense of competence, efficacy, and self-control. In other words, feeling good about oneself is reinforcing.

Bandura's hierarchy of reinforcement is helpful in understanding and planning learning experiences for our patient groups. The levels of reinforcers progress from simple to more complex as they parallel the developmental sequence.

1. Initial reinforcers refer to the external ones such as food, attention, and approval.
2. Symbolic reinforcers are internal images or messages regarding probable consequences of behavior. An example of this is a child refraining from going outside his yard because he remembers how angry his mother got the last time he did it.
3. Social contract refers to more complex or role dependent behavior such as performing a job or honoring one's marriage vows.
4. Personal satisfaction is the best and most effective reinforcer in Bandura's opinion, because it is the least dependent upon external circumstances, and therefore the least vulnerable to extinction. When feelings of self-satisfaction or self-worth result from particular behaviors, those behaviors tend to be repeated.

Since reinforcement is what motivates learning, the occupational therapist seeking to motivate a group of patients must decide what level of reinforcement the group members can respond to. Even when treating adults, we may need to fall back on external reinforcement when motivation for therapy is found lacking.

Rehearsal and Practice

A popular technique associated with the

behavioral approach is assertiveness training. This group activity requires the rehearsal and practice of newly learned assertive behaviors through group role playing, and subsequently, trying out the new behaviors in real life situations. The leader first uses self-awareness exercises to help the members analyze their own habitual responses to difficult situations as either passive, aggressive, or assertive.

- Passive—The individual does not state his feelings or stand up for his rights, and usually does not get what he wants.
- Aggressive—The individual insists on his rights, lets his feelings explode, and gets what he wants by abusing the rights and hurting the feelings of others.
- Assertive—The individual expresses his feelings and requests that his rights be honored. He may not always get his way, but his behavior encourages mutual respect and open communication.

Hypothetical situations may be presented by the leader, which are likely to be familiar, such as:

- Just as you reach the ticket counter at the movies after a 20 minute wait, someone cuts ahead of you in line.
- A group of friends with whom you are talking decides spontaneously to meet at an unfamiliar restaurant for coffee. You would like to join them, but you do not know how to get there.
- You receive a credit card bill for an item you did not buy.
- While driving you to an unfamiliar doctor's office for an appointment, your friend makes a wrong turn and becomes lost. She refuses to stop to ask directions.
- You have made your spouse/significant other a special birthday dinner,

and he shows up an hour late, with no explanation or apology.

The group discusses each situation with regard to: What would I typically do? Is my response passive, aggressive, or assertive? What would be an appropriate assertive response? The exact words of an assertive response are then practiced by each member. The key is to focus on the verbal expression of feeling or statement of legitimate rights, followed by a request for change or action. Using incomplete sentences and asking each member to fill in the blanks might be a good place to start: I feel _____ when you _____. I request that you _____. Hypothetical and real situations are rehearsed and practiced through role playing, group discussion, giving and receiving feedback, and homework. Most people have difficulty behaving assertively, and persons with disability are especially vulnerable. Assertiveness group members should be encouraged to provide one another emotional support when attempts at assertive behavior outside the group do not bring expected results. Reinforcement for assertive behavior must initially come from the group leader and members, until it is practiced often enough and with enough success to become a part of the individual's habitual response repertoire. (For further ideas on assertiveness groups, see Posthuma's *Small Groups in Therapy Settings*, Appendix A.)

Many functional skills addressed in occupational therapy require rehearsal and practice. The cognitive rehabilitation approach stresses the rehearsal of cognitive strategies in a variety of clinical contexts and practice of skills over a range of possible applications. Giving groups specific homework assignments encourages the practice of skills in real life contexts. Discussion of the results of practice allows the group leader and members to provide "reinforcement" in a controlled and predictable way.

Role Playing

According to Posthuma (1989), role playing evolved from the practice of psychodrama, in which the patient (protagonist) directs her own real life situation by choosing other members of the group to play the roles of significant others. As a behavioral technique, the structure of role playing remains the same, but the focus is slightly different. In occupational therapy groups, playing roles provides a forum for practice and rehearsal of new behaviors within a safe and supportive therapeutic environment. Members recall or anticipate difficult situations in their own lives, and bring them to the therapy setting in constructing the role play. Each role play has four parts, according to Posthuma (1989, p. 186):

1. Definition of the problem
2. Assuming the roles
3. Enactment
4. Discussion

For example, a patient anticipating a return to work after a long absence may choose others to play co-workers, supervisors, or clients/customers. The patient (protagonist) tells each member how to play his role, and the furniture in the room can be rearranged to resemble the work setting for a more realistic effect. Although the protagonist may play herself the first time through, it is often helpful for another member to play that role or to reverse roles. As a learning tool, role reversal has the advantage of helping the protagonist to see the situation from the other's point of view. The purpose of role playing is to practice new behaviors, develop insight to a situation, develop empathy with others, anticipate consequences, increase self-confidence, and/or decrease anxiety. A discussion of the role play allows the other members of the group to give feedback and support to the protagonist, and reveals its meaning for all the group members. Role plays are also models for social learning (described later, in the section on behavioral cognitive therapies).

Systematic Desensitization and Biofeedback

These techniques have elements of both behavioral and cognitive theory. Systematic desensitization has been used successfully by clinical psychologists in the treatment of phobias, such as fear of flying, and has been less successfully used to control addictions, such as drinking or smoking. The first step in desensitization is to evoke a state of relaxation, usually using some form of progressive muscle tension and release sequences combined with visualization. The "progressive" part involves the introduction of images of the feared object/situation in graded degrees of severity. For example, the person with fear of flying would begin by visualizing the drive to the airport, and gradually work up to the plane taking off, while maintaining a state of relaxation. The entire process requires a series of sessions, often over a period of several months. Psychologists are required to get special training before attempting this technique. However, the same concepts form the basis of many group activities used in occupational therapy. Progressive muscle relaxation takes on many forms, and may be used in occupational therapy groups dealing with stress management or as a coping strategy when faced with any situation that tends to evoke anxiety. Guided fantasy is a form of visualization which is useful for group treatment. Although feared images should be avoided, pleasant ones may be very powerful motivators. For example, the group may begin by members closing their eyes, breathing deeply, and imagining themselves lying on a sunny beach, listening to the rhythm of the ocean waves as they break along the shore. This visual image sets the stage for relaxation, and prepares them for learning other useful strategies for the control of anxiety, anger, frustration, and other causes of distress. A good resource for relaxation is Harlowe and Yu (1997), which contains 45 different scripts for conducting group relaxation sessions.

Biofeedback refers to the monitoring of bodily functions, such as pulse, respiration rate, heart rate, and body temperature. Stein and Nikolic (1989) suggest using biofeedback in conjunction with other stress management techniques. Mechanical monitoring devices are used to give patients information about how their mental state affects them physically. Various mental strategies can then be learned to help persons gain control over their own physiological responses to stress. Biofeedback is often combined with visualization and relaxation techniques. It is also used in the biomechanical approach to monitor the effects of movement and exercise, and as a safety precaution to prevent overexertion in any physically strenuous activity.

Biomechanical Approach

This approach is primarily appropriate for patients who lack range of motion (ROM), strength, and endurance to perform daily life tasks (Trombly, 1989). The whole is considered to be the sum of its parts: single muscles making up muscle groups or synergies; tasks divided into force and resistance, angles, and directions; and rearranged into positions and movement sequences. Therefore, behavior can be broken down into its component subskills for the purpose of easier learning. The theory draws upon the kinetic principles of human movement, and its goals are to prevent injury, restore func-

tion, and/or compensate for lost function. These are some of the same principles of strength and effort that are presently associated with work hardening.

The biomechanical frame of reference is included here because it uses the behavioral principles of conditioning, habit formation, shaping and chaining, and rehearsal and practice with the goal of restoring function. Adaptation and compensation are often required when injury or illness results in chronic physical disability. Behavioral goals and objectives are set, and effects of treatment are carefully measured. Because recovery from physical loss often requires multiple repetition, building these repetitions into meaningful group activities can be helpful and motivating.

Range of Motion

The maximum motion of every joint in every possible direction is called its ROM, or range of motion. Average ROMs for each joint in each direction have been calculated, so that deviation from the norm, or limitation of ROM, can be determined. There are many causes of limitation in ROM, including head injury, stroke, burns, fractures, arthritis, and peripheral nerve injury. ROM is measured with a goniometer, which, when applied to the joint, determines the angle or number of degrees the joint can move. For example, the typical ROM of the elbow joint is 0 to 150 degrees. The ROM can be measured actively (AROM), "Lift your arm high over your head," or passively (PROM), "Let me flex and extend your shoulder." Specific guidelines for measuring ROM for each joint may be found in Trombly (1989). In occupational therapy, activities are devised to encourage the patient to increase and/or maintain ROM. Particularly in groups of patients who are at risk, such as those with arthritis, multiple sclerosis, or post head trauma or stroke, exercise "classes" to maintain/extend ROM are common. Crafts and games can be adapted by positioning them in a way that forces the patient to reach, bend, push, pull, or grasp in order to accomplish the goal. Care should be taken to plan the right amount of movement, since overestimating it can easily cause injury. A creative activity using this approach is the "Range of Motion Dance," a supportive exercise group format originally developed for arthritis patients to maintain their ROM (Van Deusen & Harlowe, 1987).

Strength

Muscle weakness is another common problem treated in occupational therapy with physical disabilities. When illness or injury results in specific muscle weakness, or when weakness can potentially cause deformity, activities can be devised to increase muscle strength. Strength can be increased in several ways. Stress is applied to a muscle or muscle group by increase in load or weight. Lifting objects of gradually increased weight will strengthen the muscles. Duration of muscle contraction also influences strength. Holding a position or lifting and holding a heavy object for longer and longer intervals can increase strength. The rate and the frequency of contraction also affect strength; faster or more frequent exercise increases strength, even when lighter weight is used. Any combination of these parameters when applied to exercise have been found to increase strength. The challenge for the occupational therapist is to find activities that can be graded in load, duration, rate, and frequency, so that strength can be increased gradually and without injury. Craft activities, such as sanding wood or weaving on a loom, have traditionally been adapted to accomplish these goals. When treating in groups, work activities such as gardening and landscaping, cleaning and moving furniture, or stocking shelves might accomplish the goals of increasing strength.

Endurance

Endurance refers to the length of time muscles can continue to work without becoming fatigued. A person can sustain isometric contraction equivalent to 50% of maximum voluntary contraction (MVC) up to 1 minute. In normal subjects, contraction time and percentage of MVC are inversely related (Trombly, 1989). For example, if Sally carries a 50-pound bag of dog food from her car up three flights of stairs to her apartment, she will need to sustain a 50% MVC for 2 minutes. Chances are it will be necessary for Sally to stop and rest after 1 minute before continuing. However, if she carries a 25-pound bag of dog food, she can sustain a 25% MVC for the 2 minutes it takes her to walk all the way to her apartment without resting.

In occupational therapy, endurance may be increased by using moderately fatiguing activities for progressively longer periods of time. In groups, the occupational therapist can offer activities that sustain interest over the needed increases in duration. Many active games and sports can be adapted to the goal of increasing strength and endurance. Tug of war, for example, can be timed so that the length of effort progressively increases with each round. Relay races, perhaps carrying progressively heavier items, can be graded also.

Prevention, Restoration, and Compensation

Particularly in the workplace, prevention of injury and maintenance of health are important areas for occupational therapy intervention. Insurance companies, worker's compensation, and other third party payers are hiring occupational therapy consultants to organize educational groups in the use of correct body mechanics, positioning and seating, environmental adaptations, and energy saving strategies to help save the cost of worker absence and medical treatment due to preventable injuries. In addition, educational groups for persons with specific injuries, such as carpal tunnel syndrome or osteoarthritis, will help them learn good health maintenance strategies. Restoration of function is defined within the context of developing patient competence in performing occupational roles. The patient should identify the roles he will continue (e.g., worker, spouse, club member, and friend). The roles played, in turn, help define the tasks the individual must learn or relearn. The goals are specific, and occupational therapy treatment centers around accomplishing those specific goals or tasks which the patient has identified as his preferences.

The occupational therapist uses compensation strategies for patients who need to live with a disability on a temporary or permanent basis. Using this approach, the physical disability patient uses his remaining abilities to perform needed tasks. Occupational therapy helps the patient to develop strategies or use adaptive equipment that can compensate for the loss of physical capacities in order to accomplish activities of daily living. The therapist organizes the environment, then motivates and reinforces the patient toward successful completion of the task. Adaptations, compensations, and adaptive equipment may be incorporated into group activities. Competence in doing the task is achieved through repetition and practice.

Skill Acquisition—
Mosey, Denton, Trombly

The above approach to the rehabilitation of physical disabilities has previously been called "acquisitional" by Mosey (1986) and others. Denton (1987) called it

"functional performance," and Trombly called it simply the "rehabilitative approach" (1989). This refers to the process of relearning lost skills in activities of daily living, due to physical disability. Rehabilitation in occupational therapy occurs on a continuum of restoration-adaptation-compensation. That is, foundation skills of movement, strength, endurance, and perception are remediated, or brought to the highest level of recovery possible within the limitations of the illness or injury. Adaptations in everyday functioning are then made to maximize that level of recovery through use of special equipment or changes in the environment. When full recovery is not anticipated, compensatory strategies are then substituted for skills that have been lost or compromised. This practical approach to rehabilitation is so well known in occupational therapy that it has not really needed an official "name."

Two related approaches worthy of mention here are Mosey's "role acquisition" and Fidler's "lifestyle performance profile" (Robertson, 1988).

Role Acquisition

Mosey addresses the role acquisition approach to those individuals whose disability has stabilized and who continue to have difficulty in performance of tasks of their major social roles (Robertson, 1988). She identifies the basic skills common to all social roles as task skills and interpersonal skills. These basic skills are necessary building blocks for the performance of self-care (activities of daily living), family interaction, recreation, and work. Temporal adaptation, or skill in the perception and use of time, serves to organize and balance the tasks of occupational roles on a daily basis. The following lists of task and interpersonal skills may be helpful in setting group goals (Table 5-2). Skills are

Table 5-2.
Mosey's Role Acquisition: Task and Interpersonal Skills

Task Skills

1. Willingness to engage in tasks
2. Adequate posture for tasks
3. Physical strength and endurance
4. Gross and fine motor coordination
5. Interest in task
6. Rate of performance
7. Ability to follow oral, demonstrated pictorial, and written directions
8. Use of tools and materials
9. Acceptable level of neatness
10. Attention to detail
11. Ability to solve problems
12. Ability to organize task in logical manner
13. Ability to tolerate frustration
14. Ability to be self-directed

Interpersonal Skills

1. Initiate, respond to, and sustain verbal interactions
2. Express ideas and feelings
3. Be aware of needs and feelings of others
4. Participate in cooperative and competitive situations
5. Compromise and negotiate
6. Assert self
7. Take on appropriate group roles

---

separately defined for family interaction, activities of daily living, leisure, and work. Temporal adaptation, the ability to perceive and manage time, is defined as orientation, organization, planning, goal setting, and establishing a schedule. Mosey suggests that treatment in task skill development begin on an individual basis. Group treatment can be effective in learning the more advanced task skills and in working on interpersonal skills. She suggests topical or thematic groups be designed to address specific skills.

Lifestyle Performance Profile

This assessment tool developed by Gail Fidler and published in Hemphill (1982) was later presented as a frame of reference in Robertson (1988). In it, skills for self-care and maintenance, self needs/intrinsic gratification, and service to others are listed and assessed within the framework of age, culture, and biology. Figure 5-1 shows the interrelationship of skill areas/deficits, values/attitudes, and external resources/barriers so that a complete picture of the person within his current or historical context can be drawn. This profile can serve as an alternative basis for grouping patients with similar lifestyles, situations, and concerns, as well as similar deficits. Lifestyle changes and adaptations may be made more easily

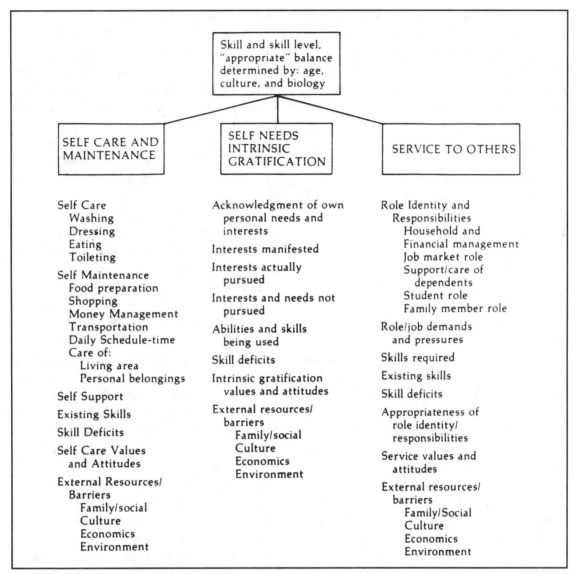

Figure 5-1. Lifestyle performance profile by Gail Fidler. Reprinted with permission from Hemphill, B. (1982). *The evaluative process in psychiatric occupational therapy.* Thorofare, NJ: SLACK Incorporated.

within a supportive, therapeutic group context.

Cognitive Rehabilitation Concepts—Toglia and Abreu

Learning theory is the foundation for cognitive rehabilitation (sometimes called cognitive-perceptual rehabilitation), according to Abreu and Toglia (1983, 1987). This training involves systematic procedures provided in each of six discrete

cognitive deficit areas: orientation, attention, visual processing, motor planning, cognition, and occupational behavior, to assist patients in the perception of stimuli and the effective solving of problems. More recently, Toglia has expanded this framework in her development of the multicontext approach to retraining and the addition of metacognition and criteria for transfer of learning. These additions do not abandon the original delineation of cognitive deficit areas, but they do alter the approach to their treatment. Toglia's recent work acknowledges the dynamic, interactive, and holistic nature of brain functioning and maximizes the likelihood of generalization of newly learned strategies or compensatory measures in restoring occupational performance.

Functional Brain Areas

The six basic areas of perception/cognition addressed by Toglia and Abreu (1983, 1987) are:

1. Orientation
2. Attention
3. Visual processing
4. Motor planning
5. Cognition
6. Occupational behavior

This organization of cognitive deficit areas has its foundation in the work of the Russian physiologist Aleksandr Luria (1980). Abreu and Toglia (1983) refer to Luria's brain region classifications in their organization of perceptual and cognitive deficits. The first brain area described includes the brainstem and the old cortex, containing the midbrain, thalamus, hypothalamus, uncas, reticular formation, and cerebellum. These are the innermost portions of the brain and are responsible for attention, wakefulness, arousal, and response to stimuli. The second brain area Luria defines includes the backmost areas and is responsible for analysis, coding, and storage of information. It receives raw data from sensory systems and assigns meaning to them. Luria's third functional area includes the frontal portions of the brain and is responsible for intentions, programs, and problem-solving. A distinction is also made between the right and left hemispheres of the brain in terms of function. The right hemisphere is responsible for diffuse representation, gestalts, and organized wholes. It deals in concepts rather than specifics, and processes visual-spatial data and nonverbal sounds. Body scheme and tactile, somatosensory integration are primarily attributed to the right side of the brain. The left hemisphere is analytic and sequential, concerned with language, specific details, and mathematical operations. While there are discrete characteristics for the two sides of the brain, functionally they work together to perform daily life tasks. Often, it is through clinical work with brain damaged patients that we learn what types of functions are lost when certain parts of the brain are damaged.

Accidents and illnesses that cause damage to discrete areas of the brain are the most likely candidates for cognitive and perceptual retraining. Abreu and Toglia (1989) have proposed an "Evaluation Model: Six Areas to Test" (Figure 5-2), as a guide in assessing the areas of dysfunction and planning strategies for retraining. Some of the theories about how cognitive rehabilitation works are outlined by Bracy (1986) as follows:

1. Lower brain areas take control and compensate for lost skills at higher levels
2. Different brain areas are utilized to replace lost skills (e.g., opposite hemisphere)
3. Normal function returns as shock effect of injury subsides
4. Function is recovered through retraining

These principles serve as the justification for the following strategies in cognitive rehabilitation.

The Multicontextual Approach

Cognitive rehabilitation with brain injured adults involves the reorganization of functional systems so that new methods of performing old behaviors are acquired. The retraining seeks to maxi-

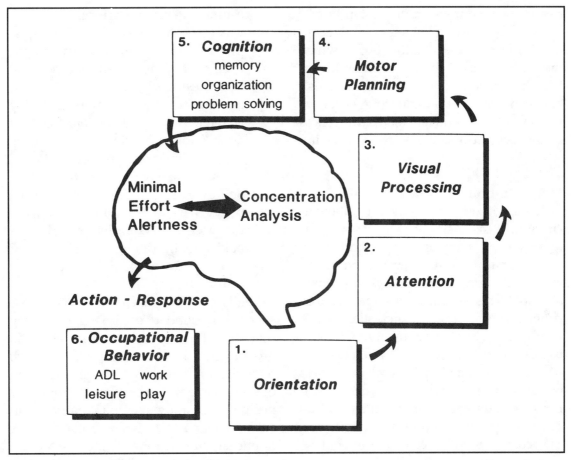

Figure 5-2. Six brain functions for cognitive rehabilitation. Reprinted with permission from Abreu, B. C., & Toglia, J. P. (1984). *Cognitive rehabilitation manual.* New York: Author.

mize the efficiency of information processing, and involves repetitive exercises that place demands on the individual to perform skills of graded difficulty. However, simply practicing each skill separately, according to Toglia (1991, 1997), does not result in the generalization of skills to life in the real world. Once cognitive strategies are relearned, they must be practiced and applied over a wide range of functional tasks, in a variety of social and situational contexts, in order to facilitate generalization of skills. For example, a client needs to learn to monitor time during task performance so that he can complete tasks more quickly and be on time to appointments. He may

begin with an individual task, writing down the time in the margin after each paragraph he reads in a magazine. In a group setting, he may complete a series of word puzzles, noting the time he started and completed each, and comparing with others to check for accuracy. He may be assigned the homework task of timing each morning task—washing, dressing, eating breakfast, shaving (or for females, applying make-up). Estimating the time it takes to get ready for an appointment may be the topic of discussion in the next occupational therapy group. In the group, time-saving ideas can be shared, and clients can learn new strategies from each other. Multiple contexts used during treatment encourage an understanding of the significance of a strategy and a recognition of properties of situations in which the strategy is applicable. The multicontext approach does not distinguish between remediation and compensation. Rather, it focuses on a person's awareness of the need to use a selected processing strategy.

Metacognition

Toglia (1991) defines metacognition as "insight, or the degree of awareness one has regarding one's cognitive or physical capacities." Impairment in metacognition results in a misjudgment of the tasks one may attempt. This misjudgment may expose patients to significant danger, such as driving with a visual impairment or failure to use a needed cane or walker when walking outdoors. Training increases self-awareness by acquiring knowledge of one's own processes and cognitive capacities and by developing self-monitoring strategies. Metacognitive skills include the ability to:

- Evaluate task difficulty
- Predict consequences of action
- Formulate goals
- Plan for anticipated problems
- Monitor one's own performance
- Recognize errors
- Demonstrate self-control

Toglia stresses that without metacognition, persons are unable to initiate and use either remedial or compensatory strategies. Therefore, these skills should be worked on significantly during therapy. Some suggested techniques for increasing metacognition are:

- Self-instruction—Person verbalizes plan before execution, then verbalizes speed and accuracy of performance during and afterward
- Self-estimation—Person rates task difficulty on a scale of 1 to 5 (very easy to very hard), then compares estimate to actual performance
- Role reversal—Patient watches therapist making errors while doing the task; patient must identify errors and hypothesize why they occurred
- Self-questioning—At intervals during actual performance, person stops and asks: "How am I doing? Am I using _____ (specific strategy)? Have I followed directions accurately?"
- Self-evaluation—After completion, persons asks: "Have I checked work for accuracy/completion? Have I paid attention or maintained focus? How confident do I feel about the results?"

Toglia suggests that metacognition has such a profound effect on new learning that this ability should be addressed in groups first, before attempting to teach remedial or compensatory strategies. In one experiment on memory training for persons with traumatic brain injury, group discussion and education about awareness of one's own performance increased accuracy of predictions by 50% on a recall task (Toglia, 1991). New research on the process of adaptation to disability suggests that for some patients, a series of shockwaves and adjustments to the reality of chronic disability, taking several months (or years), may be necessary before the kind of insight or "metacognition" Toglia suggests is actually possible (Macdonald, 1998, personal communication).

The nature of metacognitive training makes it especially well suited to group treatment for several reasons. The obvious reason is that one's performance in a group is observed by others and has the advantage of multiple opportunities for observations and feedback. The company of others who also need to work on metacognition increases the level of support and encouragement if performance is poor, while decreasing the possibility of minimizing or denying one's difficulties. Applying the above skills to any processing task in a group context can be easily planned by the occupational therapist using Toglia's guidelines.

Generalization and Criteria for Transfer of Learning

Using Toglia's dynamic interactional model, cognitive strategies are always taught in the context of an activity. The initial demonstration of a strategy may be simple and designed for clinical use. For example, an organizational strategy might be presented to the group that involves 20 picture cards in four different categories (i.e., dishes, clothing, office supplies, and furniture). Each of the four people in the group chooses one category, and takes turns picking up the cards belonging to that category. The strategy of sorting can be applied to putting away laundry (e.g., things to hang up, things for the drawer, things for the linen closet, things for long-term storage). Sorting incoming mail then follows (e.g., bills, read now, read later, throw away). Next, the group may be given a grocery list which may be sorted according to the signs in the aisles of a local grocery store, which have been photographed with a Polaroid camera. This one might be followed up with an actual trip to the grocery store to check for accuracy.

Different applications of a processing strategy represent different levels of generalization or transfer of skills. The therapist can identify a graded series of tasks that display decreasing degrees of physical and conceptual similarity to the original situation. To do this, potential tasks must be analyzed. The similarity of tasks depends on both surface characteristics and underlying concepts. Surface characteristics are as follows:
1. Type of stimuli
2. Presentation mode
3. Variables of size, color, shape, etc.
4. Stimuli arrangement
5. Movement requirements
6. Environmental context
7. Rules or directions, number of steps

The underlying concepts of tasks are:
1. Underlying skills required (eye-hand coordination)
2. Non-situational strategies (planning)
3. Situational strategies (grouping, visual imagery)

Transfer of skills may be near, intermediate, far, or very far. The closer the practice task resembles the training task, the easier the transfer. Patients in the "sorting" group example had a fairly easy time understanding how to sort the laundry items presented as pictures. They may have more difficulty if a basket of laundry is dumped on the table in front of them, because the mode of presentation and task requirement (hanging, folding) is different. The picture categories and pictures of laundry items might be considered near transfer, because only two characteristics have changed (subject of pictures and categories). In intermediate transfer, three to six characteristics have changed. Actually sorting items and putting them away adds the characteristics of three dimensions—color, texture, and necessity of manipulation and movement.

If the group takes a trip to the grocery store, members will be faced with a far transfer. Far transfer tasks are conceptually similar to the initial task, but the surface characteristics are either completely different or have only one surface similarity. In the grocery store exercise, the physical surroundings, number of people, number of steps, and variety of object properties make the application of sorting by aisle and finding items on the grocery list a much more challenging task. Very far transfer refers to generalization or spontaneous application of what has been learned to everyday functioning (Toglia, 1991, p. 508). After discharge from treatment, a person might be able to demonstrate the sorting strategy in cleaning out the attic or garage.

Dynamic Nature of Cognition

Grouping persons with brain dysfunction is based on Toglia's dynamic interactional assessment, which includes both the structural and functional capacity of each individual. Standardized pencil and paper or simulated tasks are not considered adequate for assessment. Processing skills in the six brain areas—orientation, attention, visual processing, motor planning, cognition (organization, memory, problem-solving), and activities of daily living functions—are examined and evaluated in the context of the physical, social, and cultural environment, and within the parameters and variables of everyday task performance. Often the functional capacities of brain damaged individuals can be greater in familiar social and physical contexts than it appears in the clinic. This is because a person's capacity for cognitive functioning changes in different contexts. A person's cognitive functioning is largely dependent upon familiar cues from the environment and the expectations of one's social and cultural roles.

Therapy goals are set to match as closely as possible the expected roles and requirements of the discharge environments. Persons with similar learner capabilities are grouped together for learning selected strategies which are estimated to be within their capabilities. Metacognition and multicontextual strategy training are then worked on simultaneously in these homogeneous groups. Multiple contexts for the strategy are used during treatment to encourage understanding of the significance of the strategy and a recognition of the properties of situations in which the

strategy is appropriate. For example, estimating the time needed for task performance may be applied to a variety of tasks. The group might begin by estimating the time it will take them to read a one-page article, then reading the article and monitoring the time elapsed after each paragraph is completed and totaled at the end. Estimated times are compared with actual times.

Behavioral Cognitive Concepts

Just as ego psychology was an outgrowth of psychoanalytic theory, cognitive behaviorism has advanced from the original behavioral theories. Cognitive behaviorists basically accept the principles of early behaviorism, but have added thinking to the repertoire of human behavior that can be learned and modified. The fundamental change these psychological theories have made from their predecessors is their rejection of determinism. Behavior modification is an outdated technique by which behavior of the individual is essentially controlled by the therapist through the use of external reinforcement. This technique is seldom used nowadays, except for individuals with such a low level of self-control that self-reinforcement is not possible. Just as the concept of ego autonomy implies that man can adapt and change according to his own will, cognition in the cognitive frame allows man to regulate his own behavior. This concept has important implications for treatment.

Unlike behavior modification, which puts the control in the hands of the therapist and external forces, behavioral cognitive therapies seek to modify how a person thinks. Rather than just a stimulus and response continuum, thought processes are inserted between the two. The stimulus involves a situation and an emotion or feeling state; then an analysis of both the situation and the feeling occurs in which various response behaviors are considered and their consequences anticipated. Only after such an analysis does a behavioral response occur. Cognitive therapists seek to discover the thought processes of patients and to help patients use their own cognitive abilities to dispute thinking patterns which lead to problematic behaviors.

Cognitive behavioral therapy has become firmly planted in the field of occupational therapy, as most recently described by Duncombe (1997). In reviewing the literature, Duncombe has found that the role of occupational therapy is described by Aaron Beck and colleagues as, "Occupational therapists who work in a psychiatric setting are primarily concerned with teaching skills to promote self-reliance and independence. These therapists have received extensive training on how to deal with actual physical, intellectual, or social deficits. In fact, they are probably better prepared than most psychiatrists, psychologists, or social workers to teach adaptive skills to persons with significant handicaps...The occupational therapist uses psychoeducational procedures, demonstrations, and in vivo rehearsal to build functional ability and self-esteem" (Wright, Thase, Ludgate, & Beck, 1993).

Three major contributors to the psychological cognitive behavioral theory are Albert Bandura, Aaron Beck, and Albert Ellis.

Social Learning Theory—Bandura

Bandura's work begins earliest and bridges the gap from behavior modification to cognition. Bandura's best known contribution to cognitive behavioral theory is his social learning theory (1977, p. 78). The major areas of focus in Bandura's work are: the role of internal and external reinforcers, mediating environment and person interactions, modeling and observation learning, self-control and self-regulation, and alternative sources of motivation. Bandura's hierarchy of reinforcement, mentioned earlier, spans a range of both external and internal reinforcers. Regarding reinforcement, Bandura contends that the person as well as the environment determines behavior. A social learning interaction involves three factors: person, behavior, and environment. External reinforcers are measurable outcomes from the environment, such as getting a grade on a test. The person's interpretation and expectations are considered equally important; these are the internal reinforcers. Examples of external reinforcers are money, material goods, social approval, or privileges and penalties. Self-reinforcement develops with maturity and the enactment of internal values and self-expectations.

Person-Environment Interactions

The role of cognition in mediating environment and person interactions is another important component in social learning theory. Bandura contends that behavior is an interacting determinant of the outcome or response. For example, a group member's behavior might elicit anger in the other group members. Cognition affects the person in his beliefs about himself and the group. Sam believes he is not an alcoholic, but that others in the group are alcoholics. This belief leads him to project an aloof attitude toward other members. When they ask him to participate, he refuses, and he will not respond to the comments of others. The group members interpret his behavior as critical of them— "He thinks he's better than we are." This makes them respond to Sam with anger. Sam hears their angry comments and feels rejected; he logically concludes that the group is not interested in him or able to help him. All of these processes, beliefs and attitudes, interpretations, and logical conclusions are cognitive processes that influence the person-environment interaction. In using this concept with patients, group leaders can design activities that facilitate an analysis of social interactions that encourages the uncovering of underlying beliefs and attitudes. These patients may be able to use this process to question their own attitudes and change beliefs that are troublesome.

Modeling and Observation Learning

Modeling and observation learning are types of social learning which all persons engage in throughout life. Yet people do not imitate every behavior they see. Cognition plays a major role in the analysis of observed behavior and the selection of which behavior to model. Bandura contends that this selection depends upon anticipated consequences. This means that individuals seek to model behavior which they have observed to have positive consequences. Occupational therapy group leaders can use this process to great advantage. Leaders can model positive responses to others, effective interactions, and successful problem-solving, for example. This technique helps patients to increase their own interactional and problem-solving skills. An important advantage of group treatment is the learning that takes place from watching and imitating each other.

Self-Control and Self-Regulation

Self-control and self-regulation are desired outcomes of therapy. The basic assumption is that persons are in control of their own behavior and can influence the outcome of their treatment. Cognition influences their motivation, selection of goals, and the ability to achieve them. Goals can serve as guides for self-regulation. Persons can measure their own

progress in terms of desired goals. Goals are always central in a behavioral cognitive approach to group treatment. The goals of the group are shared with patients and agreed upon at the outset. Activities of the group are directed toward the goal(s) and numbers often evaluate the group in terms of progress toward the goal. Since goals are clearly stated, progress can be easily tested and reported by the therapist. This is partly what makes this approach so useful in acute care settings, where gains are expected to be made quickly and progress is evaluated on a daily basis. This concept begins to apply at Allen's cognitive Level 4, for which goal-directed behavior is possible.

Cognition also influences the development of insight or self-understanding. Educating patients in how they might analyze their own attitudes, behavior, and consequences will enhance their ability to regulate their own behavior. When an anxious patient understands the forces in the environment and the beliefs in herself that contribute to her anxiety, that patient can more easily exercise self-control. She can regulate the situation by reconsidering the reality of her beliefs or removing herself to a less stressful environment. For example, Amy, a college student, studies in her room where her roommate constantly irritates her by playing loud music. Amy believes she cannot study with loud music playing. If she changes her attitude, she may learn to enjoy the music or she may be able to view it as a screen for other more distracting noises. If Amy cannot do this, she may choose to study in the library.

Cognitive Distortions and Automatic Thoughts—Beck

Aaron Beck developed his methods of behavioral cognitive therapy in the 1960s and 1970s through his work with depressed patients. His approach is founded in empirical investigation: he treats the patient's maladaptive interpretations and conclusions about events as hypotheses to be tested. Beck collaborates with the patient in conducting behavioral experiments, verbal examinations of alternative interpretations, reality testing, and problem-solving, with the goal of correcting cognitive distortions of reality. From his clinical findings, Beck concludes that psychological disturbances frequently stem from automatic thoughts which reflect habitual errors in thinking. This cognitive model does not assume that the cognitions operate exclusive of biochemistry or behavior symptomatic of psychopathology. Cognition is considered the problem and not the cause. The structure and process of cognitive therapy includes setting the agenda for the session, eliciting feedback, setting goals for therapy, operationally defining problems, testing hypotheses, problem-solving techniques, and assigning homework. This structure lends itself very well to occupational therapy groups which can address through activities the cognitive roadblocks to functional performance.

Exposing Irrational Beliefs—Ellis

Albert Ellis is well known for his work in rational emotive therapy (RET). Although Ellis and Beck developed their techniques over approximately the same time period, each has his own somewhat eclectic basis of which traditional behavior therapy is only a part. Like Beck, Ellis considered thinking to be a legitimate behavior which could be learned and modified using behavior modification techniques. A distinguishing feature of RET is its systematic exposition of irrational beliefs that result in emotional and behavioral disturbances. Ellis spends most of his energy looking for "unconditional shoulds" and "absolute musts." He contends that

patients take "simple preferences" such as desire for love, approval, and success and make the mistake of thinking of them as dire needs.

Ellis's view of human nature is somewhat humanistic; he believes people have inborn tendencies toward growth and actualization. He takes for granted, however, that humans are fallible and often make mistakes resulting in "crooked thinking" and "self-defeating" behavior (1973). RET has developed into a kind of structured challenging and disputing of irrational beliefs. Its confrontive methodology, such as the use of exaggeration, absurdity, and humor, is not at all humanistic.

Cognitive Restructuring

Ellis suggests a philosophical restructuring process involving a series of steps (Ellis & Harper, 1975), all of which require high level thinking. This method reflects both humanistic self-determination and the supremacy of rational thinking in controlling and directing human behavior.

1. Acknowledging our responsibility for creating our own problems
2. Accepting our ability to change our own problems
3. Seeing that emotional problems stem from irrational beliefs
4. Clearly perceiving our beliefs
5. Rigorously disputing beliefs
6. Working hard to change beliefs resulting in disturbed emotion and behavior
7. Continued cognitive monitoring and restructuring over our lifetime

Cognitive restructuring includes the process of questioning our decisions and life structures and considering alternatives. It is very much a skill development process to be used over one's lifetime. When emotional problems are identified, therapy consists of defining problems in thinking that contribute to the distressing emotions or behaviors, and finding alternative, more realistic and pragmatic ways of conceptualizing those life circumstances. The therapist acts as an educator-facilitator in collaborating with the client to achieve specific goals.

In occupational therapy groups, when we use a psychoeducational approach, our role as educator-facilitator is similar to that outlined by Ellis and Beck. Within the context of activities, occupational therapists can use cognitive restructuring principles to teach clients how to apply a scientific approach to thinking. Our goal is to teach skills that can be generalized by patients after they leave therapy groups. Groups that focus on pain management, time management, leisure planning, and health education/prevention are examples of occupational therapy groups using a behavioral cognitive approach. Discussion of the problems patients have in the performance of activities often leads to exposure of faulty thinking. In our higher functioning patient groups, occupational therapists can help the patients change their attitudes toward disability or ability as it affects performance. We can teach our group members to challenge each other and to encourage their use of rational thinking to solve problems.

Dialectical Strategies—Linehan

Dialectical behavior therapy, or DBT, was developed by Dr. Marsha Linehan (1993a) over the past 15 years as a treatment specifically for borderline personality disorders (BPD). Persons with this disorder are frequently seen in hospitals (19% of mental health inpatients, 11% of mental health outpatients); they are burdensome to the health care system because there is no effective medical treatment. It is suspected that many more "undiagnosed" BPDs enter hospitals with a host of other

diagnoses because of their tendency to exaggerate symptoms and their proneness to substance abuse and suicide attempts. Dr. Linehan translates the core of the disorder into behavioral cognitive terms by emphasizing its "pattern of behavioral, emotional, and cognitive instability and dysregulation"(1993a, p. 11). "Dialectic" is defined by *Webster's College Dictionary* (1991) as "pertaining to logical argument" and includes "conversation revealing the truth through use of logic, juxtaposition of conflicting ideas or forces, (and) debate over a constantly changing reality." Those who are familiar with BPD will recognize immediately why this term was chosen. Hallmark symptoms of this personality disorder include a tendency to distort reality, to either idolize or condemn others, to create drama and conflict in relationships, and to continually redefine their own identity. Acceptance of the nature of life as a constant struggle involving balance and imbalance of opposites is an important part of DBT. The dialectic approach to treatment meets the person with BPD on his own turf and teaches a logical approach to self-regulation. Linehan's approach to treatment is largely psychoeducational. Examples are described later in this chapter.

Function and Dysfunction

Adaptation to the environment is the common measure across behavioral and cognitive theories. Behaviorists use the terms adaptive behavior and learning, and attribute dysfunctional behavior to maladaptive learning. The emphasis is placed on concrete, observable behavior.

In the biomechanical and rehabilitation frames, a person is fully functional when she has no restrictions in ROM, strength, and endurance, and maintains the ability to perform the tasks necessary for work, play/leisure, self-care, and social roles.

Function also includes the practice of good health maintenance habits.

Function in the cognitive rehabilitation frame of reference refers to information processing skills, and their flexible use across task boundaries (generalization). Toglia and Abreu look at brain functioning as the behavior to be measured, and measure this by the outward manifestations of orientation, attention, visual processing, motor planning, cognition (memory, organization, and problem-solving), and occupational behavior. However, Toglia rejects the notion of assessing these skills in isolation and has designed and researched several "dynamic" assessments which measure these cognitive processes during functional performance (Toglia, 1997). Dysfunction in cognitive rehabilitation is characterized by limitations in the brain's ability to process information efficiently. Symptoms of poor efficiency become obvious during the performance of everyday activities when there is a mismatch between the task and the skill level of the individual. Dysfunction in metacognition is significant in that the patient's inaccurate self-perceptions cause him to misjudge the difficulty of tasks and the appropriateness of processing or compensatory strategies. Unawareness of one's own deficits prevents one from learning from mistakes and using feedback to modify behavior. Inefficiencies in organization, setting priorities, and shifting one's mental perspective or viewpoint are common areas of dysfunction to be treated from a cognitive rehabilitation perspective.

In cognitive behaviorism, a well-functioning individual has the ability to think logically and to form accurate perceptions of the self and the environment. He can use deductive reasoning to cope with problems and can logically regulate his own thoughts, feelings, and behavior. Dysfunction may be defined as faulty thinking, inaccurate self-perception, and the inability to handle one's affairs competently. Failure to adapt to the environment and to function independently in society in this frame of reference is seen as a product of cognitive disability. Therefore, it is cognitive impairments in attention, sensory awareness, perception, memory, and other thought processes that prevent efficient problem-solving, interfere with learning and application of new coping strategies, and cause problems in doing functional activities. These cognitive functions, therefore, should be the focus of treatment in occupational therapy.

In designing groups with persons of similar cognitive ability, many assessments are available to use as guidelines. Claudia Allen (1997, workshop materials) has prepared a comparison chart of some of the most commonly used assessment scales, which may be helpful in selecting group membership (Table 5-3). Allen's Cognitive Levels scales are further defined in Chapter 6, *Allen's Cognitive Disabilities Groups*. The Medicare Physical Assistance and Cognitive Assistance Scales are taken from Medicare Part B Guidelines. For other scales, readers can refer to Katz (1997) *Cognition and Occupation in Rehabilitation*.

Change and Motivation

Following the guidelines of learning theory, the basic strategy for change is reinforcement. Change occurs when behavior is reinforced in some way. In behavior modification, behavior may be controlled and shaped by the therapist (or other person) using external reinforcement. The type of reinforcement that can be effective will vary from patient to patient. Some patients do not seem to have the internal motivation to learn new skills. For these patients, external reward is most appropriate. This can be anything the

Table 5-3.
Comparison of Various Medical Scales

Allen Cognitive Level	Medicare Cog. Assist. %	Medicare Physical Assist. %	Rancho Head Trauma	Global Deterior-ation Scale	Global Assess Scale	GAF DSM-IV Axis V	Age (Bayley Maturational) *approx.
0.8	100	100	I				
1.0	99		II				0-1 mo.
1.2	98		III				1-5 mo.
1.4	96	75					4-8 mo.
1.6	92						4-10 mo.
1.8	88	50					6-12 mo.
2.0	84	25	IV	7			9-17 mo.
2.2	82	15					10-20 mo.
2.4	78	10			1-10		
2.6	75						12-23 mo.
2.8	70					1-10	
3.0	64		V		11-20	11-20	18-24 mo.
3.2	60				21-30		
3.4	54			6	31-40	21-30	
3.6	50				41-50		3 yr.
3.8	46					31-40	
4.0	42	8	VI	5	51-60		4 yr.
4.2	38						5 yr.
4.4	34				61-70		6 yr.
4.6	30		VII	4		41-50	
4.8	25				71-80		
5.0	22	6					7-10 yr.
5.2	18	4			81-90		11-13 yr.
5.4	14	2		3		51-60	14-16 yr.
5.6	10	0	VIII	2	91-100	61-80	17 yr.
5.8	6					81-90	
6.0	0			1		91-100	18-21 yr.

patient is willing to work for, such as praise, extra attention, candy, cigarettes, or privileges. Bandura expanded the definition of reinforcement to include a range of internalized reinforcements. Some patients respond to social reinforcement, such as the praise and acceptance of their peers, family, or friends. At a higher level, patients will strive to learn skills or improve functioning in order to gain the approval of society or meet the expectations of their cultural group. The highest form, self-reinforcement, spontaneously emerges as the individual strives to measure up to his own internal standards. In occupational therapy, simple skills are mastered before more difficult ones are attempted. Thus, the patients can develop feelings of competence as each new skill is mastered. The feeling of competence gained from successful occupational performance, in itself, provides reinforcement. This is known as self-reinforcement, the highest form of motivation patients can achieve.

In the behavioral cognitive approaches,

people change by changing the way they think. For adults with acquired brain injury, cognitive rehabilitation produces change by training in the use of remedial or compensatory processing strategies in the context of a broad range of tasks. To the extent that they are capable, persons use metacognitive strategies, increasing awareness and monitoring of their own cognitive capacities and limitations. The occupational therapist can use a psycho-educational approach to teach patients to apply logic to produce adaptive change in persons with intact processing skills (e.g., persons with disorders of substance use, eating disorders, obsessive compulsive disorders, or personality disorders). In DBT, becoming aware of beliefs and attitudes that result in problem emotions and behaviors is the first step. Patients are sometimes asked to sign a contract, agreeing to try out new thinking and self-regulation strategies for a defined period of time. Challenging their "faulty thoughts" can often convince patients to change or replace them, and this will lead to a change in behavior.

Current cognitive approaches assume that people have a natural drive toward competence and mastery and to achieve a better position in life. People wish to be self-directed and to have an effect on others and on the environment. To achieve these goals, most people are willing to learn and try new coping strategies for problem-solving and for self-improvement/regulation.

A difficulty with this approach may be to find effective reinforcements for those patients who do not seem to be motivated or are unaware of a social pressure to improve their status.

Group Treatment

Groups are homogeneous in this frame of reference. This does not mean, however, that all the members have the same diagnosis. Since a broad range of functional levels, verbal and reasoning abilities, and diagnostic categories is being addressed, assessment of the critical abilities for group involvement is an important prerequisite. In planning group treatment, patients with similar needs or deficits are usually grouped together, and goals are set to address their common deficiencies. They should be grouped together, no more than eight at once, to focus on learning a particular skill. Members should be at approximately the same level cognitively, so that they will be able to learn at the same pace and through similar modes of presentation. Groups working on perception and memory skills in cognitive rehabilitation, for example, might be given several memory games during a therapy session. All the members should be able to understand the verbal directions if the activity is to be successful in accomplishing its goal. In a psychoeducational problem-solving group, the goals might be to master each step in the problem-solving process. Patients will be able to:

1. Clearly state the desired outcome of the problem
2. Gather relevant information
3. Analyze and interpret the data
4. Devise a plan to solve the problem (describe the actions that need to be taken and sequence the steps)
5. Implement the plan
6. Evaluate the outcome

The goals in the behavioral cognitive frames of reference are always very specific, observable, and measurable. This is because the treatment approach is very goal directed. Problems are generally addressed narrowly and specifically, and the learning, rehearsal, and practice of specific skills are usually the goals. The most closely aligned to behavioral theory is the biomechanical/rehabilitative frame of reference. When planning groups in this model, exercises to increase ROM, strength, and endurance are demonstrated, imitated, and practiced in the groups within the context of functional activities. Groups may be designed around the need for training in the use of adaptive equipment or in techniques of energy conservation. Biofeedback and monitoring techniques during exercise groups allow individual members to participate at different levels, while having the advantage of group support and socialization. For the sake of clarity, any group examples that include elements of physical rehabilitation or the monitoring of physical attributes, such as relaxation, will be called biomechanical/rehabilitative, even though it may also draw upon behavioral techniques.

In cognitive rehabilitation, Toglia and Abreu's six cognitive areas (orientation, attention, visual processing, motor planning, cognition, and occupational behavior) may be used as guidelines for the selection of group activities. Persons who share similar functional problems may be treated in groups of three to six, or up to eight with a co-leader. The group should be structured so that at several different contexts are presented for using the same strategy. For example, attention-sustaining strategies may be practiced with pencil and paper tasks, like alternating numbers and letters in a sequence when connecting dots on a page. Done in a group, partners can take turns monitoring and giving each other cues. Attention must be used when playing group board games, card games, or word games. Likewise, many visual processing, motor planning, memory, and problem-solving strategies may be learned and practiced in the context of group activities. There are numerous workbooks and collections of exercises that exist in the literature that are most helpful in planning

groups (Dougherty & Radomski, 1987; Toglia & Abreu, 1987). Some of the advantages of working on cognitive strategies in groups are:

1. Group "games" can be motivating and fun
2. Groups provide a real-life context for the use of skills
3. Therapeutic groups allow practice with guidance and safety
4. Feedback on performance from others increases self-awareness
5. Observation of a variety of group responses encourages generalization of skills
6. Possible applications of skills can be discussed and explored

Psychoeducational groups, based on behavioral and behavioral cognitive principles may be designed for skill training, such as assertiveness, social skills, or stress management. Occupational therapists often use a psychoeducational approach involving the imparting of information and the use of structured learning exercises. In *Dialectical Behavior Therapy*, Dr. Linehan has identified specific issues that need to be addressed by persons with BPD, which she defines as a "disorder of self-regulation"(1993a). These are dysregulation of emotion, interpersonal relationships, behavior, cognition, and sense of self. Group treatment has traditionally been the treatment of choice for individuals with BPD, because of their difficulty with authority, their need for peer feedback, and the desirability of avoiding the power struggles that are inevitable in one-to-one relationships, therapeutic or otherwise. Linehan (1993b) has designed a workbook for psychosocial skills training, which outlines specific group exercises in four major categories.

1. Core mindfulness. Teaches the mind to focus on one thing at a time, to pay attention to all the information avail-

able in a situation, and to refrain from quick judgments or jumping to conclusions or acting on the basis of emotional responses. A useful technique is writing; taking time to describe conflict situations in words delays the response and leads away from the emotional and into the rational, analytical mind. Awareness of beliefs and attitudes one typically uses, and analyzing these applying logic, labeling behaviors and emotions as harmful and destructive or helpful and productive in accomplishing one's objectives in the conflict situation, are also a focus of group exercises in the mindfulness category.

2. Interpersonal effectiveness. Skills for achieving specific objectives in relationships, getting and keeping good relationships, and maintaining self-respect in relationships are learned and practiced in these group exercises. Recognition of the factors that interfere with relationships, strategies for challenging these negative factors, and self-reinforcing positive responses are also included. Exercises for expression of feelings and opinions, negotiating, reciprocating, and making specific requests help to build a repertoire of skills for building and maintaining healthy interpersonal relationships.

3. Emotion regulation. This series of exercises begins with challenging beliefs about emotions and their importance. Describing and naming the emotions (love, joy, shame, fear, sadness, and anger are major categories) becomes the first step toward a rational approach, reducing vulnerability to the negative effects of emotions. Exercises in effective self-interventions when emotions threaten to overwhelm or take over include

strategies for evoking positive emotion, building positive experiences, and steps to reduce painful emotions.

4. Distress tolerance. These exercises for groups teach techniques for crisis survival. The goal is to stop the negative behavioral responses typical of BPD, such as substance abuse and self-destructive or suicidal acts. Strategies for distracting, self-soothing, and improving the moment (prayer, relaxation, deep breathing, brief escape) allow time for reason to gain control. Attitude change from "This is awful" to "I can survive this" is practiced. This is followed by exercises in the application of logic: listing the pros and cons for tolerating the distress and directing "willfulness" (imposing one's will on reality) toward what works, and not what interferes with survival. Developing an awareness of the pleasures of ordinary tasks, and cultivating a "half-smile" of acceptance, lead group members toward the expectation that it is OK for life to be ordinary, and that life circumstances are not always going to be ideal.

Care is taken to address each of these psychosocial skill areas in positive terms, avoiding the least hint of criticism (which commonly evokes anger and thus interferes with learning). The exercises use a variety of cognitive restructuring techniques to modify dysfunctional assumptions and beliefs, and other behavioral and cognitive techniques mentioned earlier, including practice and rehearsal, therapist reinforcement, feedback and coaching, modeling, and role playing. Groups of six to eight members are suggested for skill training, and these are offered in 8-week modules, complete with worksheets, handouts, and homework. Linehan offers workshops for training in DBT, which are open to occupational therapists as well as other professionals. Her *Skills Training Manual for Treating Borderline Personality Disorder* includes handouts that may be photocopied for use with client groups (for more information, call The Guilford Press at 1-800-365-7006).

Role of the Leader

The occupational therapist's role is more directive in this frame of reference than it is in most others. In a hospital setting the focus is often on evaluation. The therapist typically chooses the activity or task, and structures the group for concentrated work toward a specific goal. Efficiency in goal attainment is all-important, and the occupational therapist structures the group and the environment with this in mind. The therapist's role is active during the group, giving assistance, providing cues, and asking questions that will guide group members to improve their performance. Discussion may require frequent redirection to remain focused, with the guiding principle of reinforcing the learning of specific skills and achievement of specific goals. The occupational therapist should carefully monitor interaction to make sure the feedback given by members to each other is of a therapeutic nature.

Goals of the Group

Goals are behaviorally defined, specific, observable, and measurable. Occupational therapy goals are practical in nature, focusing on increasing functional performance. This fact alone makes the behavioral cognitive approach the best fit in the current health care atmosphere. Measurable goals are easy to document and justify the need for treatment. In working with the physical or cognitive/perceptual dysfunction, the therapist sets goals for the group based on her best assessment of the patients' potential. Norms are helpful in setting goals in

the biomechanical areas, such as "resume normal strength in the injured right leg," or "increase ROM from 160 to 180 degrees in a spastic elbow." In patients with temporary cognitive impairment, Allen's Cognitive Level 6 or Rancho Los Amigo's head trauma Level VII may be an appropriate goal. For patients with the capacity for rational thought, the goal is insight. Only when a patient understands the impact of his cognitive distortions and irrational beliefs is he able or willing to change them. It is assumed that a change in thinking will produce a change in behavior. Therefore, goals will generally address the thought processes rather than the affective or overt behavioral components.

Current literature in occupational therapy has emphasized the importance of culture and individual values in goal selection. For this reason, the patient's own preference and social expectations may play a part in determining the goals. Research has shown that a meaningful task increases motivation and elicits a patient's best effort. Long-term goals may be set collaboratively with each patient, based on his expected environment, culture, and social roles. Within the group, limited choices can be offered, so that individual interests and preferences may become incorporated into the group experience.

Activity Examples

In psychoeducational groups, occupational therapists use and adapt many specific behavioral techniques to enhance group learning. Some of these techniques should be recognized as very powerful and therefore dangerous to use without specific training. Some of the techniques occupational therapists should avoid unless specifically trained are flooding, paradoxical intention, and systematic desensitization. These techniques involve vivid imaging of much-feared and disturbing situations, and the management of patients who have been so aroused requires more advanced therapeutic skills.

However, in moderation, imaging and visualization may be incorporated into a structured activity or may be expanded into drawing, sculpture, or dramatic role play. The use of images or visualization is a technique many occupational therapists have found helpful. For example, the guided fantasy can enhance relaxation and foster creativity and self-awareness. Once goals are set, visualizing images of their successful achievement is often motivating. Drawing images of various kinds is one way to structure our groups to work on specific goals.

The concepts of group problem-solving, keeping journals, and giving homework are also useful ideas in occupational therapy groups. Behavior rehearsal may be useful in the learning and practice of social skills. Some other techniques are contracts with oneself or with the group to change certain thoughts and behavior, self-reward or self-punishment, writing beliefs in words and then deciding if the statements are true or false, and positive or negative labeling of thoughts, feelings, and behavior. The reader is referred to McMullin's *Handbook of Cognitive Therapy Techniques*, Linehan's *Skills Training Manual for Treating Borderline Personality Disorder*, Moyers' *Substance Abuse: A Multi-Dimensional Assessment and Treatment Approach*, and Precin's *Living Skills Recovery Workbook* for more ideas. Following are some examples of behavioral cognitive groups (Activity Examples 5-1 through 5-8). They will be identified as belonging to the following categories: biomechanical/rehabilitative, cognitive rehabilitative, or psychoeducational. All of these categories use behavioral and cognitive principles, techniques, and strategies.

Group Leadership

The seven-step group format is not changed in structure. If anything, in this frame of reference, groups become even more structured. The beginning of the group places an emphasis on defining specific problems and collaborative goal setting. The therapist may do this individually before the group begins.

Introduction

This kind of group will dispense with the warm-up and get right down to business. A more complete explanation of the goals and purpose will substitute. Expectations are spelled out in behavioral terms, and the group is told how the members' progress will be evaluated. The timeframe of the group should coincide with the members' level of cognitive functioning.

Activity

Behavioral cognitive groups focus on learning coping skills and improving task performance. There is usually didactic instruction given in the form of short lectures or demonstrations of the steps in doing a task. The activities are learning experiences and opportunities for practice. In a leisure skills group, for example, members learn to do a series of specific activities: how to knit, how to cook, how to catch a fish, or how to play card games. In a stress management group, the occupational therapist gives mini-lessons in cardiovascular fitness, high nutrition diets, and progressive relaxation in conjunction with activities. The experience may take longer, up to two thirds of the session, leaving the rest for discussion/demonstration.

Sharing

If members have done an individual activity, such as a worksheet, this is the time for reading it aloud or holding it up for the group to see. The leader should give recognition and feedback, and encourage other group members to do the same. In the cognitive rehabilitation groups, this is an opportunity to discuss self-evaluations and compare results. Leaders should be cautious not to encourage competition, but to place emphasis on how well each member was able to predict and monitor his own performance. For behavioral cognitive and psychoeducational groups, feedback from others is an important social reinforcement to learning and should be offered to all members. Feedback comes mostly from the therapist in the lower level groups, and from fellow members in higher level groups.

Processing

Discussion of the underlying dynamics of the group is also not an area of focus. Most of the interaction should be between the leader and each member, just as a teacher interacts with a class. However, when the feelings or the implicit forces of the group begin to interfere with group learning, then the therapist must temporarily make group process the focus. This is not to say, however, that feelings about the activity should be ignored. This part of the discussion should invite honest expression of emotions, both positive and negative, as they pertain to the issues addressed by the activity. The group energy may be rallied in support of members who are discouraged with their progress or having difficulty adapting to residual or permanent dysfunction. Group leaders need to beware of the offering of false hope or flattery by members, and discussion should be kept focused and controlled.

Generalizing

Inductive reasoning is encouraged in the members to come up with general principles to be learned from the experience. Inductive reasoning involves collecting evidence from many specific examples to build a general principle or theory. Members can do this best when they have heard several responses to the experience from other members, which has hopefully been done in the sharing and processing steps. In a well-planned group, the general principles suggested by the members will coincide with group goals. If this does not happen spontaneously, the therapist should help the group to make the connections. In cognitive rehabilitation groups, for example, members may take this opportunity to verbalize the specific strategies they have worked on, take note of what they learned about their own ability to process information, and summarize insight they have gained.

Application

There is more emphasis here than in any other part of the discussion. An effective group will include a carry-over of behavior change from the clinic to the community environment. An open group discussion of how newly learned strategies may be concretely applied in everyday life will increase the likelihood of carry-over. Members should know before they leave the group exactly how they will apply their new knowledge or skill. Application requires deductive reasoning, the application of theoretical ideas to specific, individual situations. Often the therapist must structure this reasoning with thought-provoking discussion questions and concrete examples. Members may then share ideas on how to do this. The activities done by the group are usually planned to address specific problems, so the application is generally built into the group experience at the outset. If patients leave the group consciously aware of the usefulness of certain skills, they may communicate this to family members and caretakers, and they may initiate the process of self-reinforcement. Homework may be given by the therapist to support the application of what is learned. When homework is given, a timeframe should be included, and members should know when and where they will be asked to report on the results of the homework activity.

Summary

A verbal summary by the therapist is a tradition to be continued throughout the frames of reference. In this one, its major purpose is to reinforce learning. It is best done by the therapist in most cases. Emphasizing the important points of the session and giving positive feedback to members are the important elements. The few minutes it takes to summarize may make the difference between forgetting and remembering what was learned. Reminders about homework and announcements about what is planned next are also appropriate.

Bibliography

Abreu, B., & Toglia, J. (1983). Cognitive rehabilitation: A model for occupational therapy. *American Journal of Occupational Therapy, 41*, 439-453.

Abreu, B., & Toglia, J. (1989). Cognitive rehabilitation: A model for occupational therapy. *American Journal of Occupational Therapy, 41*(7), 439-448.

American Psychiatric Association. (1994). *Diagnostic & statistical manual of mental disorders* (4th ed.). Washington, DC: Author.

Bandura, A. (1977). *Social learning theory.* Englewood Cliffs, NJ: Prentice-Hall.

Beck, A. (1976). *Cognitive therapy and emotional disorders.* New York: International University Press.

Bracy, O. (1986). Cognitive rehabilitation: A process approach. *Journal of Cognitive Rehabilitation, Mar/Apr,* 10-17.

Bruce, M., & Borg, B. (1993). *Frames of reference in psychosocial occupational therapy* (2nd ed.). Thorofare, NJ: SLACK Incorporated.

Denton, P. L. (1987). *Psychiatric occupational therapy: A workbook of practical skills.* Boston: Little, Brown and Co.

Dougherty, P., & Radomski, M. V. (1987). *The cogni-tive rehabilitation workbook.* Rockville, MD: Aspen.

Dryden, W., & Golden, W. (1986). *Cognitive-behavioral approaches to psychotherapy.* London: Harper & Row.

Duncombe, L. (1997). Cognitive behavioral model in mental health. In N. Katz (Ed.), *Cognition and Occupation in Rehabilitation.* Bethesda, MD: American Occupational Therapy Association.

Duncombe, L., & McCraith, D. (1997). *Cognitive approaches for psychosocial evaluation and intervention.* Paper presentation. AOTA, SIS Practice, Phoenix.

Ellis, A. (1973). *Humanistic psychology: The rational emotive approach.* New York: McGraw-Hill.

Ellis, A., & Harper, R. (1975). *A new guide to rational living.* North Hollywood, CA: Wilshire Book Co.

Fidler, G. (1982). The life-style performance profile. In B. Hemphill (Ed.), *The Evaluative Process in Psychiatric Occupational Therapy.* Thorofare, NJ: SLACK Incorporated.

Fidler, G. (1988). The life-style performance profile. In S. Robertson (Ed.), *Mental Health Focus: Skills for Assessment and Treatment.* Rockville, MD: American Occupational Therapy Association.

Greenfield, J. M., & Godinez, M. (1989, April 20). Stroke clients learn independence by leading their own therapy group. *OT Week.*

Harlowe, D., & Yu, P. (1997). *The ROM dance: A range of motion exercise and relaxation program* (2nd ed.). Madison, WI: Uncharted Country Publishing.

Hemphill, B. (1982). *The evaluative process in psychiatric occupational therapy.* Thorofare, NJ: SLACK Incorporated.

James, W. (1985). Habit: Its importance for psychology. *OT in Mental Health, 5*(3), 55-67.

Katz, N. (1997). *Cognition & occupation in rehabilitation: Cognitive models for intervention in occupational therapy.* Bethesda, MD: American Occupational Therapy Association.

Linehan, M. (1993a). *Cognitive-behavioral treatment of borderline personality disorder.* New York: The Guilford Press.

Linehan, M. (1993b). *Skills training manual for treating borderline personality disorder.* New York: The Guilford Press.

Luria, A. (1973). *The working brain.* New York: Basic Books.

Luria, A. (1980). *Higher cortical functions in man.* New York: Basic Books.

McMullin, R. E. (1986). *Handbook of cognitive therapy techniques.* New York: Norton.

Mosey, A. (1986). *Psychosocial components of occupational therapy.* New York: Raven.

Mosey, A. (1988). Role acquisition: An acquisitional frame of reference. In S. Robertson (Ed.), *Mental health focus.* Rockville, MD: American Occupational Therapy Association.

Moyers, P. (1992). *Substance abuse: A multi-dimensional assessment and treatment approach.* Thorofare, NJ: SLACK Incorporated.

Posthuma, B. (1989). *Small groups in therapy settings: Process and leadership.* Boston: Little, Brown & Co.

Precin, P. (1998). *Living skills recovery workbook.* MA: Butterworth Heinemann.

Robertson, S. (1988). *Mental health focus.* Rockville, MD: American Occupational Therapy Association.

Skinner, B. F. (1953). *Science and human behavior.* New York: Macmillan.

Stein, F., & Nikolic, S. (1989). Teaching stress management techniques to a schizophrenic patient. *American Journal of Occupational Therapy, 43*(3), 162-169.

Toglia, J. (1991). Generalization of treatment: A multicontext approach to cognitive perceptual impairment in adults with brain injury. *American Journal of Occupational Therapy, 45*(6), 505-516.

Toglia, J. (1997). A dynamic interactional approach to cognitive rehabilitation. In N. Katz (Ed.), *Cognition & Occupation in Rehabilitation: Cognitive Models for Intervention in Occupational Therapy.* Bethesda, MD: American Occupational Therapy Association.

Toglia, J., & Abreu, B. (1987). *Cognitive rehabilitation.* New York: Author. Contact J. Toglia, OT Dept., Mercy College, 555 Broadway, Dobbs Ferry, NY 10522.

Trombly, C. (1989). *Occupational therapy for physical dysfunction* (3rd ed.). Baltimore: Williams & Wilkins.

Van Deusen, J., & Harlowe, D. (1987). The efficacy of the ROM dance program for adults with rheumatoid arthritis. *American Journal of Occupational Therapy, 41*(2), 90-95.

Webster's College Dictionary. (1991). New York: Random House.

White, R. H. (1967). Competence and the growth of personality. In *Science and Psychoanalysis, Vol. XI, The Ego.* New York: Grune and Stratton.

Wright, J., Thase, M., Ludgate, J., & Beck, A. (1993). *The cognitive milieu: Structure and process. In cognitive therapy with inpatients.* New York: The Guilford Press.

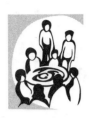

Behavioral Cognitive
Activity Example 5-1
I Can Remember (Cognitive Rehabilitation)

Materials: Twenty objects on a tray, selected from three different categories (e.g., things normally found in the kitchen, things normally found in an office, and grooming items normally found in a bathroom cabinet), towel to cover items from sight, pencils and paper for each member, and a printed list of 10 commonly known names of objects (e.g., telephone, ruler, picture frame, mailbox, baseball, lamp, pitcher, teddy bear, stool, boat) for each member.

Strategies: Repetition and rehersal, grouping and counting.

Directions: There are many reasons why we might need to be able to remember things. What are some things that are important for you to remember? Today we will practice two strategies to assist you in remembering things.

Repetition and Rehersal

When you encounter something you want to remember, say it over and over to yourself. For example, when you meet someone new, say the person's name to yourself four or five times. Look at the person as you are doing this so that the name and the face will be connected in your brain. To practice this, turn to the person next to you and introduce yourself. (If they already know each other, making up a new name or using their middle names may suffice.) Using his name in the next sentence of conversation is another way to practice: "Nice to meet you, Henry" or "Henry, how are you feeling today?"

Next, we will use the same strategy to memorize a list of words. (Give out printed list.) You will note that the worksheet lists common objects numbered 1 to 10. Before we start, I would like you each to predict how many of these items you think you will be able to remember after 1 minute of practice. Write this number down on the top of your paper. Now begin memorizing, using repetition and rehearsal, repeating the words over and over. (Time for 1 minute.) Time is up. Please turn you paper over and write on the back as many words as you can remember. No looking at each other's papers is allowed. How does the result compare with your prediction? Look back at the list and correct your errors. This can be repeated if desired.

Next, we will practice remembering objects that we see. I will show you a tray full of objects, and you will have 1 minute to look at them. During that minute, you should say the name of each object to yourself. When I cover the tray of objects, you will write down as many names of objects as you can remember, so get your pencils out. Paper will be given out as soon as the objects are covered. No note-taking is allowed. (Place the tray in the center of the table, uncover it for 1 minute, then re-cover it.) How did everyone do? How many objects did you list? How many were there all together? Did anyone count?

From Cole, M. B. *Group Dynamics in Occupational Therapy, Second Edition.* © 1998 SLACK Incorporated.

Grouping and Counting

The second strategy we will use is counting the items you wish to remember and then grouping them into categories. When we try this again, count the objects first, then try to remember items together that are associated in some way. This strategy is used in addition to the repetition and rehearsal we have already practiced. There are objects from three categories on this tray. Did anyone notice what those might be? (Discuss and clarify the strategy as needed. Give out blank paper.) Before we begin, we will predict how many items we can remember this time, and write that number down in the corner of your paper. Now we will begin. (Uncover tray and time for 1 minute, then re-cover.) Write down as many as you can remember. (Pause.) How many items were there? (20) How many were in each category? Let's make a master list. (Have someone volunteer.) Write the three categories, then have group list the items. When finished, uncover tray once again to self-correct errors. How did people do in comparison with last time? Did the grouping help you to remember more items? Now compare with your predictions.

Application discussion follows, in which members discuss two or three ways they can use these strategies during the next week. Homework may be given as needed.

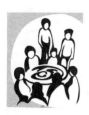

Behavioral Cognitive
Activity Example 5-2
Setting Priorities (Psychoeducational)

This activity has been used as the first session of a time management workshop for substance abuse patients. It serves as an ice breaker for patients who do not know each other well, and also helps the therapist to formulate goals for the group.

Materials: Values Survey Worksheets and pencils.

Directions: Often the things we spend our time doing are not the things we want most to do. Setting priorities means deciding what is important to us and doing that first. As a first step in helping to plan our time better, we will look at what we value.

(Pass out Values Survey Worksheet.) Take the next 10 minutes to think about the values listed, and number them according to their order of importance to you. Put number 1 next to the most important item, number 2 for the next level of importance, and so forth, up to number 8 for the least important. Do not use the same number more than once.

(Ask each member to share their top three values and discuss in what way these values are a part of his life right now.)

Write your top three values on the lower section of the Values Survey Worksheet, and below each write one specific goal that reflects that value. For example, if "freedom to do what I want" is one of your values, your goal might be to move out of your parents' house and get your own apartment. You have 5 minutes for this part.

Looking at your goals, choose one to work on this weekend. At the bottom of the worksheet, write down one activity that you can plan this weekend to help you accomplish the goal.

From Cole, M. B. *Group Dynamics in Occupational Therapy, Second Edition.* © 1998 SLACK Incorporated.

Values Survey Worksheet

Directions: Eight commonly held values are listed here. Think about your own life in relation to these values. Then give each a number, beginning with number 1 for the most important to you, number 2 for the second most important, and so forth, up to number 8 for the least important. Do not use any number more than once.

_____ A good love relationship
_____ Financial security
_____ A satisfying religious faith
_____ Freedom to do what I want
_____ Meaningful family life
_____ Success at my chosen career
_____ Excitement and adventure
_____ Making lots of money

First most important value:

Goal:

Second most important value:

Goal:

Third most important value:

Goal:

Planned activity to work on goal:

From Cole, M. B. *Group Dynamics in Occupational Therapy, Second Edition.* © 1998 SLACK Incorporated.

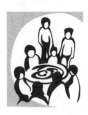

**Behavioral Cognitive
Activity Example 5-3
Telling Others About Your Illness
(Psychoeducational)**

This behavioral cognitive activity has been part of a patient group on coping with illness. The group is given short lectures each week on a different aspect of coping with illness, followed by participation in a related activity. This one uses role playing and behavioral rehearsal, and the support of the group serves as social reinforcement.

Materials: Two chairs placed in the center of the group.

Directions: Each patient will take a turn sitting in the chair in the center. First, the patient will tell the group what her illness is, and why it is difficult to talk to others about it. Then the patient will choose another member to play the part of a relative or friend. The therapist is the "director" and directs as follows:

Friend or relative: Ask how the patient is and ask follow-up questions.

Patient: Answer him as if it were a real conversation.

Patient: Now change places with your friend and respond for him. Now change places again and be yourself again. Try to tell your friend how you "feel" about being ill. Try to keep each conversation going for about 5 minutes. Members should volunteer for this and no one should be forced.

After each discussion, the group is asked to respond and to discuss the role play. Were the players being "genuine?" Were feelings being expressed freely? What are other ways to make the discussion helpful?

From Cole, M. B. *Group Dynamics in Occupational Therapy, Second Edition.* © 1998 SLACK Incorporated.

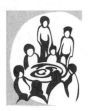

Behavioral Cognitive
Activity Example 5-4
Relaxation Fantasy Activity
(Biomechanical/Rehabilitative)

This activity has been a part of a stress management group in which members use the techniques of visualization and guided fantasy to control their state of tension.

Materials: Carpeted open space, patients wearing sweatsuits and sneakers or other comfortable clothing, and pillows for each person.

Directions: Members sit in a circle on the floor, pillows in their laps. They should be far enough apart that all can lie down and reach out their arms without touching one another.

1. Introduction—Relaxation is as much in your mind as in your body. Therefore, if you want to be relaxed and free your body from stress, your mind must take the lead. It is very difficult to feel relaxed when your mind is preoccupied with worry. As you do this exercise, try to concentrate on the visual images that come into your head. Instructions will be given for you to move your physical position as well as parts of your body. Try to do these with your eyes closed, so you will not lose the mental images created.

2. You are about to take a 30-minute relaxation break from your busy, stressful, or boring day. Maybe you have a lot of work to do or a difficult situation to face. Put that out of your mind for the next 30 minutes. Afterward, when you are relaxed, you will have more energy to cope with life's hassles.

3. Begin by reaching both arms up over your head in a big stretch. Open your mouth wide and yawn. Now place the pillow behind your hips and lean back on your elbows. Close your eyes and imagine a door far across the room in front of you. Without moving your position, imagine yourself walking toward the door. Move your feet, your ankles, your knees, and your hips as if you were walking. When the right leg is tense, allow the left one to relax. Now point your toes each time you take a "step." Slow down your steps and inhale as you tense your right leg, then exhale as you tense your left leg. As you approach the door, your steps become slower and slower (2 minutes). When you reach the door, stand in front of it and continue breathing slowly.

4. Push yourself up with your arms to a sitting position. With your eyes still closed, lean forward and peek through a small hole in the door. You see a welcome view. It is a lovely, sunny patio with a sparkling in-ground pool. It is surrounded by clean, comfortable lounge chairs. Keep your hands behind you on the floor as you lean forward to get a better view. Stretch your back and push yourself forward with your arms until you feel the stretch behind your thighs. Keep breathing slowly.

5. With eyes still closed, bend your knees up to your chest. With one hand gripping each knee, imagine that your knees are the handles of the door. Pull gently on the "handles," straightening your back as you pull. Then let go as the door opens wide. As you pass through the door, you leave behind all the worries of the day. On the other side of the door there are no worries, no stress, so let them all go.

From Cole, M. B. *Group Dynamics in Occupational Therapy, Second Edition.* © 1998 SLACK Incorporated.

Relaxation Fantasy Activity
(Biomechanical/Rehabilitative) (continued)

6. Without opening your eyes, straighten your legs and move the pillow under your head as you lie down on one of the comfortable lounge chairs. The sun feels good as it warms you. Imagine you are wearing a bathing suit under your sweatshirt. While still lying down, pretend to take the sweatshirt off. First, put hands near hips and push down on elbows to raise hips slightly off the floor. Then raise hands up to chest level, elbows still on the floor. Push head back into the pillow as you raise shoulders slightly off the floor. Pause here and breathe. Now raise your head off the pillow as you pretend to lift the sweatshirt off over your head and let it drop to the ground behind your pillow. This done, slowly return arms to your sides while breathing out slowly. Just lie there breathing slowly, enjoying the warm sun (2 minutes).

7. Check your body to be sure it is relaxed. Wiggle your fingers and your toes. Roll your head to the right, then roll your head to the left. If there is tension anywhere, shake it out. Put your hand behind your neck and massage your neck muscles. Keep breathing slowly. It feels so relaxing to lie here in the warm sun (2 minutes).

8. The sun is getting hot now. Maybe it is time to go for a swim. Raise yourself up to a sitting position again and bring your knees up to your chest. Now imagine you are sitting on the edge of the pool. Dangle your legs into the pleasantly cool water. Turn around to the left and look behind you; turn around to the right and look behind you. The signs say "Good Swimming Today," so turn over slowly onto your stomach as you lower yourself into the water.

9. As you float on your stomach, your pillow has become a life preserver. Hold onto the pillow as you kick your legs slowly, floating around the pool. Your feet need not even leave the floor. It takes almost no effort at all to move you through the water. Your body does not feel heavy. Now inhale as you kick your right leg, exhale as you kick your left leg. As you reach the edge of the pool, push away again, continuing to hold onto the life preserver with one hand, then the other.

10. Now lift up on your elbows and push the pillow down under your ribcage, so it supports your chest as you lean on your elbows. Continue to breathe slowly. Shrug your shoulders up toward your ears, then release. Shrug away your last bit of tension. Now you are relaxed, refreshed, and energetic. Now you are capable of resuming your day without feeling tension and stress. Miraculously, you are out of the pool, dry and dressed again, standing in front of the door. Now you feel prepared to go back through that door and take on the world. When you are ready, open your eyes.

From Cole, M. B. *Group Dynamics in Occupational Therapy, Second Edition.* © 1998 SLACK Incorporated.

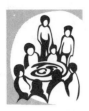

Behavioral Cognitive
Activity Example 5-5
Building Our Community
(Psychoeducational)

This activity is part of a psychoeducational group focusing on independent living skills with chronic schizophrenic patients. The goal of this session is to help the group become aware of community resources. My thanks to D.M. Hancock, occupational therapy student at Quinnipiac College, for this creative idea.

Materials: One square of 1/4-inch plywood, approximately 30 x 30 inches, a variety of small blocks of scrap wood with rough edges and splinters sanded off, jars of poster paint in several colors, brushes, and wood glue. This project may take two sessions to complete.

Directions: The group begins by discussing the communities they live in and what services and resources are available there. The occupational therapist helps the group develop a list of services members need to have available in their community. A typical list includes a hospital, grocery store, department store, drug store, police department, fire department, school, and movie theater. Why they need each one and how they would use it is discussed.

Next, the group members build from the blocks a community they would like to live in. Each member chooses one or more community resources to build, and constructs a school, a movie theater, etc. by gluing blocks together. The "buildings" are then painted and colored signs are painted on to label them. Buildings are then placed and glued onto the plywood square, something like an architect's model city. Streets, parking lots, parks, or bodies of water may be painted directly on the plywood if desired (Figure 5-3).

Discussion/Summary: Sharing has already been done during the activity. Members are asked how they felt about doing the activity and about the result. Some generalization was done earlier, in the choices of structures and organizations to be included in the community, and their uses and importance. This may be reinforced and elaborated here, with an emphasis on how to contact and use community resources appropriately to meet one's needs. Each member then compares the "model" they have built to his own neighborhood or community. Application includes each member's plans for using his own community resources, now and in the future.

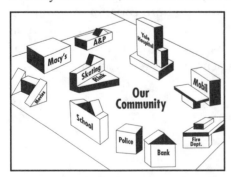

Figure 5-3. Our community.

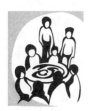

Behavioral Cognitive
Activity Example 5-6
Exercise Groups
(Biomechanical/Rehabilitative)

Exercise to music or dance activities have good potential as therapeutic tools. Circle or group dancing is usually best suited to our purpose in occupational therapy. In physical disability areas where goals involve maintaining and increasing strength and ROM, group activities that accomplish these goals are more enjoyable and motivating than individual exercise programs. A good example of this type of group is the "Range of Motion Dance," an exercise program for patients with rheumatoid arthritis developed by Diane Harlowe and Patricia Yu at St. Mary's Hospital Medical Center in Madison, Wisconsin (Van Deusen & Harlowe, 1987). This is a guided fantasy done with groups of arthritis patients seated in chairs. The exercises, while following the story, go systematically through the ROM for nearly every joint in the body. Once the sequence of motions is learned, it can be repeated by the patients at home by listening to the story on an audiotape.

Greenfield and Godinez have introduced a similar group for stroke patients, called "Self Range of Motion Exercises" (1989). They have defined eight skill levels for these exercises, ranging from complete dependence on the therapist leader to independence in performing the exercises.

In doing such groups, it is important to use the potential of the group to provide mutual support, encouragement, and feedback. Do not let the activity speak for itself; combine it with verbal reinforcement, progress checks, and education about how and why it is helping. It is generally the social and emotional aspects of a group that keep members coming back.

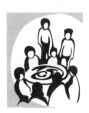

A group of cognitively impaired patients has the goal of improving skills in visual perception and verbal communication. They are given a map of their community, and a worksheet with a list of 10 locations. The following are examples of their tasks.

1. Write directions from Merritt Park Way to the Trumbull Shopping Mall on Main Street.
2. Write directions from the corner of Madison and Stonehouse Roads to Trumbull High School on Stroebel and Daniels Farms Roads.
3. Describe two alternate routes to get from the golf course on Tashua Road to Main Street at the Bridgeport line.
4. Direct someone from Teller and Whitney to the dog pound on Church Street.
5. Plan a route to pick up three friends, on Indian Ledge Road, Brittany Road, and Autumn Ridge Road, and take them to the Town Hall meeting room on Quality Street.

To change the context, other maps or diagrams can be introduced and directions given verbally or in writing. Each patient in the group should have at least one location to find on his own, and then communicate the directions to the rest of the group. The therapist should encourage members to give each other feedback about the accuracy of the directions and clarity of communication.

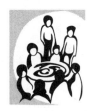

**Behavioral Cognitive
Activity Example 5-8
Design Duplication
(Cognitive Rehabilitation)**

This activity appears in *The Cognitive Rehabilitation Workbook* by Dougherty and Radomski (1987). The goals are to give and follow verbal directions. The objectives are to develop vocabulary to give precise directions, increase accuracy in conveying detailed information, and develop a tolerance for the pitfalls in making oneself understood. Followers of directions are expected to increase their accuracy, develop skills in clarification and confirmation, and increase speed of processing verbal directions.

A group of six is divided into pairs. One from each pair acts as the direction giver and holds a line drawing of several lines and shapes. The other half of each pair sits with his back to his partner and holds a clipboard with blank paper and a pencil with an eraser. Both partners are provided with rulers. Partner 1 must verbally describe the line drawing so that Partner 2 can draw an exact duplicate of the drawing being described. Attention must be paid to shapes, spacing, and dimensions. The pair has 20 minutes to accomplish the task. Then a new drawing is given to each pair and roles are reversed.

It is very important that a feedback session follows each trial. The pairs should discuss the results and analyze any errors in communication in order to correct these on the next trial. This activity can be fun as well as useful, and the therapist should try to create a relaxed atmosphere for the group.

Chapter 6

Allen's Cognitive Disabilities Groups

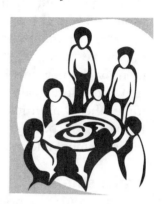

The group approach discussed here is the cognitive disabilities theory of Claudia Allen. Allen has been developing this theory since the early 1970s. Her basic premise is that functional behavior is based on cognition, and that in order to produce a more functional behavior, the thinking process must change. Group activities combine assessment and treatment in this approach, and these usually occur concurrently. Therapist observation of behavior during group activities leads to new assumptions about how information is being perceived and processed. Allen has developed a hierarchy of six cognitive levels, and described typical behaviors of each, based on clinical observation. Using her guidelines, we can easily evaluate our patients and place them in activity groups that are appropriate for each's cognitive level.

Many of the patients we will treat in occupational therapy are cognitively disabled. Examples of some disorders that involve a cognitive disability are: stroke, traumatic brain injury, schizophrenia and other psychotic disorders, anxiety and substance abuse disorders, personality disorders, Alzheimer's and other dementias, mental retardation, autism, and learning disability.

Some of these disorders can be successfully treated. For those cases, Allen groups provide one of the most accurate measures we have for documenting progress. However, for many persons with these disorders, a plateau will be reached beyond which no further cognitive development is possible. These patients need ongoing care, protection from danger, and assistance with many activities of daily living. For these patients, an assessment of cognitive level during a group activity will provide useful guidelines for the level of assistance that will be needed after discharge.

Focus

The cognitive disabilities approach is broadly applicable for both chronic and acute care settings. Allen provides a pragmatic approach to living with the consequences of illness or injury. Some theorists have been critical of the Allen approach because it focuses on "disability" and seems to emphasize weaknesses rather than strengths. This is a misinterpretation. In fact, it is by acknowledging and understanding disability that Allen gives us the profession's most precise guidelines for utilizing a patient's remaining ability to maximize function. "Therapists should identify the person's best ability to function and select treatment goals that maximize these abilities" (Allen, Blue, & Earhart, 1995, p. 1). The focus of therapy is on assessment and management.

Assessment

Perhaps Allen is best known for Allen's Cognitive Levels Screen (ACLS), which uses leather lacing to assess the precise cognitive level of the patient (from 3.0 to 6.0). This test has become increasingly standardized over the past decade, and is widely used by occupational therapists as a screening tool. It gives a quick estimate of the patient's current capacity to learn (Allen & Earhart, 1992). Other standardized tests of cognitive level developed by Allen are the Routine Task Inventory (RTI) and the Cognitive Performance Test (CPT) (Allen & Earhart, 1992). These assessments use everyday activities to determine the cognitive level. The *Allen Diagnostic Module* (ADM), the most recently developed test, takes motivation and socialization into account and uses a dynamic approach to assessment of cognitive level. (The latest updates of these assessments may be obtained from S&S Worldwide, 1-800-566-6678.) The ADM uses a group format to observe performance while doing a variety of standardized craft activities. Crafts, which make an effective evaluation at Levels 3.0 to 5.8, are motivating because they are meaningful across the spectrum of cultures. Observation of an individual's

response to instructions and sensory cues from the materials and tools of the craft provides the basis for predictions about many other aspects of human performance. Examples of these crafts are given later in the chapter in the section on activities.

In the past few decades, science has dictated a standardized, rigid approach to assessment. In this context, neither crafts nor routine daily activities have face validity. There are too many variables and too many individual differences for scientific accuracy to be applied. Therefore, therapists should use caution in making judgments about cognitive level based on the observation of these activities. Allen's levels and modes should never be considered labels, which prejudice others and limit the person's options or autonomy. Rather, they should be used as guidelines, upon which to plan initial activities, or make tentative discharge arrangements, which will only become valid when the person with cognitive disability has an opportunity to demonstrate his best ability to function.

Since the Allen approach advocates that patients be treated in groups of similar cognitive level, the initial screening becomes an important part of group planning. The approximate cognitive level must be determined in order to place patients appropriately in occupational therapy treatment groups.

Management

Once the patient's best ability to function (ACL) has been determined, decisions about lifestyle and discharge placement need to be made. The occupational therapist's role is to make recommendations about the level of assistance the patient will need in the immediate future.

Management of the patient involves two aspects: assistance from caregivers and adaptation of the environment. The guiding principles for management come from the cognitive modes of functioning within each level. Goals for expected behaviors in activities of daily living are defined, along with the amount of physical and cognitive assistance needed at each mode/level (Allen et al., 1995).

Environmental adaptation flows from the amount of conscious awareness the patient has at his disposal. To elicit a person's best effort in doing a task, the usable task environment must be defined. Supplies needed for a task to be done must be placed within the limits of conscious awareness, for example, within arm's reach at Level 3. Concurrently, all distractions and unsafe items should be removed. Think about how hard it is to get anything done when your desk is piled high with junk mail or your kitchen is stacked with dirty dishes. Our patients need our help to remove the clutter and help them focus on what is necessary to perform essential tasks.

Another essential component of patient management is providing needed assistance. Allen also builds into the cognitive levels and modes the quality and quantity of assistance needed. To elicit the patient's best performance, the caregiver must first observe the patient's response to the task environment, and then intervene as needed in a variety of ways. Four of the possible ways to give cognitive assistance suggested by Allen are:

1. Facilitate—Give sensory cues appropriate to the level
2. Probe—Ask focused questions to encourage problem-solving
3. Observe—Allow patient time to process cues and questions and try out new behaviors
4. Rescue—When frustration arises, correct error or do a step for the patient

The experienced therapist should never do for patients what they can do for themselves.

For example, the person at Level 3 responds best to tactile cues. The caregiver, therefore, facilitates by using touch to get the patient's attention and demonstrates the use of necessary objects. To assist with dressing, the caregiver hands the patient a shirt and touches the right hand to be inserted in the sleeve. Probing or asking questions that suggest the next step might then be tried, "How can you get your arm in the sleeve?" Observing the response determines if more assistance is needed. If the response is unproductive, a third attempt might be a direct verbal instruction, accompanying the demonstration, "Hold it by the collar with this hand, and put the other arm in here." The "rescue" is always a last resort; if the patient shows significant signs of frustration, put the arm in the shirt for him.

In general, the amount of assistance needed to do a task decreases as the cognitive level increases. Table 6-1 is a general guideline for the amount of cognitive assistance needed at each level.

Basic Assumptions

Cognitive Disability Defined

Allen (1987b) defines cognitive disability as "a limitation in sensory motor actions originating in the physical or chemical structures of the brain and producing observable and assessable limitations in routine task behavior." Allen accepts the concept that a person's cognitive level has biological and chemical determinants. There is a distinction made between an impairment and a disability. An impairment, according to the *International Classification of Impairments, Disabilities, and Handicaps* (World Health Organization, 1980), is "any loss or abnormality of psychological, physiological, or anatomical structure or function." Impairments, in the medical model, are called diagnoses,

Table 6-1.
Allen's Cognitive Assistance for Levels 1 Through 6

Level	Cognitive Assistance Needed	Compensation Provided for the Following Cognitive Functions Which Are Lacking
1	Total	Sensory stimulation (and 2 to 6)
2	Maximum	Prevent getting lost or into unsafe areas (and 3 to 6)
3	Moderate	Help with self-care (and 4 to 6)
4	Minimum	Maintaining the home (and 5 and 6)
5	Standby	Planning, advising, supervision
6	None necessary	None

names of diseases, or injuries with clusters of associated "symptoms." A disability, according to the same source, is "any restriction or lack of ability to perform an activity in the manner or within the range considered normal for a human being." Impairments often cause a disability. For example, mis-shaped lenses of the eyes (an impairment) can cause near-sightedness (a disability). A handicap is defined as "a disadvantage for a given individual, resulting from an impairment or disability, that limits or prevents the fulfillment of a role that is normal for that individual"(1980). Following the above example, if an airline pilot were to develop near-sightedness, he would not be able to continue the role of "pilot." For the pilot, near-sightedness is a handicap. An accountant with the same impairment might obtain a pair of glasses to overcome the subsequent disability, and continue in that career as before, without a handicap. Glasses are the "adaptive equipment" which corrects the disability and prevents it from being a handicap. For cognitive disabilities, assessment and management in occupational therapy serve a similar purpose: accepting the impairment, using assistance and environmental adaptation to overcome disability, and as much as possible, using our understanding of the limita-

tions in task behavior to predict appropriate placement, thus preventing handicap as a social consequence.

Being unable to work, care for others, or maintain a home are some of the roles that are commonly lost as a result of cognitive disability. However, there are other roles that may be acquired, such as volunteer, hobbyist, family helper, and organization participant, with the appropriate cognitive assistance.

Allen's Task Analysis

Task analysis is defined as a method of determining the functional complexity of an activity by separating the activity into steps and determining the physical and cognitive functional abilities required to do each step. In recent years, Allen has developed a more dynamic approach to task analysis, which includes factors such as culture, motivation, and situational context, as well as the basic ability to process information. This approach is visually outlined in Figure 6-1, and this serves as the basis for planning and interpreting craft activities such as those used in ADM.

Cues

Cues consist of the environment itself, the materials needed for a task, and all forms of verbal, written, or demonstrated

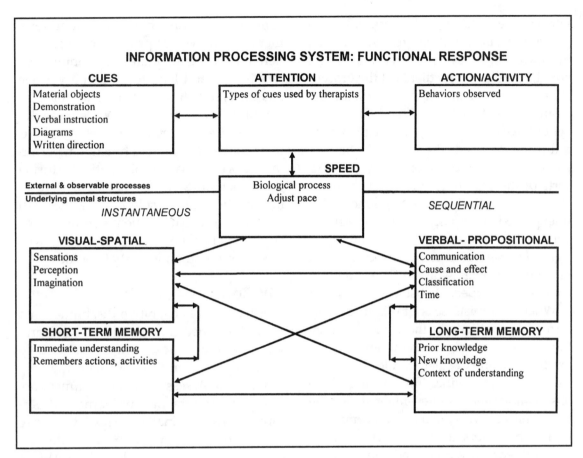

Figure 6-1. Allen's task analysis. Copyright Claudia Allen, conference materials, 1997. Adapted with permission.

instruction. In normal everyday activity, when we find ourselves in a kitchen at mealtime, the cues we use are the food in the refrigerator or cabinets, the recipe or preparation we have in mind, and the equipment available for preparing a meal (e.g., bowls, baking pans, dishes, knives). Visual, olfactory, and gustatory memories may guide and motivate us.

Attention

Attention to cues is necessary for functional activity to occur. How our brain receives or screens out cues may depend on many psychological, physiological, social, and cultural factors. In cognitive disability, the limitations of attention and

sensory screening need to be evaluated in order to plan appropriate treatment. When using cues in treatment, Allen advocates careful planning of the environment (clinic or home setting), thoughtful selecting and placing supplies and equipment to be used for a task, and varying the amount and type of assistance given, according to the specific guidelines at each cognitive level or mode.

Action/Activity

The combination of cues and a person's ability to attend and focus will hopefully result in an action or response (the performance of functional activity). Continuing the kitchen analogy, when I go home to my kitchen after a hard day's work, my meal preparation task will be greatly enhanced by how well I have prepared ahead. If I bought the right ingredients at the grocery store, if the pots and pans and dishes are clean and ready to be used, and if I remember or have easy access to the recipe or procedure to be used, the meal will be prepared correctly and in a timely manner. All sorts of things can go wrong, even in the absence of disability—telephone calls, unexpected company, key ingredients being eaten by another family member, the right size baking pan borrowed and not returned. Problem-solving is needed to cope with unexpected obstacles.

When therapists select tasks to be performed by patients in the clinical setting, the patient's problem-solving ability may be observed and evaluated. Allen has given us specific guidelines for making these observations and for interpreting them. The six cognitive levels are based on compiling typical behaviors at each cognitive level (and subsequently, each mode) in response to a variety of tasks (cues). From these sample behaviors, cognitive disability theory makes inferences about the thinking processes which produced them. These inferences explain how the person's brain processes the information being presented.

Speed

The speed of response depends upon the speed with which the brain processes information. Biological factors, such as brain chemicals, are responsible for setting the rate of thinking and behavior. Persons functioning below Level 5 generally have a difficult time adjusting the speed of their performance.

Underlying Cognitive Processes

Information processing involves visual-spatial components (right hemisphere) in conjunction with short- and long-term memory, and verbal-propositional components (left hemisphere) in conjunction with short- and long-term memory. Allen has analyzed these components for each cognitive level and mode. While these differences are too detailed to describe here, their contribution to the functional performance we observe in our patients during group activities should not be underestimated. In activity selection, a therapist should consider the patient's prior knowledge, experience, and preferences, as well as sensory motor and verbal abilities.

Six Cognitive Levels

Allen divides cognitive disabilities into six well-defined cognitive levels, and provides several assessment tools to help occupational therapists evaluate the cognitive level. Assessment and treatment are based on how the patient learns and performs tasks. Originally, the six levels were derived from Piaget's work on intellectual development. However, based on Allen's clinical observation, the cognitive levels are largely presented as descriptions of typical behaviors at each level.

For the purposes of understanding how cognition impacts task performance, three dimensions of task performance are outlined at each level: attention, motor action, and conscious awareness.

Attention

In observing people interacting with their environment, the first thing noted is what sensory stimuli capture their interest. The sensory systems most utilized at each cognitive level seem to more or less follow a developmental sequence, beginning with body sensation (position and movement), and proceeding to incorporate touch and vision, and then integrating these and using them together.

Table 6-2.
Allen's Cognitive Levels 1 Through 6

	1. Automatic Actions	2. Postural Actions	3. Manual Actions	4. Goal-Directed Actions	5. Exploratory Actions	6. Planned Actions
Attention to Sensory Cues	Subliminal	Proprioceptive	Tactile	Visible cues	Related cues (all senses)	Symbolic cues
Motor Actions						
Spontaneous	Automatic	Postural	Manual	Goal-directed	Exploratory	Planned
Imitated	None	Approx-imations	Manipulations	Replications	Novelty	Unnecessary
Conscious Awareness						
Purpose	Arousal	Comfort	Interest	Compliance	Self-control	Reflection
Experience	Indistinct	Moving	Touching	Seeing	Inductive reasoning	Deductive reasoning
Process	Habitual or reflexive	Effect on body	Effect on environment	Several actions	Overt trial and error	Covert trial and error
Time (Attention Span)	Seconds	Minutes	Half hours	Hours	Weeks	Past/future
OT Activities	Sensory stimulation	Gross motor, games, dance	Simple, repetitive tasks	Several-step tasks	Concrete tasks	Conceptual tasks

Motor Action

Second, motor actions are observed in the context of task performance. The therapist uses observations of a person's movements and verbalizations to make some assumptions about her perception, understanding, and intention, all part of cognition.

Conscious Awareness

Finally, conscious awareness of the surroundings is observed. The scope or range of awareness, and the ability to use that awareness to determine appropriate action, increases with each level. Table 6-2 describes a simplified description of attention, motor action, and conscious awareness at each of the six levels. For a more complete understanding of these levels and their assessment, the reader is referred to Allen's books (Allen, 1985; Allen & Earhart, 1992).

Level 1—Automatic Actions

The Level 1 patient is in most cases bedridden. He is conscious but responds mainly to internal or subliminal cues (sensations from within the body), such as hunger or pain. Behavior is largely habitual or reflexive. Arousal and response to others may be elicited for a few seconds at a time. Most daily needs (dressing, grooming, feeding) have to be done by caretakers. Occupational therapists at this level are most helpful in providing appropriate sensory stimulation and attempting to elicit motor responses of any kind.

Level 2—Postural Actions

At Level 2, patients can be stimulated to perform postural actions (changes in position) in response to proprioceptive (sense of motion and position) cues. Patients can imitate gross motor actions, and can assist a caregiver in bathing, dressing, and grooming. Usually Level 2 patients can feed themselves, although this may be messy. Twenty-four hour nursing care is required. Engaging the patient in any self-care tasks is an appropriate intervention at this level. Movement or exercise groups using imitation of position can be done, however, patients cannot benefit from interactive group treatment until they are at Level 3. A good quick test to determine whether a patient is at Level 2 or 3 is to administer the Lower Cognitive Levels test. Ask the patient to watch you while you clap your hands three times loudly (approximately one clap per second). If the patient starts before you finish three, stop him and ask him to watch you first. If the patient is able to imitate three claps, he is probably a Level 3, and therefore should be considered for group treatment.

Level 3—Manual Actions

At this level, patients perform manual actions (movements with their hands) in response to tactile cues (touch). Actions based on interest in objects found within arm's reach may be repeated many times. Attention can be maintained up to 30 minutes. Basic daily grooming tasks may be done independently with reminders; patients can walk to familiar places but get easily lost in new surroundings. Repetitive work tasks can be done at Level 3. Some of the tasks requiring supervision are care of belongings and clothing, money management, preparing meals, following a schedule, and use of a telephone. Care should be taken to place potentially dangerous items out of reach or locked away, as a person at Level 3 cannot discriminate items by their intended use (i.e., paper napkins in the toaster). Tool use must be supervised, as it may be inappropriate (i.e., using a hammer to shut a window). However, with proper instruction, familiar repetitive actions can be fairly skilled, such as using a peeler to peel a potato or a paring knife to cut an apple. Tools that are an "extension of the hand," such as a fork, paintbrush, or nail

file, are usually safe to use with supervision at Level 3. Steps in a task can be imitated one at a time, when demonstrated.

Level 4—Goal-Directed Actions

Becoming goal directed represents a major step toward independent functioning. It is goal directedness that makes activity purposeful; therefore, actions below this level are generally random or habitual. At Level 4, basic living skills are intact—grooming, dressing, toileting, bathing, and feeding. In addition, Level 4 patients perform goal-directed actions in response to visual cues. In other words, if they see a toothbrush, toothpaste, and a cup next to the bathroom sink, these visible cues will remind them to brush their teeth. These patients are able to complete short tasks such as making a sandwich or washing the dishes. Attention is up to 1 hour and steps toward a goal can be imitated in short sequences. Patients perform most daily self-care activities but need assistance in coping with new events, anticipating needs, and managing money. Visual stimuli are the focus, but non-visible properties in the environment, like heat and electricity may pose a danger (e.g., a hair dryer near the bathtub, paper towels near a hot stove). Directions for getting places or doing tasks must be demonstrated visually, since verbal and written directions are not followed. Familiar routine tasks should be reinforced as new routines are established only by repetitive "drilling." Because persons at Level 4 are aware of the goal, they are able to ask for assistance, and this plays a major role in keeping them safe and functional.

Level 5—Exploratory
Actions/Independent Learning

Use of trial and error is the hallmark of Level 5. Here, for the first time, persons use inductive reasoning and are capable of new learning. Patients at Level 5 can imitate new procedures and remember several steps at a time. In task performance, novelty is sought and variation explored. In choosing group projects, this is the first level at which choices may be given. Deficits at Level 5 are in functions that require anticipation and planning. Persons at Level 5 are concrete thinkers primarily, and have trouble imagining the long-term consequences of their actions or inactions. Hence, preventative measures are often not taken. In the home, for example, needed repairs may be neglected (a broken step is neglected until someone trips and falls). Cooking presents a problem when timing is involved; burning is not anticipated, for example. Money management is a major problem since Level 5 patients seldom save for emergencies or anticipate future expenses. Also neglected are purchasing needed items for a meal, cleaning or laundering clothing, and getting prescriptions refilled. The lack of abstract thinking prevents these patients from understanding the nature of their illness or the effects of medication. Jobs and social relationships may suffer because of failure to anticipate the consequences of self-centered behavior. Positive interventions at this level are activities that increase social awareness, reciprocation in relationships, and accepting the supervision of others in helping to avoid negative consequences.

Level 6—Planned Actions

This is the highest level and represents the absence of disability. The main distinguishing characteristic is the ability to use deductive reasoning and to plan ahead. Future events are anticipated and behavior is organized. Verbal and written directions can be followed without demonstration and the person is able to use symbolic cues (Allen, 1988).

The Principle of Brain Conservation

It is natural to think of ourselves as Level 6, which is Allen's representation of "normal." However, everyone has a flow of effort within the entire range of cognitive levels over the course of the day. We may indeed be functioning at Level 6 when we are listening to a lecture and rapidly taking notes in class. But there are many tasks we engage in that do not require that much effort. Bathing and dressing for the day are routine activities that may only require a Level 3 effort. Jogging around a track for exercise allows our brain to take a break and sink to a Level 2. Our brains have a tendency to conserve energy whenever possible. The difference between "normal" and "disabled" is that in disability, no amount of effort can evoke a higher level of cognitive functioning. This limitation is what puts cognitively disabled persons at great risk when they encounter unexpected problems in everyday life. For example, Margaret, at Level 4, could drive a car from her home to a familiar nearby grocery store. But when road construction necessitated a detour, she ended up lost. She was unable to alter her usual route or to locate the necessary resources to find her way home. She wandered around on unfamiliar streets until someone noticed and called a policeman to escort her back home.

The Usable Task Environment

Allen's theory tells us that as the cognitive level increases, awareness of the environment also increases. Specific guidelines are included in Figure 6-2.

For example, a new patient, Sam, is being observed eating a meal. If he is being fed by an aide at his hospital bed, most likely he is at Level 1. If piece of bread is placed in his hand, and he brings

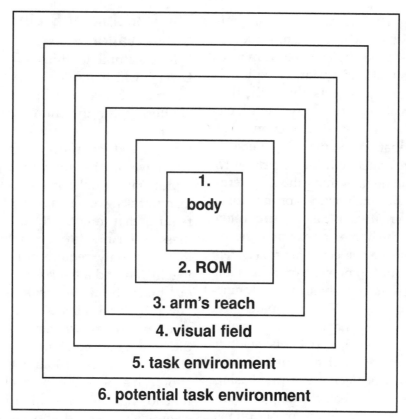

Figure 6-2. The usable task environment. Adapted with permission from Allen, C. K. (1985). *Occupational therapy for psychiatric diseases: Measurement and management of cognitive disabilities.* Boston: Little, Brown and Co.

it to his mouth and takes a bite, he is at least a Level 2, because he is able to use movement functionally. If Sam reaches for the pitcher of juice in the center of the table, an Allen therapist knows he is at least a Level 3, because his attention extends to everything within arm's reach. If Sam asks that the catsup on the opposite side of the table be passed, the therapist will know immediately that Sam is at least a Level 4; he is using his visual system to look for what he wants, and his attention is projected beyond arm's reach. If he likes barbeque sauce, and he gets up and goes to get it out of the refrigerator, he is probably at least a Level 5; he looks for items he cannot see in places where they are typically kept, an action that integrates sensation, perception, and memory. At Level 6,

Sam may remember he is out of milk, and go to buy some next time he is out shopping. At each level, Sam's usable task environment has expanded.

Principle of Task Equivalence

Many people wonder why Allen uses crafts in her group assessment activities (ADM). The answer lies in the principle of task equivalence. The cognitive processing necessary in doing a craft activity is presumed to be equivalent to a variety of everyday tasks which a patient will choose to participate in after discharge from an acute setting. The careful observation of the patient doing a craft activity in a group allows the trained occupational therapist to determine the patient's level of cognitive processing. A patient who paints a wooden box on the top and three sides, but does not turn the project to paint the back, the bottom, or the inside, is showing some important limitations in her ability to process information and apply it to task performance. This patient is only attending to what is immediately visible. Before she goes home, the therapist will be able to predict equivalent tasks that are likely to be problems for her there, such as personal grooming, keeping clothing clean, appropriate food preparation and storage, and many other aspects of home safety and maintenance. Because of task equivalence, recommendations for the level of assistance, supervision, and environmental adaptation needed for the best function and safety of the individual at home can be made more accurately. The usefulness of task equivalence, however, depends on the accuracy of the therapist's task analysis, using Allen's principles.

Function and Dysfunction

Allen gives the profession its best defined system for measuring the impact of cognitive dysfunction. Not only are there six levels, ranging from comatose (1) to highly functional (6), but there are 52 modes of performance in between. Modes are identified by the decimal points after the level. Scores on the ACLS are expressed as 3.0, 4.4, 5.8, etc. Each mode has implications that guide the occupational therapist in observing a progression of cognitive skills from one level to the next. A recent publication (Allen et al., 1995), "Understanding Cognitive Performance Modes," describes each mode from 1.4 to 6.0 with regard to expected cognitive abilities, functional goals, treatment methods, and safety. This text incorporates the most current research on cognition and provides excellent guidelines for accurate assessment, caregiver education, and discharge planning or placement. It requires some training and experience to learn to use the modes in assessment, treatment, and documentation.

For the purposes of students and therapists who are not previously familiar with cognitive disabilities theory, just identifying the low and high end of each level makes a good starting point for placing patients in groups. Table 6-3 outlines some simple behavioral observations that can be used to approximate the cognitive level for the purposes of group placement and initial activity selection. The level can then be confirmed by observation of task behaviors during the group itself.

The function-dysfunction continuum of cognitive abilities fluctuates in every individual, including those without a diagnosed disability. For this reason, treatment in the cognitive disabilities frame of reference cannot really be separated from ongoing evaluation. Treatment groups are primarily used, not so much for cognitive skill training, but as an opportunity for the patient and therapist to discover the optimal environmental conditions necessary for the patient to safely engage in purposeful activity. The patient's response to a group activity may be understood as one example of the way he will respond to similar activity situations outside the treatment environment. The observation of group behaviors, together with Allen's modes of performance, allows the occupational therapist to make reasonable predictions about the difficulties patients are likely to encounter in everyday activities. This information is invaluable to medical teams who must document the need for services, as well as to families who must take appropriate safety precautions and provide needed guidance. In this regard, Allen uses group treatment as an ongoing evaluation.

Allen has been concerned with competence, which legally means the ability to handle one's own affairs. There is no cutoff cognitive level for defining compe-

Table 6-3.
Quick Overview of the Allen Cognitive Modes

ACL	Common Behavioral Descriptions
1.0 - 1.4	Bedridden; stimulus/response of head
1.6 - 1.8	Sits with support; moves trunk/limbs; says "no"
2.0 - 2.4	Stands, righting actions, walks; names body parts, bed, toilet
2.6 - 2.8	Steps up/over; pushes/pulls; holds for support; sings; names target of action
3.0 - 3.4	Spontaneous grasp/release; repetitive actions; speaks in short phrases
3.6 - 3.8	Looks at effects of actions and follows cues to do the next step in self-care; understands waiting a minute, being done (finished with activity)
4.0 - 4.4	Independent in doing routine activities; identifies and sustains goals for 1 hour; speaks in sentences
4.6 - 4.8	Looks around and gets supplies; learns new procedure inflexibly; "Is this right?"—needs help now!
5.0 - 5.2	Discovers how to improve actions through overt trial and error; normal intonation and expression in speech; impulsive and poor judgment
5.6 - 5.8	Understands safety precautions; uses information gained by reading
6.0	Compares hypothetical plans, anticipates consequences

tence. Determination of competence or incompetence are generally based on the ability to make sound judgments and reasonable decisions about those activities that the individual intends to do.

Change and Motivation

Cognitive change occurs when the brain physiology or chemistry changes. We see an increase in cognitive level through activity when the brain recovers from acute illness, or the brain chemistry is affected by a change in activity level, hormones, diet, or medication. Using Allen's cognitive levels, the therapist verifies the presence or absence of a functional disability. If a patient's cognitive ability stabilizes below Level 6 ("normal"), the occupational therapist assists the patient and caregivers in making the necessary adjustments in daily living required by a residual cognitive disability. However, even when cognitive processes are irreversibly damaged by trauma or disease, Allen suggests that we can still produce changes in adaptive functioning by manipulating the

environment. Allen's updated writings and presentations acknowledge the importance of culture and context in motivating a patient to put forth her best effort. Offering a choice of craft projects, as well as including socialization in the selection of activities, helps to engage patients in group treatment. In doing a task, there are several factors to be manipulated. The task environment includes the placement and storage of materials, lighting, seating, facilities available, and assistance available. The task demand is the supplies, steps and instructions, and physical and cognitive abilities necessary to complete the task. Allen suggests that both the task environment and the task demand can be altered in ways that allow the patient to perform more independently within her cognitive level. In planning activities, therapists should give group members a "just right challenge," that is, the task should match but not exceed the members' capabilities. For example, Level 4 patients can reach their maximum adaptive functioning when presented with a three- or four-step task, setting out all the necessary materials within their visual field, demonstrating the instructions, and providing a completed sample for them to copy. Successful performance of a task that is perceived as socially positive will reinforce the patients' sense of well-being and increase motivation. Level 4 patients will be motivated to perform most self-care tasks at home with appropriate assistance and a suitable and safe environment.

Group Treatment

Treatment group membership in occupational therapy is based on cognitive level. Patients are treated in homogeneous groups of similar cognitive level. Level 2 is the lowest that can be treated effectively within a group. Level 3 is the lowest level at which group interaction can be expected. Earhart (Allen, 1985) suggests that in a large facility a variety of groups should be offered for Levels 2 through 6. Some patients will move up a level or two as their acute symptoms remit. Others will stabilize at a lower level and will require a variety of tasks within that level. Activities appropriate for each level are suggested. Table 6-4, which describes the cognitive abilities of patients at each of the six levels, can serve as a guide for planning activities. The table is based on an earlier chart by Allen, revised by Mary Brinson and Mary Ann Mayer.

Role of the Leader

The leader must be more directive in this approach than in most others. In a hospital setting, the focus is often on evaluation. The therapist typically chooses the activity or task, or limits choices. The occupational therapist must use expertise in activity analysis, controlling or adapting the environment, and instructing the group members in the procedures of the task. The therapist's role requires skill in assisting patients in acquiring and demon-

strating cognitive skills at increasing cognitive levels. The size of groups should not exceed eight members when led by one occupational therapist. However, when assisted by one or more COTAs, groups of up to 12 members can still be effective. One OTR assisted by one or more COTAs may be ideal in using the Allen approach, since skilled observations of task performance are necessary for ongoing assessment. The most significant factor in determining group size is the members' need for assistance. The lower the cognitive level, the more frequently members need assistance with the task. However, at Levels 4 and 5, verbal interaction consumes a larger portion of group time, and more individual attention is needed for social and emotional support. For higher cognitive levels, groups should be limited to eight members so that group leaders can facilitate group discussion to reinforce learning. Therefore, the occupational therapist needs to weigh several factors before deciding on the size of an Allen group.

Structures and Goals

Allen's goals for patients have to do with function and adaptation. Specific goals might be set to encourage a patient to progress to a higher level or to provide the ideal environmental support and assistance so that a patient can maximize function within a given cognitive level. Allen has designed several excellent evaluation tools and specified many behaviors that indicate progress toward higher cognitive levels.

The structure and goals for an Allen group are different for each level. For this reason, groups at each level will be discussed separately, with examples of appropriate activities.

Level 2 Groups

Movement activities are suggested to meet the needs of the Level 2 patients

Table 6-4.
Task Analysis for Cognitive Disabilities

	LEVEL 1: Automatic Actions	LEVEL 2: Postural Actions	LEVEL 3: Manual Actions
Setting	Reduce the number of stimuli when possible. Patients do not screen out external stimuli.	Open space. Patients enjoy planned gross motor actions.	Clutter free. Patients are engaged in doing simple tasks which have repetitive actions.
THE THERAPIST'S DIRECTIONS			
Demonstrations	Looks at demonstrated directions but does not imitate them.	The therapist may need to physically guide the action.	Patients will follow a demonstration of a familiar action on an object.
Verbalizations	Verbs, introjections.	Pronouns, names of body parts, simple verbs reinforce demonstration.	Names of material objects, repeated simple nouns and verbs.
Number of Directions	One action or direction, repeated	One action or direction, repeated	One action or direction, repeated
TASK SELECTION			
Structure of the Activity	Alerting stimuli. The most important tasks are eating and drinking.	Familiar, repetitive gross body movements.	An activity which has one step or one scheme repeated.
Choice and Sample Provided		The therapist plans movements and demonstrates actions. The therapist may respond to patient's suggestions or actions.	Activity is pre-planned by therapist. Choices limited to two or three material items/objects.
Tools	Stimulated use of body parts	Spontaneous use of body parts. Objects which are associated with gross body movements eg, softballs, jump ropes.	Hands: Some use of familiar tools.
Storage of Materials/ Projects	Taken care of by the therapist.	Taken care of by the therapist.	Taken care of by the therapist.
Preparation by the Therapist		Plan movements and obtain any needed equipment.	Supplies are laid out in advance. Do any preliminary or finishing steps which are not repetitive or familiar.

Copyright Mary Ann Mayer and Mary H. Brinson. Information gathered from Claudia Allen's 1988 ACL workshop at the Institute of Living, Hartford, Connecticut.

(Level 3 patients may also be included). Activities consist of imitation of gross body movement such as clapping, bending over to touch toes, and passing or tossing a large, soft ball. Simple movement games such as bean bag toss or foam basketball may be useful, although Level 2 patients are apt to disregard directionality. Setting limits in Level 2 groups may be difficult because disruptive behaviors of

Table 6-4. (continued)
Task Analysis for Cognitive Disabilities

	LEVEL 4: Goal-directed Actions	LEVEL 5: Exploratory Actions	LEVEL 6: Planned Actions
Setting	Other patients working on the same task, a shared goal. Setting conducive to production of immediate end product.	Clutter can be present, and others performing variations on similar tasks. Setting fosters exploration, trial and error.	Free access to materials and supplies to stimulate covert problem-solving, sharing of plans with others.
THE THERAPIST'S DIRECTIONS			
Demonstrations	Patients will imitate single steps in a series and moderately novel actions which expand familiar schemes.	Patients can learn through serial imitation, so a number of steps may be demonstrated. Unfamiliar steps assimiliated.	Not required. Patients learn through serial imitations so directions may be retained.
Verbalizations	Simple adjectives, adverbs nouns and verbs; avoiding open-ended questions or discussions.	Adjectives and prepositions may be used in explaining variations.	Conjunctions, conjectures, images.
Number of Directions	One step at a time.	Several steps at a time.	Unlimited. Images, diagrams, written directions may be followed.
TASK SELECTION			
Structure of the Activity	Simple quick tasks with a tangible end product. Avoid childish connotations.	An activity which permits variation, and which allows results to be easily seen and corrected.	An activity which permits variation in the selection and planning of steps.
Choice and Sample Provided	Avoid confusion by limiting the decisions and materials. The opportunity for exact replication of a sample is present.	Several choices in materials, tools and activity selection. Demonstrate and clarify tangible possibilities.	Several choices in materials, tools, and activity selection. Discuss the hypothetical possibilities.
Tools	Hand tools limited to familiar objects. No power tools.	Simple tools which are a linear extension of the hand and arm.	Patients learn how to use unfamiliar machines and tools.
Storage of Materials/Projects	Patients will place and/or find supplies when clearly visible or very familiar.	The patient will search for things in probable locations and can place/find things in labeled drawers or cabinets.	The patient will follow verbal directions to place or find materials
Preparation by the Therapist	Supplies are laid out in advance. Provide an exact sample of the end product. Do those steps which require unfamiliar tools or schemes.	The sample of the finished product need not be exact. Patterns and procedures are supplied by the therapist.	Materials, designs, and/or pictures are provided to assist covert problem-solving.

Level 2 or 3 patients are oblivious to verbal direction (but often responsive to demonstrated direction). Movement at this level provides a pleasurable sensory experience, as well as needed stimulation and exercise. However, motor skill is likely to be limited. See Activity Example 6-1 for a sample activity for Level 2 patients.

Level 3 Groups

The guiding principles in choosing appropriate activities for Level 3 are repetition and manipulation. Persons at this cognitive level are not goal directed. The process must interest them in order for them to be drawn to participate in an activity. Therapists should think of activities that focus on these attributes as strengths.

Many of our daily activities have the attributes of manipulation and repetition. Washing the dishes, sewing a button, clipping fingernails, and eating a bowl of cereal are examples. It is timing, knowing when to begin and when to end, that is difficult for Level 3 patients. For example, in doing a woodworking project, Level 3 patients may keep on sanding long after the wood is smooth. They will apply much more glue than is necessary. They will string beads until they get to the end or all the beads are used up. They may place tiles in a row along the edge of a frame, without regard for color or spacing. The therapist must be responsible for structuring the activity into steps and keeping track of time to move the group along.

The ADM identifies a variety of craft projects that are appropriate for Level 3 groups. Some of them are tile trivets, ribbon mugs, sticker cards, canvas placemats, bargello bookmarks, whale note holders, and recessed tile boxes. (All of these projects have standardized materials which are available from S&S Healthcare, and a free catalog may be obtained by calling them at 1-800-243-9232.) Standardized

materials are desirable to increase reliability of the therapist's observations in assessing the mode of performance within each cognitive level. The ADM is recommended for groups in acute care or other settings where the accuracy of assessment is important in planning for discharge.

However, in chronic care settings, such as group homes or skilled nursing facilities where functional maintenance programs are needed, more interactive group activities can be planned using Allen's guidelines. When selecting activities for Level 3 groups, repetition and manipulation should be the guiding principles. For example, one therapist who works with Level 3 dementia patients may have them make long chains with yarn and crochet hooks and attach balloons to decorate for a party, or string popcorn and cranberries for a Christmas tree. An occupational therapy aide or recreation aide may be taught to use Allen principles in executing such activities.

The timing of a Level 3 group should not exceed 30 minutes, as that is the limit of their attention according to Allen. Many work tasks are ideal for Level 3, for example, stuffing envelopes, attaching labels and stamps, or collating multiple-page documents. Such tasks have successfully been assigned to sheltered workshops. The workshop might be contracted to assemble packets of plastic utensils, napkins, salt, pepper, sugar, and powdered creamer in plastic bags for serving meals on the airlines. In a hospital or day treatment setting, a Level 3 group might be assigned the task of copying and distributing an in-house newsletter or invitations to an event. Again, the principles of repetition and manipulation should guide selection of appropriate work tasks. All materials should be within arm's reach for each Level 3 participant, and the task should be structured so that one step at a time can be performed repeatedly.

Activity Examples

Two examples of activities are included here. First, the "Recessed Tile Box," a standardized craft activity selected from the ADM (1993) is described in Activity Example 6-2. Although this craft is also used to assess Level 4 patients, only instructions for Level 3 have been given here. An ADM craft activity should be used for groups when assessment of the level and mode of functioning is desired. Activity Example 6-3 is an interactive skill maintenance activity called "Summer Salad," which uses the same Allen Level 3 principles, but is not set up as a standardized assessment.

Level 4 Groups

At Level 4, activities are goal directed. Sequences of steps toward a goal are now possible. Having a goal in mind represents an important step toward problem-solving. However, attention is still limited, and group activities should not be planned to last for more than 1 hour. Projects are either completed in one session, or separate steps may be done in two sessions. For example, the wooden tile trivet may be sanded and painted in the first session, and tiles selected and glued in a second session.

Craft projects are ideal experiments in problem-solving. A woodworking kit with three pieces, such as a napkin holder, can be structured into a simple sequence: sanding, painting, and gluing. A finished sample must be available to represent the goal. This takes advantage of Level 4's tendency to attend to visual cues. Some ADM crafts suggested for Level 4 are tile trivets, Indian key fobs, ribbon cards, hug-a-bear, and various bear clothes. Many other crafts may be structured in a more group interactive way, using similar Allen Level 4 principles of goal orientation, several-step sequences, and visually stimulating colors and contrasts.

The environment is of special concern to Level 4 groups because their usable task environment now extends beyond arm's reach to the entire visual field. Items necessary for the task to be accomplished should now be placed in plain view. But more importantly, all irrelevant items should be placed out of sight or they will cause major distraction. If a work room is small, lacking in storage space, and/or has multiple uses, getting rid of visual "clutter" is easier said than done. Considerable preparation time must be spent setting up the room before a Level 4 group begins. Likewise, the storage of objects is guided by the principle of visibility. What cannot be seen, for all intents and purposes, does not exist. Once this is understood by the therapist, it is clear what must be done. Level 4 patients will not go searching in cabinets and drawers. The same principle holds true for the home environment.

Assistance needed at Level 4 will be with processes that are not visible, such as the drying of paint or the changing of color or glaze as it dries. Although many food preparation tasks are ideal for this level, processes that involve heating or cooling are not understood or considered. Verbal direction alone is not enough when giving instructions for a task; demonstration should accompany verbal instruction. Written instruction is not at all useful, but sometimes pictures or diagrams can assist the patient in progressing through the steps of a task that is familiar. Patients at Level 4 have a tendency to come to the end of a step, and then ask "What do I do now?" They know there is a goal they are working on, a completed project or a meal on the table, but they are not sure how to get there. Probing or asking leading questions can encourage the patient to think about the sequence and use available cues, such as the sample or the work of other members, to learn to problem solve at a higher level. If the task is too difficult, or the patient's cognitive abilities are lower than what is required, the therapist may need to "rescue" by correcting an error or completing a step for the patient. The information gathered from patient-therapist interactions is then used for selecting a more appropriate activity for the next session. Activity Example 6-4 is an activity for Level 4 patients.

Level 5 Groups

At this level, the focus is on safety. The difficulties requiring treatment usually involve impulsivity and a lack of planning or anticipation. For this reason, Level 5 patients are introduced to more complex tasks in groups. Some activities suggested are clay and mosaics, cooking, and advanced crafts. While one-step, demonstrated directions are not necessary, the safe use of tools and procedures must still be demonstrated at Level 5. Several steps can be taught at one time, and patients are capable of selecting projects and varying colors and designs. Planning is involved and projects may continue for more than one session. The occupational therapist still needs to monitor safety and check understanding of directions, especially with regard to the intangible variables of time and temperature.

The ADM includes the following activities for Level 5: sewing Raggedy Ann and Andy dolls and doll clothes, constructing and stenciling of multiple piece woodworking projects, and an assortment of projects using stenciled designs or iron-on decals. The cautious use of hot irons, power tools, ovens, or hot plates under supervision is suggested so that the occupational therapist might observe the patient's knowledge and use of caution when handling these items. Group projects involving cooking, grilling outdoors, or participating in recreational activities such as hiking, swimming, boating, or fishing can also be used therapeutically to learn and evaluate safety in Level 5 groups. A craft for Level 5 patients is detailed in Activity Example 6-5.

Persons functioning at Allen's Level 6 may be placed in craft groups for assessment purposes, or included in Level 5 groups if possible decline is suspected.

Group Leadership

Introduction

Names are mentioned around the table for acknowledgment, and the therapist introduces herself. The leader explains the purpose of the project in concrete terms. Each member has materials for the activity set up at his place in advance. The purpose of the group is different from its goals. Because each member's mode of functioning is different, the goals for each member are individual. However, the goal of the group is to provide a practical example in problem-solving, which serves as both practice for the members and ongoing assessment for the therapist.

The purpose should be stated so as to elicit each member's best effort. The therapist should use concrete terms in explaining the purpose, the structure, and the procedure, in language known to be understood by the members at their cognitive level. Projects are to be kept by the patients once completed. The usefulness and desirability of the project should be emphasized, and this can be individualized. Social recognition is an important component when motivating patients to select and begin to work on a project. For example, the tile box may be a gift for someone special, so "you should do your best to make it look nice." Timing is mentioned for Level 4 and higher, and it should be stressed that anyone needing assistance may signal the therapist at any time during the group.

Activity

The structure of groups described by Allen resembles Mosey's "Project Groups" (see Appendix A). Interaction occurs mainly between therapist and each member. Doing the activity really takes the entire session. Demonstration will be given according to the cognitive level, and the project sample can be referred to as the goal. Even for those not yet goal oriented (Level 3s), the sample is an important learning tool to use for error recognition and correction, imitation, and encouragement of higher level thinking. Cleaning up, as appropriate to the task, may take up the last 5 or 10 minutes of the session.

Sharing

No formal sharing takes place in Allen groups. However, informal comments about the projects of others by group members can provide needed social recognition for members.

Processing

A brief discussion at the end may focus on processing. Persons at all levels should have an opportunity to express their feelings about doing the task. The concrete end product is usually the focus of this discussion. Leaders should be careful not to give false praise, but limit comments to appropriate, reality-based feedback.

Generalization

Generalization by patients is really not possible until Level 5. For lower levels, therapist comments reflecting the purpose and the goal can be made when appropriate. Level 5 groups should be encouraged to find meaning in the activity at hand, and appropriate discussion questions by the leader will elicit this response.

Application

Applying new learning to everyday life can be reviewed at the end of the session. The therapist is directive in individualizing application. However, no individual feedback is given during the session regarding problem behaviors. The occupational therapist may choose to give feedback to patients individually after having an opportunity to score the activity (using ADM worksheets), or to determine the most useful response to specific situations.

At Level 5, application focuses on task equivalence and discussion of safety issues in the home or work environment. The use of peer discussion may help group members to accept critical feedback or the need for change.

Summary

The therapist ends with instructions about the project itself; it may be taken (if completed) or it may be picked up later (e.g., after paint is dry). Names on projects should be dealt with if projects are to be left. More interpersonal issues are mentioned as the level of the group increases.

Bibliography

Allen, C. K. (1982). Independence through activity: The practice of occupational therapy (psychiatry). *American Journal of Occupational Therapy, 36,* 731-739.

Allen, C. K. (1985). *Occupational therapy for psychiatric diseases: Measurement and management of cognitive disabilities.* Boston: Little, Brown & Co.

Allen, C. K. (1987a). Eleanor Clarke Slagle lectureship—1987: Activity, occupational therapy's treatment method. *American Journal of Occupational Therapy, 41,* 563-575.

Allen, C. K. (1987b). Measuring the severity of mental disorders. *Hospital & Community Psychiatry, 38,* 140-142.

Allen, C. K. (1988). Cognitive disabilities. In S. C. Robertson (Ed.), *Focus: Skills for assessment and treatment.* Rockville, MD: American Occupational Therapy Association.

Allen, C. K. (1991). Cognitive disability and reimbursement for rehabilitation and psychiatry.

Journal of Insurance Medicine, 23, 245-247.

Allen, C. K. (1994). Creating a need-satisfying, safe environment: Management and maintenance approaches. In C. B. Royeen (Ed.), *AOTA Self-Study Series: Cognitive Rehabilitation.* Rockville, MD: American Occupational Therapy Association.

Allen, C. K. (1997). Cognitive disabilities: How to make clinical judgments. In N. Katz (Ed.), *Cognitive Rehabilitation: Models for Intervention in Occupational Therapy.* Rockville, MD: American Occupational Therapy Association.

Allen, C. K., & Allen, R. (1987). Cognitive disabilities: Measuring the social consequences of mental disorders. *Journal of Clinical Psychiatry, 48*(5),185-190.

Allen, C. K., Blue, T., & Earhart, C. A. (1995). *Understanding cognitive performance modes.* Ormond Beach, FL: Allen Conferences, Inc.

Allen, C. K., & Earhart, C. A. (1992). *Occupational therapy treatment goals for the physically and cognitively disabled.* Rockville, MD: American Occupational Therapy Association.

David, S. (1988). Allen cognitive level and sensorimotor treatment in acute care. *Sensory Integration SIS Newsletter, 11*(1), 1-3.

Earhart, C. A., Allen, C. K., & Blue, T. (1993). *Allen diagnostic module instruction manual.* Colchester, CT: S&S Worldwide.

Heinmann, N. E., Allen, C. K., & Yerxa, E. J. (1989). The routine task inventory: A tool for describing the functional behavior of the cognitively disabled. *Occupational Therapy Practice, 1,* 67-74.

Josman, N., & Katz, N. (1991). Problem-solving version of the Allen Cognitive Level (ACL) test. *American Journal of Occupational Therapy, 45,* 331-338.

Kehrberg, K. *Large Allen cognitive level test manual* (with kit included). Colchester, CT: S&S Worldwide.

Levy, L. L. (1997). The use of the cognitive disability frame of reference in rehabilitation of cognitively disabled older adults. In N. Katz (Ed.), *Cognitive Rehabilitation: Models for Intervention in Occupational Therapy.* Rockville, MD: American Occupational Therapy Association.

World Health Organization. (1980). *International classification of impairments, disabilities, and handicaps.* Geneva, Switzerland: Author.

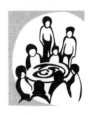

Materials: 12-foot-long piece of white nylon rope, 1-inch thick, with ends tied in a over-hand knot; and a cassette player with instrumental music in a variety of rhythms (e.g., John Philip Sousa marches, Strauss waltzes, the overture from "The King & I").

Participants: Six maximum.

Directions: Start the music to alert members and get their attention. Therapist stands inside the rope circle and motions members to come toward her. Therapist greets each member and places each member's hand or elbow around the rope, approximately 2 feet apart. Begin by walking in a circle to the right, marching to the rhythm of the music. Turn to face the rope and hold with both hands or elbows. Therapist leads group in raising rope up high, then down low, to the rhythm of the music. Group imitates the therapist in doing a variety of in/out motions with arms and legs, while holding the rope. Have members take turns ducking under the rope and standing inside the circle. Two members can hold the rope bending over so that rope is 1 foot high, while therapist leads other members in stepping over it. Teams of three then take each end and pull each other back and forth slowly, changing their force when pulled or pushed gently by the therapist. Action ceases when the music ends (approximately 20 minutes). Therapist says "good-bye" to each member by shaking hands, saluting, or other gesture of recognition and farewell.

No verbalizations are needed to direct this group. However, proprioceptive cues are used as needed to direct the actions of the group and to recapture attention of straying members.

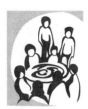
Materials: Box with lid, 3/8-inch tiles, two colors separated into bins, sandpaper, brown wood stain, brush, rag, glue, and one completed sample for every two patients (checkerboard pattern in two contrasting colors). See Figures 6-3a and 6-3b. Access to a sink and water for clean-up is preferred. Glue bottles should be opened, and stain uncovered and stirred.

Participants: Six to eight members. Seat persons at table, each with individual set of supplies. Figures 6-3c and 6-3d depict the standardized set-up for evaluation.

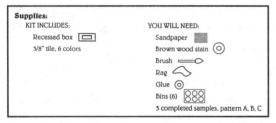

Figure 6-3a. Key for supplies needed. Copyright Claudia Allen, Allen Diagnostic Module. Reprinted with permission.

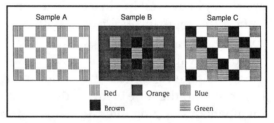

Figure 6-3b. Sample designs. Copyright Claudia Allen, Allen Diagnostic Module. Reprinted with permission.

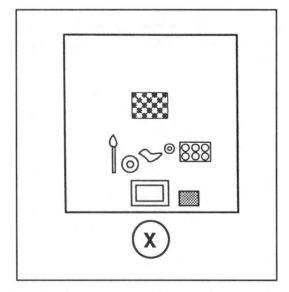

Figure 6-3c. Supplies set-up for each individual. Copyright Claudia Allen, Allen Diagnostic Module. Reprinted with permission.

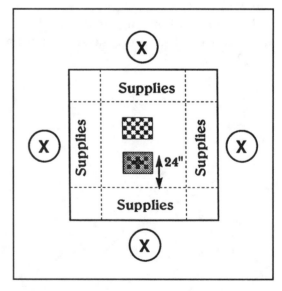

Figure 6-3d. Table set-up for four individuals. Copyright Claudia Allen, Allen Diagnostic Module. Reprinted with permission.

Recessed Tile Box (Levels 3 and 4) (continued)

Timing: Introduction and purpose—5 minutes

Sanding, staining, and gluing tiles—20 to 30 minutes

Processing and summary—5 minutes (does not include clean-up)

Since the maximum attention span for Level 3 is 30 minutes, progress must be monitored and timing adjusted accordingly. If more than half the group has not finished staining at the end of 15 minutes, it is recommended that gluing the tiles be done in a second session.

Directions: Introduce group and explain purpose of the activity. Instructions are taken from the ADM (1993, pp. B2-5). "This is a tiled box which can be used to store jewelry, medicine, change, or other small items. All the supplies needed to complete it are in front of you. In order for me to see how you are doing today, it is important for you to try to make your box look as much like...the sample as possible."

Provide steps as indicated below as needed. Observe performance, provide appropriate prompts or assistance, and rate behavior for each step (see rating criteria) (p. B3). Move to the next step when the last one has been abandoned, or when a person says "I'm done" or requests next step.

Step 1: Sanding—"The first step is to sand the wood on all sides until it is smooth." Pick up sandpaper and demonstrate sanding with the grain and feeling for smoothness.

Step 2: Staining—"This is stain. It may need to be stirred. It is painted on with the brush and then wiped off with the rag like this." Demonstrate painting and wiping one side. "Do all the sides."

Step 3: Gluing tiles—"The tiles are glued on in rows like this." Demonstrate placing glue on the back of a red tile and placing it in the corner of recess in lid. Repeat with a white tile along short side. Space the tile but do not comment on this. "Try to make a pattern like...this sample" (p. B3). Critical observations of each member's sanding, staining, wiping, gluing, and placing tiles are given, and rating is done by the therapist to assess the mode of functioning for each member according to the rating criteria. The critical observations for sanding are feeling/looking for smoothness, altering pressure and direction, turning box to access all surfaces, altering the shape of the sandpaper, and noting effects.

Rating Criteria: The ADM specifies detailed rating criteria for each step: sanding, staining, and gluing tiles. Table 6-5 shows behaviors expected at each cognitive mode (3.0 through 4.8) for the first step (sanding). Refer to Allen (1993) for ADM criteria for this and other steps of the craft.

	Table 6-5. Sanding
3.0	Reaches for and grasps object; holds, feels, may name object
3.2	Sands randomly; may not look at box while working; stops and starts on command; may comment with short phrases
3.4	May begin before instructions given, fail to stop when asked; actions sustained 1 minute or longer, may change suddenly; looks at object inconsistently, does not note effects
3.6	Begins before instructions are given, stops when told; copies demonstration one step at a time; notes effects, moves location; may miss all/part of visible surface
3.8	Stops between steps after visible surfaces are sanded and says "I'm done"; sands all visible surfaces but misses inside surfaces
4.0	Does not spontaneously refer to sample within 24"; sands all large visible surfaces; may miss or refuse to sand small or hidden surfaces
4.2	Refers to sample when only cued; may miss hidden surfaces or ask if inside/bottom should be done
4.4	Refers to and compares work to sample; may ask for verification before going on to next step; bends over box to reach back, still misses small edges
4.6	Scans environment to locate sample or supplies in plain sight; varies pressure/force/duration for better effects; may attempt to fold/tear sandpaper to do inside of box
4.8	Rotates/examines all surfaces after sanding is completed; may not note grain of wood; may ask for help for best way to access small edges

Processing and Summary: A brief discussion about how members liked the activity follows. All generalizations must be done by the therapist. Members may be asked questions about possible uses for their box—a gift, to keep jewelry, to store coins, etc. In summarizing, feedback from the therapist about the strengths of each member in following directions, responding to cues, and general workmanship is often helpful and appreciated, and ends the session on a positive note.

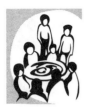

Cognitive Disabilities
Activity Example 6-3
Summer Salad (Level 3)

This Level 3 group activity represents a functional maintenance activity that uses the same Allen guidelines as the standardized craft previously described, but is more interactive. Up to eight members whose functioning has stabilized at Allen's Level 3 may be placed in groups like this, which are designed by an OTR or COTA using the principles of repetition and manipulation. Other staff members may be instructed by the OTR or COTA in leading these groups. The activity should not exceed 30 minutes, and sharing of tools and materials should not be required at this level.

Materials: One serrated plastic knife, one heavy plastic fork, and one cutting board or thick paper plate for each member. One big bowl in the center of the table is filled with as many pieces of fruit as there are members. Good choices are apples, pears, bananas, oranges, peaches, cantaloupe halves (wrapped in plastic), and pineapple slices (wrapped in plastic).

Participants: Six to eight members are ideal, with a co-therapist. Members should wash their hands before starting this group.

Directions: The therapist explains that the group will make a delicious fruit salad. The ground rules are that no one eats anything until all the fruit is cut, put back in the bowl, and mixed with a coconut and yogurt dressing. Each member introduces self and selects a piece of fruit from the bowl. Covering eyes and identifying fruit by touch may be an interesting variation. Members should be reminded not to eat the fruit, but to wait for a therapist to demonstrate to each member how their specific fruit should be prepared and cut into bite-size pieces. Approximately 15 minutes are spent cutting and trimming. A plastic-lined trashcan is passed around to throw away cores, pits, and peels with the help of the therapist. A volunteer mixes one pint of plain yogurt, one scoop of brown sugar, and half a cup of coconut flakes. Other volunteers take turns stirring the dressing into the fruit. Other volunteers scoop the fruit salad into bowls and pass them out to the members. Eating the fruit is a well-deserved reward for all their hard work.

*From Cole, M. B. *Group Dynamics in Occupational Therapy, Second Edition.* © 1998 SLACK Incorporated.*

201

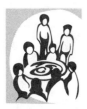

Cognitive Disabilities
Activity Example 6-4
Falling Leaves (Level 4)

This is a basic craft group for Level 4 patients. It is a group project following the guidelines of goal orientation, visual cues (colors and shapes), and short sequences of steps, in this case, leading to a common end product.

Materials: The table is set up by the therapist for six to 10 patients. Half of the patients have a sheet of colored paper, a pencil, a pair of paper scissors, and a cardboard pattern of a leaf. Leaf shapes used are maple, elm, oak, ash, tulip, and birch. Real leaves can be traced to produce these patterns, however, this is done by the therapist. The other half of the patients have a piece of white posterboard with a tree trunk and branches traced in black magic marker and the name of the tree outlined in black. Chunky capital letters are best, saying OAK, MAPLE, etc. with the centers to be colored in. Patients with the tree trunks also have two wide-tip markers, brown or gray and another color, and a small bottle of glue.

Directions: The therapist should demonstrate the processes.
1. Leaves. Place the leaf pattern on the colored paper and trace around it with the pencil. Fit as many as you can on the paper without overlapping any lines. When finished cut out each leaf along the lines you have traced.
2. Tree trunks. Color in the tree trunk with the appropriate color. Then color in the letters with another color. When finished, glue the appropriate leaves on the tree branches. Patients may work in pairs, so that maple leaves are glued to the maple tree trunk, etc. Colors of the leaves should be appropriate for autumn. For variation, two autumn shades may be used for each leaf to create a more interesting pattern.

Processing and Summary: Feelings about the craft activity and its end result are then elicited. Generalization discussion will center around the autumn season, what happens in the fall, and what kinds of tasks must be done to prepare for the autumn/winter season. Application can concretely be interpreted in discussing where to display the posters, and what other decorations might be desired. Therapist feedback may be given in summary. The tree posters make a good decoration for the ward.

From Cole, M. B. *Group Dynamics in Occupational Therapy, Second Edition.* © 1998 SLACK Incorporated.

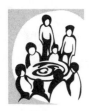

Cognitive Disabilities
Activity Example 6-5
Straw Hats with Potpourri (Level 5)

This is an appropriate activity for spring, and utilizes the strengths of Level 5, trial and error exploration in creating a pleasing result with the materials provided, utilizing more than one sensory system (visual and olfactory). It also includes a safety check, as members are supervised in the use of the hot glue gun and advised of the need for caution as needed.

Materials: 6-inch straw hats for each member, four rolls of thin satin ribbon (one each in pink, baby blue, red, and white), a variety of 1/2-inch silk flowers (daisies, roses, etc.), scissors, a glue gun with glue sticks, bags of potpourri in floral and herbal scents, nylon netting, spool of thread, and several colorful samples of finished hats.

Timing: Introduction—5 minutes
 Activity—30 minutes
 Processing/summary—20 minutes
 Clean-up—5 minutes

Directions: The leader introduces members, and explains the project and its purpose. It could be a door decoration, a gift, or a preparation for the Easter holiday. Doing the craft will be a way to monitor the skill level of members and to observe how they deal with limited choices, verbal instructions, and safety precautions. The goal is for each member to design and decorate one straw hat.
 Step 1: Potpourri—Cut a circle of nylon netting about 6 inches in diameter. Fill this with enough poupouri to fill the interior portion of the straw hat. Gather in the edges of the netting and tie it with a piece of string. Set this aside to be glued in later.
 Step 2: Decoration—Choose ribbons to tie around the center portion of the hat. Ribbons may be tied with bows or knotted with streamers hanging down. Each member may choose two to four flowers to glue around the ribbon cluster. One piece of ribbon should be cut about 10 inches long, with the ends tied in an overhand knot to serve as a hanger.
 Step 3: Gluing—The therapist should have the glue gun plugged in and heated to the correct temperature. A separated area with a fireproof surface and nothing flammable nearby should be maintained for gluing. Members can approach the gluing area several times during the session. First the ribbons should be stabilized with a blob of glue right under the bow or knot. Next, the silk flowers are attached with glue. The nylon packet of potpurri is glued with the "tail" tucked inside the hat. Finally, the ribbon hanger loop is glued on the back, so that the hat may be hung from a hook on the door or wall.

Discussion and Summary: Feelings about the craft are elicited, followed by generalization of what other spring tasks around the house have similar attributes (i.e., getting out spring clothes, fixing up the house, making it smell nice). Discussing the use of the glue gun may be a good lead-in for reinforcing safety precautions around their homes. Other tasks involving heat and electricity (e.g., cooking, ironing, or using hair dryers, curling irons, or electric razors) should be discussed with each individual member with regard to safety. The straw hat activity may also trigger discussion of planning ahead for spring, the importance of spring cleaning, storage of winter clothes, care of lawns and gardens, or other tasks requiring anticipation, a typical problem area for Level 5. Summary should include feedback from the therapist. Hats are kept by the members to use however they like.

Chapter 7

A Developmental Approach

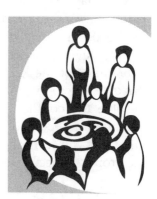

This chapter focuses on developmental theory as it applies to adults. Although some of the theorists deal primarily with children, it is assumed that disease and injury interfere with development in ways that affect them as adults. The guiding principle of all developmental theories is that there is a developmental sequence from birth to maturity and throughout life to death. This sequence is determined by both biological and environmental forces. This development occurs in stages, which are specific, progressive, and hierarchical. Development is divided into stages for the benefit of our understanding. In reality, the transition from one stage to the next is gradual. Each stage, however, is subdivided into specific skills, issues, or conflicts and each has characteristics that distinguish it from other stages.

Progressive stages refer to the idea that each stage increases in complexity and represents, in some way, progress toward maturity. It is assumed that maturity is the highest stage, and therefore the goal. Maturity is seen in both an individual and a social context. In other words, the goal of maturity may be the survival and success of the individual, but maturity also involves cooperation with others and the survival and flourishing of humanity. Hierarchical stages mean that each stage builds on the next. It reinforces the idea that there are foundation skills upon which higher level skills are built. According to developmental theory, skills that are deficient must be learned in the same sequence in which they normally develop. This idea seems common to all the theorists reviewed here.

Focus

The developmental frame of reference is best used as a guidepost by which to measure the effects of illness, and thereby set realistic goals for recovery. Age is never a true measure of development. However, by viewing persons with disability through the perspective of developmental stages, discrepancies between developmental and chronological age can help the therapist to appreciate the true impact of disability on a person's life.

Most developmental theories define points of change, crises, or conflicts to be resolved before the person moves up to the next stage or level. These points of stress may be instrumental in bringing about the onset or exacerbation of illness. If the occupational therapist pays attention to developmental theory, she can take advantage of the knowledge that specific tasks need to be mastered, in order to resolve the conflicts or crises which are really normal parts of development. These life tasks can form the basis for therapeutic groups in occupational therapy.

Basic Assumptions

There are many different theories of human development, some ending with adolescence (Freud) and others continuing right through old age (Erikson, Jung). Those discussed here are chosen because they help clarify our thinking about occupational therapy groups. Included are Jung, Erikson, Levinson, Kohlberg and Wilcox, and Gilligan. Some of the theories of physiological and cognitive development, such as Ayres and Piaget, have been eliminated here and are covered instead in the next chapter on the sensory motor frames of reference.

Jung

Jung, who wrote in the 1940s and 1950s, might be considered the father of adult developmental theory. He differed from Freud in extending the developmental process throughout life, and acknowledging the contribution of external factors to growth and adaptation. Jung divided life into four basic stages:
1. Childhood
2. Youth
3. Mid-life
4. Old age

In Jung's view, childhood is spent in blissful ignorance. Although influenced by many inherited predispositions, children develop with no doubts, unaware of their own growth processes. Youth is marked by the onset of consciousness, of doubts, problems, contradictions, and responsibilities. Jung described the second half of life as beginning between ages 35 and 40, when the essential character of life changes and energy becomes rechanneled. Before age 40, the individual has put his energy into external events such as establishing occupation, community position, marriage, and family. After age 40, Jung believes the individual turns inward, focusing more on the spiritual (Schultz, 1976).

Middle age is described by Jung as the "afternoon of life." Polarities are opposite tendencies of the self present in an individual, such as introversion vs. extroversion, rationality vs. intuitiveness, aggressiveness vs. sensitivity, and action vs. contemplation. At mid-life, Jung contends that whatever sides of the self were expressed in the person's youth, the opposite sides will prevail in mid-life. It was Jung who identified individuation as the true goal of life, a concept much in question in the 1980s. Individuation is a kind of enhancement of identity which involves further definition of the self it continues through each of the stages in greater depths and in different ways. The end result of individuation was thought to be integration, a uniting of all parts of the self into a qualified whole.

Old age is the final stage. As a person ages he faces physical decline, removes himself from positions of authority and responsibility, and faces the inevitability of his own death. Jung assumed a belief in the presence of an afterlife, and began the idea that all individuals ultimately contribute to a "collective unconscious," and so live on through others (Table 7-1).

Table 7-1.
Jung's Stages of Development (Spiritual)

Age	Stage
Birth to Puberty (Childhood)	Blissful ignorance, inherited predispositions
Puberty to Age 35 (Youth)	Conscious and doubting, taking on responsibility
Age 35 to old age (Midlife)	Change in direction to express latent parts of self individuation and integration
Infirmity and Death (Old Age)	Infirmity, acceptance of death, afterlife and collective unconscious

Table 7-2.
Erikson's Eight Stages of Development (Psychosocial)

Age	Stage
Birth - Infancy	Trust vs. Mistrust
2-4 Toddlerhood	Autonomy vs. Shame and Doubt
5-7 Early childhood	Initiative vs. Guilt
8-12 Middle child	Industry vs. Inferiority
13-22 Adolescence	Identity vs. Role Confusion
23-35 Young Adult	Intimacy vs. Isolation
35-50 Adulthood	Generativity vs. Stagnation
50-Death	Integrity vs. Despair

Erikson

Erikson also built on Freud's psychosexual stages, and extended his theory to include adolescence and adulthood. His ideas are compatible with Jung's, but more social in nature and based on the central issues of each stage as conflicts to be resolved. The stages which most impact our adult patient groups are:

- Identity vs. role confusion (ages 13 to 22)
- Intimacy vs. isolation (ages 23 to 35)
- Generativity vs. stagnation (ages 35 to 50)
- Integrity vs. despair (ages 50 to death)

Erikson's stages are well-known and referred to often in occupational therapy literature. The conflict areas can guide our choice of activities in occupational therapy and can serve as a basis for setting goals at the various age levels. For example, trust issues can be worked on through movement activities, such as "falling" and "being caught," or through verbal activities, such as giving and receiving emotional support (Table 7-2).

Levinson

Levinson (1978) has published the most extensive (although admittedly controversial) research study to date on the developmental stages of adulthood. He based his findings on a longevity study of 40

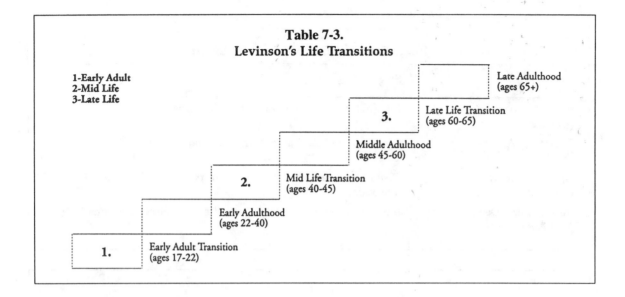

Table 7-3.
Levinson's Life Transitions

1-Early Adult
2-Mid Life
3-Late Life

Late Adulthood
(ages 65+)

3. Late Life Transition
(ages 60-65)

Middle Adulthood
(ages 45-60)

2. Mid Life Transition
(ages 40-45)

Early Adulthood
(ages 22-40)

1. Early Adult Transition
(ages 17-22)

men. Levinson presents adulthood as periods of stability alternating with periods of transition. The three life transitions he identifies are:

1. Early adult (ages 17 to 22)
2. Mid-life (ages 40 to 45)
3. Late life (age 60 to 65)

These periods of conflict are interspersed with periods of relative stability in which the individual lives within an established life structure and stays more or less on course (Table 7-3).

Levinson contends that each transition period occurs during specific age ranges and each transition has its own developmental tasks. Like Erikson, he saw each transition as requiring the resolution of conflicts before the person can move on to the next stage.

Primarily the tasks of each transition period are to re-evaluate the existing life structure, explore the possibilities of change, and make choices that will restructure life in the next era. Eras are in between stages of stability described as young, middle, and late adulthood. In the Levinson study of 40 men, work was considered to be a "base for life in society" giving the man his life structure in a cultural, class,

and social sense as well as occupational (Levinson, 1978, p. 9). Since the thrust of the study was to examine the mid-life transition, subjects selected were age 35, from four different occupational groups, and were followed to age 45. Biographical information collected from these subjects forms the basis of the young adult transition. The late adult transition is only briefly covered by Levinson and is considered to parallel the preceding transition.

Levinson's theory has been selected for focus because it presents a good structure around which to understand life problems of patients and to plan occupational therapy groups.

The Early Adult Transition

The essence of this transition is the separation from the family of origin in order to establish a new home base. The separation is both geographical and emotional, and generally creates a sense of loss, yet the excitement involved in establishing oneself in the adult world provides a sense of satisfaction. Exploration in the early adult transition quickly pushes toward commitment as the young man is required to take on adult responsibilities. Balancing exploration with the need for structure is an ongoing struggle. The major tasks of the early adult transition are: forming the dream, finding a mentor, forming an occupation, and starting a marriage and family.

Forming the Dream

The first task which plays a powerful role in early adulthood is called forming a dream. Levinson states that the dream emerges during the early adult transition where the boy/man imagines himself settled in the adult world. This may be connected with concrete reality or far removed from his actual world. The ability to play make believe in early childhood is the forerunner of this imagining in early adulthood. The dream is a vehicle for exploring his image, and "provides a source of hope, self-esteem, and personal integrity" (1978, p. 93). The young adult's task includes forming relationships with others who can facilitate his work on the dream and find ways of living it out in his life. If the dream is unconnected with choices made in this stage, it will resurface during the mid-life transition and demand a place for self-expression then.

The Mentor Relationship

According to Levinson, the mentor relationship is very complex and extremely significant for a man during early adulthood. The mentor is a transitional figure in a person's life, serving as a teacher, sponsor, guide, and adviser. The most important function of the mentor is "to support and facilitate the realization of the dream" (1978, p. 98). Offering expertise and counseling to a young man, yet not being parental, the mentor is usually older than his protégé by a half generation. All men in the study had male mentors, although Levinson's own mentor was a female, and it is expected that as more women enter currently male-dominated fields, they too will serve as mentors to both men and women.

In a study made by Margaret Hennig of 25 high-level women executives, it was shown that all had found male mentors early in their careers (Sheehy, 1976). Interestingly, these successful women chose careers rather than marriage in their 20s, yet realized around age 35 that something was missing and began to explore their feminine sides. Levinson reports a similar happenstance for men who become less involved with their mentors by age 40, and face the task of reintegrating the feminine side of their personality.

Choosing an Occupation

The process of choosing an occupation extends throughout the entire life cycle, beginning in childhood with make-believe games like "doctor" or "teacher." As Levinson remarks about other important life choices, "The great paradox of human development is that we are required to make crucial choices before we have the knowledge, judgment, and self-understanding to choose wisely" (1978, p. 162). Transforming one's early interests into an occupational choice during young adulthood is a complex psychosocial process, and a pattern usually emerges with some definition by the early 30s. An occupation often serves as an index of an individual's worth in society, both economically and socially, and defines his role in the community. For many of the men in Levinson's study, establishing an occupational identity is often tied up with parental expectations, and the nurturing given to the dream concept with or without the presence of a mentor. There are enormous differences between individuals regarding the meaning of success and failure, and concepts around these values change as growth occurs throughout their lifespan.

This stage has important implications for occupational therapy. Because illness almost always interrupts the work role of the patient, values around self and work need to be reconsidered. Group activities dealing with values around the work role, and the exploration of alternate roles in the home and community, are appropriate for a wide variety of patient populations.

Marriage and Family

The developmental task of forming a marriage and family also involves making premature choices. It is unusual to have integrated the many components of a stable adult relationship in the early adulthood stage. Sexuality, dependency, emotional intimacy, friendship, and the capability for commitment are but a few of the issues that extend beyond this phase. Actually, the ability to relate to the feminine or masculine aspects of self is a lifetime task, one of the many polarities that both Levinson and Jung give importance to in adult development. Undertaking the obligation to marry and have children does not necessarily mean one is prepared for the responsibilities and commitments. Often this step is intricately bound up with the other tasks of early adulthood, such as separating from parents and finding support for the dream pursuit. Levinson describes a "special woman" (1978, p. 109) who facilitates a man's entry into the adult world by providing boundaries within which his aspirations can be realized and giving nourishment to his occupational journey. If the marital choice is made in such a way as to be antithetical to the dream, the relationship may suffer conflicts at a later date. Obviously, the relationship will be modified over time to accommodate the dreams of both the man and woman, and there are endless possibilities for creating a family pattern that is suitable for both. The importance of fatherhood may not emerge until the individual has outgrown his occupational mentor and is prepared to provide those types of functions himself to his younger associates and to his own offspring.

The Mid-Life Transition

This period is said to provide the bridge from early to middle adulthood. It brings a man to question, search, and re-examine his life and his values. For the great majority of men in the Levinson study (80% of subjects), this great struggle within the self and the external world may reach crisis proportions. Often several years are needed to go through the process and come to some resolution. A culminating event often signifies success or failure in the man's fantasy, and this self-judgment may be all-encompassing. If he fails to get a promotion, he may regard himself as a failure in other aspects of his life as well. This transition period begins when a man realizes that he cannot go on as before, that he cannot "become his own man" under his existing life structure, and that changes will be necessary in order to advance sufficiently in any chosen direction. Three main tasks are defined by Levinson for this stage of development:

1. To terminate the era of early adulthood (reappraising the past)
2. To take the first steps toward middle adulthood (modifying life structure)
3. To deal with the polarities that are the sources of deep division in his life (individuation)

Each of these broadly defined tasks has many specific aspects to consider.

Reappraising the Past

Recognition of his own mortality gives a man a renewed sense of urgency about the use of his remaining time. He examines his accomplishments in relation to earlier hopes, values, and expectations, asking "Have I accomplished all that I set out to do?" Because of the nature of a dream, which is essentially fantasy, many ideas, assumptions, and beliefs associated with the dream do not withstand the comparison with actual experience. Levinson defines "de-illusionment" as "a recognition that longheld assumptions and beliefs about self and the world are not true" (1978, p. 192). The process of de-illusionment is accompanied by emotions of disappointment, joy, relief, bitterness, grief, wonder, freedom, and pain. At this stage a man may ask, "What have I done with my life? Is what I'm doing now what I want to be doing in the future? Have I reached success at my job? Am I fulfilled by my marital relationship? What are my present values and priorities? Am I spending my time on the things I really value? Is what I have done really meaningful? How have I been fooling myself? What is my true worth in my eyes and society's?" Occupational therapy groups can focus on some of these issues to help patients who are facing a mid-life transition to answer some of these questions.

Modifying Life Structure

Having taken stock of the past, the man now begins to plan for the next phase. Exploration of new patterns for living occurs. Some changes are externally motivated. The realities of growing families, aging parents, and changes in spouse and the marriage require certain changes in role and point of view. Experience of world politics, economy, and cultural and social values also influence the planning of man's new life structure.

But whether or not visible change occurs, one's outlook, values, and expectations of life are essentially different as a result of the developmental tasks of the mid-life transition. Questions to be asked are: "What do I want to change in my life? What are my options for change in occupation, marriage and family roles, roles in the community? What are the external changes in my life that put pressure on me to change? What pressures do I feel from society, friends, associates, and family, either to change or to remain the same? How can I feel more fulfilled? What parts

of myself have gone undeveloped that I would now like to give expression? What faults do I see that I would like to eliminate? What new character traits can I work on developing? How can I set a more realistic goal for the future? What new beliefs can be adopted to replace the delusions of the past?" The possibilities of occupational therapy activities to help with the planning process are endless. Furthermore, the potential for self-discovery and exploration of options are maximized in group treatment.

Individuation at Mid-Life

At mid-life, individuation is a continuation of past processes. An increasingly separate existence has been evolving since birth, gradually forming clearer boundaries between the self and the outside world. This individuation plays a part at each transition. Levinson takes his cue from Jung in describing the mid-life individuation tasks as resolving four polarities:

1. Young/old
2. Destruction/creation
3. Masculine/feminine
4. Attachment/separateness

Every life structure necessitates giving high priority to certain aspects of the self while minimizing others. In young adulthood, youth, creativity, masculinity, and attachment often outweigh their counterparts. At mid-life, neglected parts urgently seek expression.

The Young/Old Polarity

Young and old are viewed as relative terms, not specifically tied with any age. Young takes on such meanings as birth, growth, possibility, initiation, openness, energy, potential, promise of spring, fertility, and vision of things to come. Conversely, old represents termination, fruition, stability, rigidity, completion, impotence, senility, and death.

The issues of the young/old dichotomy at mid-life are realization of one's own death, fear of loss of youth, decline in bodily and psychological powers, realization that one's time is limited, wish for immortality and fear that man is not immortal, loss of omnipotence, and acceptance of limitation. Out of the recognition of one's own mortality comes the imagery of the legacy, or what a man will pass on to future generations. Among possible legacies are children, teachings or discoveries, concrete and social structures, objects of lasting value, written documents, and artistic works.

The Destruction/Creation Polarity

A new awareness of the destruction as a universal process takes on several forms in the mid-life transition. A man must come to an understanding of his grievances toward others for their destructiveness toward him. This typically results in anger toward loved ones—parents, wife, mentors, and friends whom he sees as having hurt him. He must also look at his own destructiveness in terms of how he has hurt others. It is necessary for him to accept destructiveness as a natural part of life and to take responsibility for it. Taking action in any direction always has consequences, some creative and some destructive. "If he is forced to maintain the illusion that destructiveness does not exist, he will also be impaired in his capacity for creating, loving, and affirming life" (Levinson, 1978, p. 224).

The Masculine/Feminine Polarity

Levinson refers to the terms masculine and feminine as going beyond the biological and social differentiation. Masculinity refers to bodily prowess and toughness, homosexuality, rationality, achievement and ambition, and an intolerance of weakness. Femininity refers to motherhood, caring and emotionality, artistic creativity, softness, and lack of strength and stamina. The masculine and feminine are really both aspects of the same person, and are

seen as poorly integrated in early adulthood, due to immaturity, cultural tradition, and the necessity for aggressive pursuit of one's occupation and social position. In middle adulthood, however, man comes to new terms with this polarity, seeing masculine and feminine as less rigidly divided within the self and combining them more creatively in work, personal relationships, and acceptance of self. Aggressiveness may give way to a more nurturing and sensitive side of the personality without really injuring the masculine role identity. The resolution of the masculine/feminine dichotomy opens new possibilities for the man in both love relationships with peer women and mentor relationships.

In occupational therapy, we are constantly faced with the masculine and feminine identities of our patients. In doing activity groups with male and female patients, it is important to consider their values and expectations. For example, male patients, especially those of Hispanic origin, may refuse to do activities like cooking or sewing, which they consider to be "women's work." Female patients may have negative feelings about doing money management or using power tools. In using developmental theory, the age and gender of our patients as well as their disability will determine what activities they are willing to try.

The Attachment/Separateness Polarity

Attachment is defined by Levinson as "to be engaged, involved, needy, plugged in, seeking, and rooted" (1978, p. 239). Separateness is distinguished from isolation and loneliness in that it refers to a person's involvement in his inner world, his fantasies. In early adulthood, with marriage and mentor relationships, typically attachment takes precedence at the expense of separateness. At mid-life, developmentally a more equal balance between the two must be achieved. This generally means the man at mid-life moves further into himself, and through this process is able to examine his own feelings, values, and goals apart from external and social expectations.

The Late Life Transition

Levinson positions the late life transition at ages 60 to 65. The tasks of this period are to reappraise the past, create a new life structure, and make choices that are relevant to the final stage of life. Levinson's study does not extend beyond mid-life and must be viewed as speculation. The issues facing the older adult are physical decline, loss of a productive role, and coming to terms with death, both of self and loved ones. According to some theorists, changes in perception of time begin at mid-life, from "time since birth" to "time left to live." In the late life transition, the approach of death can no longer be ignored. The limited time remaining must be devoted to resolving old conflicts, finishing unfinished business, deepening important relationships, and arranging to leave one's legacy. These life tasks lend themselves very nicely to group activities in occupational therapy. Life review groups are one example of how occupational therapy can address these issues.

Physical Decline

By the year 2020, the average life expectancy will be 77 years and 20% of the population in the United States will be over age 65. As people live longer, the effects of normal physical decline become more prominent. At the most basic level, aging cells begin to degenerate and die. Loss of neurons in the brain are the cause of senility and occur naturally, but more rapidly in degenerative diseases such as Alzheimer's. Brain cell loss causes functional loss of memory and personality changes as well.

Functioning of vital organs, including heart and lungs, slows down. Anatomic changes result in loss of hearing, decline in eyesight, loss of height, and lower muscle mass and tone. Most people are familiar with the graying of hair and the general loss of strength and endurance. Osteoporosis (brittle bones) and osteoarthritis (painful joints) are common.

Changes in the immune system often make older persons more susceptible to disease. Longevity has been shown to be related most closely to heredity. However, regular medical check-ups and a healthy lifestyle are still the best preventive measures. Vulnerability to stress also increases with age. Despite the skills accumulated over a lifetime, change at older ages is still more difficult and more stressful.

Coping with bodily decline requires an acceptance of a more passive role with respect to the environment. Changes in lifestyle that limit physical demands while providing a sense of worth and satisfaction are preferable. Occupational therapy groups can center around energy conservation, setting goals and priorities, exercise and fitness, health education and maintenance, and exploring activities that encourage continued use of skills and maintenance of self-esteem and social recognition.

Loss of Productive Role

Retirement may be voluntary or mandatory between ages 60 and 65. Either way, the changes produced by it are many and show mixed responses in individuals. For some, the increased time to relax and pursue leisure interests is welcome. But for many, retirement is a negative experience that lowers self-worth and leaves them socially isolated. The economic impact of retirement is very real, and those without pensions or retirement plans may find themselves having to accept a lower income and lower socioeconomic status. Retired persons need to find a new structure to replace the work role and new interests to give them a sense of self-worth. Occupational therapy groups dealing with retirement issues can address time management, financial management, leisure planning, community involvement, volunteering, socialization, new skill development, and many others.

Coming to Terms with Death

Loss is a predominant theme in the lives of older people. Erikson's view of the final conflict to be resolved may be helpful in understanding how loss can be accepted. His eighth stage, integrity vs. despair, suggests that contentment in old age results from the view of "a life productively lived" (Kaplan & Sadock, 1998). The late adult transition necessarily includes reviewing one's life experiences and reappraising them to sum up their worth. The results of this reappraisal may determine how an individual copes with the later years. At best, in later life, grandparents enjoy spoiling their grandchildren and retired workers enjoy knowing that the younger generations will benefit from their life's work. Teachers may enjoy watching the success of their students, for example. According to Erikson, peace and contentment in old age occurs only if one has previously achieved intimacy and generativity. An older person needs to know that his life has been productive and he has passed on his wisdom to others in some way. Without this belief, there is only despair. Despair, according to Erikson, is indicated by a fear of death, and the realization that it is too late to start over.

Preparation for death is another necessary prerequisite of integrity in old age. As life is reappraised, old conflicts and unfinished business may be recalled. It is not unusual to wish for reconciliations with estranged friends or relatives. Often there are old wrongs to be forgiven, apologies to make, and unkept promises to be reconsidered. These are important emotional concerns of the elderly, and should not be prematurely dismissed. Those who are physically or cognitively impaired may need help in dealing with these issues. Even when actual reconciliations are not feasible, a great deal can be done through group experiences incorporating role play and other creative activities. Developing a point of view about death is a spiritual and philosophical concern. Carl Rogers, psychotherapist and major spokesman for humanistic psychology, described a new interest in his 70s as he explored the world of the paranormal with his wife. His experiences changed his understanding of death. Whereas in his 50s and 60s he regarded death to be the end of the individual, he now considers it possible that the spiritual essence of man continues to live after death. He mentions the views of Arthur Koestler about each individual's consciousness being a part of the "cosmic consciousness" (Rogers, 1980, p. 88), a view which echoes Jung's ideas regarding the collective unconscious. Zemke and Gratz (1982) point out that for the aged, illness and disability tend to renew earlier crises. "The (occupational) therapist must acknowledge and work toward resolution of these just as she would with any other disabled adult. Only then can the ego integrity crisis be faced. Techniques such as remotivation or life review provide a basis for the thoughtful review and acceptance of life experience necessary for resolution at this final stage of life" (Zemke & Gratz, 1982, p. 61).

Kohlberg and Wilcox

Kohlberg and Wilcox built on the work of Piaget, who developed stages of intellectual development. They looked at the

Table 7-4.
Kohlberg and Wilcox Development of Moral Reasoning

Age	Stage

2-4	**Preconventional level: decisions made on the basis of punishment and reward**
	Stage 1 - person is egocentric
	    - no ablity to empathize
	Stage 2 - reciprocity
	    - makes deals with authority

6+	**Conventional level: decisions based on pleasing others**
	Stage 3 - confirms identity as good
	    - authority is fair
	    - good people get best treatment
	Stage 4 - law and order orientation
	    - rules necessary to maintain social structure
	    - only one system is "right"

11-12	**Post-conventional level: fairness is free standing logic**
	Stage 5 - individual rights and human dignity can override rules
	    - empathy influences decisions
	    - right and wrong is separate from rules
	Stage 6 - ideal stage, rarely encountered in reality
	    - unconditional value of rights of humanity
	    - empathized with all participants in a moral dilemma
	    - creatively resolves polarities and contradictions

way logic was used in the development of moral reasoning. How people get along in society, their view of themselves, and the social structure depend on how they make decisions about right and wrong. Kohlberg and Wilcox suggest three levels and six stages of moral development (Table 7-4). This perspective is useful in planning groups with patients who are not psychotic, but have problems with society or in dealing with authority figures or rules. Motivation to move up to the next level is having experiences which contradict one's former beliefs, and cause them to question their own reasoning. According to Kohlberg, all of the stages can be brought into adulthood. Many adults have been found to operate at the preconventional and conventional levels. Therapists should look for lags in moral reasoning as a possible explanation of behavior in patients (and staff).

Bruce and Borg (1993) suggest that occupational therapy group leaders encourage growth in moral reasoning by creating dissonance. Therapists do this by exposing the group members to reasoning at a slightly higher level and encouraging role taking and role reversal. Introducing moral dilemmas for a group to discuss and problem solve might provide an appropriate setting for this kind of developmental learning.

Gilligan—"A Different Voice"

Gilligan (1982) challenges previous theories of development in two respects. She sheds doubt on the "age and stage" concept of development, and she suggests that women have a different way of thinking about life than men do and that their developmental stages may also be fundamentally different. Gilligan points out that prior theorists, including Erikson,

Kohlberg, and Levinson, have based their beliefs primarily on observations of men. A professor at Harvard, Gilligan performed her own research regarding men and women from childhood through maturity, regarding their identity and moral development, rights and responsibilities, and the role of conflict in development.

In relation to Kohlberg, Gilligan suggests that these stages relate more to men than women and do not consider the variables of culture, time, occasion, and gender. She observes that events of women's lives and of history promote the view that concern with individual survival is "selfish" or "bad" as opposed to the "responsibility" of a life lived in relationships. For women, life is caring in relationships. When the focus on individuation and individual achievement extends into adulthood and maturity is equated with personal autonomy, concern with relationships appears as a weakness of women rather than a human strength.

The stereotypes of adulthood or maturity suggested by Levinson and Erikson favor separateness or self-sufficiency over connection to others, primarily a "male" point of view, according to Gilligan. According to these theorists, young adulthood is characterized by a conflict of commitment in which either identity or intimacy wins out. The male believes that separation empowers the self and permits full self-expression; intimacy, the choice of women, represents immaturity and impedes expression of the self. Gilligan states that "the silence of women in the narrative of adult development distorts the conception of its stages and sequence" (1982, p. 156).

Gilligan does not suggest an alternative sequence of developmental stages, nor does she describe how pre-established stages are different for women. Yet her points are well-taken and encourage us, in using this frame

of reference, not to accept the proposed ages and stages as absolute reality.

In considering Gilligan's message for occupational therapy groups, we need to consider more carefully the role of relationships for our patients. There is no better place than a group to explore and work on the skills that affect relationships.

Function and Dysfunction

If one uses an age and stage theory, then healthy functioning is having achieved the appropriate developmental tasks for one's age. For example, a 23-year-old will have separated from his parents, chosen a career, and if not married, at least developed a support system of peers with whom to identify. Conversely, dysfunction may be looked at as failure to develop age-appropriate skills, a failure to achieve the tasks of an age-appropriate stage. The stages of childhood and adolescence have been studied historically in much greater detail than those of adulthood. So as Gilligan implies, it is better to use the ages given for developmental tasks as approximate guidelines. Furthermore, as illness interferes with normal development, the discrepancy between age and developmental level may be so great that the term "age-appropriate" becomes meaningless. It is the developmental stage that we as occupational therapists are concerned with, since that is what determines the level of function and adaptation to the environment. Dysfunction can be seen as a lack of adaptive skills necessary for effective and satisfying interaction with one's environment. It can be caused by a failure to develop these skills (e.g., developmental delay), a loss of these skills (e.g., due to brain trauma), or a regression to an earlier stage of development (e.g., that caused by depression or schizophrenia).

In adult development theory, just the normal tasks at each transitional stage may be enough to cause a crisis situation. If Levinson speaks of the mid-life transition as a potential crisis for 80% of the population, think of the impact it must have on those with physical or mental disability. If Levinson is right, the stress produced by this kind of crisis is likely to contribute to physical and mental breakdown, even in those without previous illness.

Development is almost always affected by illness. As disabled patients are referred to occupational therapy, the assessment process is likely to uncover missing skills that patients have failed to learn in earlier stages of development. The difficulty in coping with illness in the present is often due to the inadequacy of earlier skill development. Because the stages of development are hierarchical, occupational therapy cannot address issues of the patient's current age until earlier skills are learned. For example, a 20-year-old may not be expected to work on career choice and separation from parents if her illness has resulted in a lack of ability to form peer relationships and her own identity is not developed. Because of discrepancies between chronological and developmental age in persons with illness and disability, groups in occupational therapy often include patients of varying ages. Occupational therapists organize treatment groups by developmental levels (not age levels), so that members can work together on similar skills.

Change and Motivation

Motivation comes from an individual's natural desire for mastery of age-appropriate skills. The drive toward mastery is, at least in part, biologically determined. However, as a person matures, the environment plays a greater part in motivation. If a person's attempts to progress developmentally are met with success, motivation will likely remain intact.

Repeated failures to keep up with peers, on the other hand, may discourage a person from continuing to try. Occupational therapy may encourage the rediscovery of the drive toward mastery by creating a "just right challenge." This is a task or situation that encourages a patient to use higher level skills, but one that is not beyond her reach.

When there is a developmental lag or loss of skills, they must be learned or relearned in the correct developmental sequence. Mosey called this "recapitulation of ontogeny" (1970). If the patient is more than one level behind, the change process may be slow, but it follows a more or less predictable pattern. Since developmental stages are hierarchical, the earlier skills must be mastered before the learning of later developing skills is possible.

Consider a group of individuals with chronic mental illness. The age of onset for several chronic mental illnesses is the early 20s. Often patients have achieved at least some of the developmental tasks of the young adult transition before becoming ill. Many have vocational or educational training in a chosen career, some have begun working and have moved out of their parents' homes, some have married and had one or two children. These are accomplishments beyond the capacity of most patients with chronic mental illness. One might see these patients as regressed. Because of their illness, they have gone backward to an earlier, less mature stage of development. In treating these patients, the occupational therapist needs to determine the correct level at which to begin. This will be the level at which mastery is possible and growth and change can be motivated.

Mosey's concept of the six adaptive skills is helpful in identifying a patient's correct developmental level, as well as determining which skills need work.

These skills are:
1. Perceptual-motor
2. Cognitive
3. Dyadic interaction
4. Group interaction
5. Self-identity
6. Sexual identity

Each adaptive skill has several subskills whose typical ages of development are identified. These are described more fully in Appendix C.

Change occurs through the learning of new skills. This can be encouraged by setting up a growth-facilitating environment. The occupational therapist looks carefully at the physical environment in terms of safety. The emotional environment may best be set through the patient-therapist relationship and through the use of groups. Mosey's concept of the developmental groups is useful here. The hierarchy of group structure and leadership requirements in these groups can help occupational therapists to plan treatment groups for patients that are appropriate to their level of development (see Appendix B).

However, the benefits of group treatment go beyond the learning or relearning of group interaction skill. All six adaptive skills identified by Mosey may be effectively learned in a group context through occupational therapy activity. At the higher developmental levels, the tasks of adult development may be facilitated through group activities in occupational therapy.

Group Treatment

It has been implied that groups in this frame of reference are best organized along the lines of developmental level. Occupational therapy groups would be primarily homogeneous. At lower levels, patients in a parallel group may be participating in activities that promote sensory motor or cognitive skill development. At higher levels, groups may use interaction skills to work on career choice in the young adult transition, re-examine their values in the mid-life transition, or participate in retirement planning in the late life transition. The structure of occupational therapy treatment groups is organized according to the developmental level, and this guides the occupational therapist's choice of activity as well.

The limitations for use of this frame of reference are minimal. Patients of every age and almost any type of disability are appropriately treated within its bounds. The theories of adult development described in this chapter, however, are most helpful in planning groups for the later stages of development. Guidelines for the earlier stages, dealing with sensory motor and cognitive development, are described in Chapter 8.

Role of the Leader

In developmental groups, the occupational therapist takes a directive role. Knowledge of the predictable conflicts and skills in each developmental stage guides the use of activities and setting of group goals. She evaluates patients' skills to determine their developmental levels and attempts to predict their potential for further development. When placed in appropriate groups, patients can work together on their mutual tasks with the leader's guidance. Because the sequence of learned tasks is hierarchical, the occupational therapist cannot give too many choices to the group. If the groups are planned appropriately, their area of interest should coincide with the developmental tasks of their level. Occupational therapists need to challenge their groups to develop further by consistently introducing higher level activities at appropriate times.

It is also the responsibility of the leader to create and maintain a growth-facilitating environment (Mosey, 1970). In the treatment setting, patients should be supported and rewarded for growth, not discouraged. If a group is ready to take on more responsibility, this should be allowed. If growing requires a stage of upset and turmoil, and it has to get worse before it gets better, this should also be met with patience and support.

The occupational therapist should be on the lookout for signs of developmental transitions in patients with physical disability as well as mental illness. Even when the illness is physical, addressing developmental issues can be the most beneficial in helping the patient to cope. Coping with illness or developmental crises often requires the learning of enabling skills. These are specific cognitive, psychosocial, or sensory motor learned behaviors that make it possible for the individual to meet his developmental needs (Bruce & Borg, 1993). Examples are reading and writing, communication skills, and the ability to empathize with others. Mosey's adaptive skills might be used as a guide.

Examples of Activities

Those activities chosen should address issues to be resolved or specific skills appropriate to the developmental level of the patient group. The theorist, the specific stage to be addressed, and the specific task or skill within that stage should be identified. Since most of the theorists have an identified hierarchy of issues, tasks, or skills to be learned at each level, these can easily serve as guidelines for activity choice. When designing group activities, leaders should note the specific developmental theory that relates to it, as well as the stage of development being addressed. See Activity Examples 7-1 through 7-10 at the end of the chapter.

Group Leadership

The seven stages of groups can remain intact when working with most adult groups in this frame of reference. The introduction is done according to the guidelines offered in Chapter 1.

Activity

Activities and goals are chosen using specific guidelines from the ages and stages of development. The learning exercise in Worksheet 7-1 may be helpful in identifying the theory and stage which is appropriate for your particular patients. Fill in the chart by writing under the various chronological ages the appropriate information from the theories reviewed at the beginning of this chapter.

It is especially important to plan an environment that incorporates safety, support, and challenge. The goals for these groups are to help members progress to higher levels of development. The timing of groups may be altered to suit the group, the activity, and the goal. Many of the tasks of adult development are quite complex, and there are many aspects to be explored. Activities, such as those listed previously, may take several sessions, depending on how they are planned and how much discussion seems appropriate. If patients are motivated by a particular activity, it may be desirable to give homework. Patients may be asked to think about the issues discussed between sessions, to explore options for change, or to try out new behaviors with family and friends.

Sharing and Processing

Sharing, including self-expression and feedback, is an important part of the developmental group. However, while members are working on similar tasks, there is no expectation that they will produce similar results, since each person

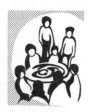

Directions: Using information from this text and others, fill in the developmental stages for each of the theorists. Estimate the chronological age range for each stage and fill in on the chart below.

Chronological Age				Years			
	0-1	2	5	10	15	20	
Jung (Spiritual Stages)							
Erikson (Psychosocial Stages)							
Levinson (Life Transitions)							
Kohlberg (Moral Development)							
Mosey (Appendix C) (Adaptive Skills)							
Perceptual-Motor, Cognitive							
Dyadic Interaction, Group Interaction							
Self-Identity, Sexual Identity							
Physical Milestones/ Attributes Typical of Age							

From Cole, M. B. *Group Dynamics in Occupational Therapy, Second Edition.* © 1998 SLACK Incorporated.

Developmental Theories
Comparative Chart (continued)

Chronological Age				Years			
	25	30	40	45	50	60	65
Jung (Spiritual Stages)							
Erikson (Psychosocial Stages)							
Levinson (Life Transitions)							
Kohlberg (Moral Development)							
Mosey (Appendix C) (Adaptive Skills)							
Perceptual-Motor, Cognitive							
Dyadic Interaction, Group Interaction							
Self-Identity, Sexual Identity							
Physical Milestones/ Attributes Typical of Age							

must complete a developmental task in his own way.

Processing the group may uncover many feelings about both past and present experience. This is one frame of reference in which talking about past events is not discouraged. Relationships among members evidenced during processing can be helpful in supporting patients through many traumatic memories, as well as stressful present day realities. Group cohesiveness in this frame is desirable and encouraged.

Generalizing and Application

Generalizing an experience should be somewhat predictable, since most of the activities will address specific developmental issues. The therapist really has to take the lead, to guide the discussion of general principles along developmental lines.

Application is a particularly important aspect of developmental groups, since the group experiences are designed to have a specific impact on development. If there is a focus to the discussion of developmental groups, it should be the application of learning to each individual's everyday life. The summary can be shared by members and leader, depending on the ability of the group, and this should also stress application of learning.

Bibliography

Bruce, M. A., & Borg, B. (1993). *Frames of reference in psychosocial occupational therapy* (2nd ed.). Thorofare, NJ: SLACK Incorporated.

Cole, M., & Gross, M. (1982). *Structured group experiences for life's adult transitions.* (Unpublished.)

Gilligan, C. (1982). *A different voice.* Cambridge, MA: Harvard University Press.

Greenfield, J. M., & Godinez, M. (1989, April 20). Stroke clients learn independence by leading their own therapy group. *OT Week.*

Kaplan, H., & Sadock, B. (1998). *Synopsis of psychiatry* (8th ed.). Baltimore: Williams & Wilkins.

Levinson, D. (1978). *The seasons of a man's life.* New York: Ballentine Books.

Mosey, A. C. (1970). *Three frames of reference for mental health.* Thorofare, NJ: SLACK Incorporated.

Mosey, A. C. (1986). *Psychosocial components of occupational therapy.* New York: Raven.

Rogers, C. (1980). *A way of being.* Boston: Houghton Mifflin.

Schultz, D. (1976). *Theories of personality.* Monterey, CA: Brooks/Cole.

Sheehy, G. (1976). *Passages: Predictable crises of adult life.* New York: E. P. Dutton.

Viorst, J. (1986). *Necessary losses.* New York: Ballentine Books.

Wilcox, M. (1979). *Developmental journey.* Nashville, TN: Abbington Press.

Zemke, R., & Gratz, R. R. (1982). The role of theory: Erikson and occupational therapy. *OT in Mental Health, II*(3), 45-63.

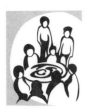

Developmental
Activity Example 7-1
Ideal Man/Ideal Woman

This activity addresses Levinson's early adult transition, specifically, the tasks of finding a special woman or man and finding a mentor.

Materials: 12- x 18-inch sheets of white drawing paper, pastels, pencils, erasers, and tissues.

Directions: First look into your fantasy, and envision a person of the opposite sex whom you consider to be ideal, having all the qualities you would wish for in a mate, companion, and friend. What does that person look like? Notice hair, eyes, facial expression, stature, clothing, style of movement. What is that person doing? Perhaps he or she is sitting across from you at dinner, participating with you in an active sport, sitting by the fireside planning a new project with you, having lively interactions with others at a party, seriously engaging in a business venture, or walking alone on a deserted beach. When an image has come to mind, try to capture its essential qualities by drawing them.

Fold the paper in half and draw your first picture on the left half of the page. Never mind if your drawing does not look exactly like your mental image—just do the best that you can. You have 15 minutes for the drawing. After 10 minutes, next to your drawing make note of any particular personality traits, habits, attitudes, values, and other internal attributes possessed by the person you drew. Is this person sensitive, strong, energetic, intellectual, responsible, gentle? What talents and abilities does the person possess?

Now imagine a person of the same sex, whom you consider to be ideal. Maybe the person is someone whose accomplishments you admire or whose lifestyle seems appealing. Perhaps the person holds a position in life you aspire to or has talents you desire to develop in yourself. Do not think too much about this, but allow images to enter your mind, remembering that this will be a person you create, not necessarily someone you know. You may combine attributes of several people or just make up new ones. Keep in mind the images you consider most ideal and when the image crystallizes, begin to draw it on the second side of your paper. Do the same as you did for the first part, considering physical appearance, activity or situation, and both external and internal traits. Write down those elements which cannot be defined by drawing (15 minutes).

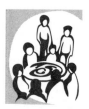

Developmental
Activity Example 7-2
Times of Your Life Collage

This activity addresses Levinson's mid-life transition in providing an opportunity to review past accomplishments as well as unrealized expectations. It will assist patients in re-evaluating the past and present life structures in preparation for making changes in middle adulthood (Figure 7-1).

Materials: Variety of magazines suitable to patients, large posterboard, glue, scissors, and marker for each patient. If patients in the group are of similar or known ages, the posterboard may be set up ahead of time to provide a space for every 5 years of their lives up to their present ages.

0-5	5-10	10-15	15-20
20-25	25-30	30-35	35-40

Figure 7-1. Times of your life collage. Draw format on large posterboard. Adapt ages for each member.

Directions: The object of this exercise is to get a temporal perspective on our lives, and to see how the parts fit into the whole to make us the people we are today. The posterboard will represent the whole. Our life will begin on the upper left and proceed to the lower right, divided into time intervals of 5 years. Leave one space for the present. (Show example.) Now think about the events that occurred in each segment of your life, what you were like then, people who were in your life then, places where you lived or traveled, accomplishments you made, decisions you made. Then look through the magazines and find pictures, words, and phrases that best describe the major event or aspect of each segment of your life up to and including the present.

This activity can take up to 2 hours. Depending on patient group, the project can be done on one day, discussed the next, or it can carry over several group sessions. Discussion should center around evaluation of events and account for spaces left blank. High and low points may be identified. Emotional responses to events or patterns may be identified. Are there patterns? Were there changes? How were the changes made? Markers may be used to identify highs, lows, and emotions surrounding events.

Change options should then be explored. What accounts for the decisions in your life? Were they made impulsively? Influenced by others? Done with careful planning? If you

From Cole, M. B. *Group Dynamics in Occupational Therapy, Second Edition.* © 1998 SLACK Incorporated.

could go back and change parts of your life, what would you change? What do you wish you could add or delete? What was missing in your life development that you wish had been there?

A follow-up drawing can be added to this exercise, entitled "The Future." Planning the next 5 or 10 years can be done using the same collage techniques.

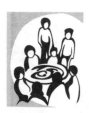

Developmental
Activity Example 7-3
Fabric of Life

This simple weaving activity addresses the life review task of Levinson's late adult transition. It is in keeping with the views of Erikson and Jung as well. The use of colors, patterns, and materials encourage the incorporation of emotional as well as substantive memories or essences, as well as marker events (Figure 7-2). This exercise requires two or three 1-hour sessions for most groups.

Materials: Pencils, paper, and a medium paper bag for each group member to plan his project. A heavy wire circle (loom) 12 to 18 inches in diameter (warped with strong yarn dividing the circle into 16 equal parts, tied together in the center) and one pair of sharp scissors should be provided for each person. A large variety of fabric remnants (can be scraps from a seamstress or cut from old, donated clothes, curtains, sheets, tablecloths, etc.), trimmings, ribbons, and several colored balls of yarn. Fabrics should be cut into long 1-inch strips.

Directions: Fabrics are, for most of us, associated with clothing, home furnishings, draperies, bedsheets, and the like. They are adorning and surrounding us constantly, and although often not the focus of our attention, they influence our sensory experiences and our mood and color our lives in ways of which we may be unaware.

In this exercise, we will associate key events, places, and persons in our lives with a sensory awareness of the fabrics that may symbolize them. We will choose fabrics, trimmings, or ribbons to represent both events and significant others in our lives. In addition, each of us will choose one special yarn or fabric to represent ourselves. Begin by writing down any of the following which apply most to you. As you choose fabrics, trimmings, and ribbons for each memory, cut an arm's length of it and place it in your paper bag.

1. Birth and young childhood—Envision your room or most memorable environment as a child. What do you see? What can you feel? Is there a favorite blanket or stuffed toy? What color is there? How does the texture of the fabric feel to your touch? Choose a fabric or material from the collection to represent this association as closely as possible.
2. Parents—Envision each of your parents, either separately or together, doing whatever they ordinarily were doing when you were a child. How were they dressed? What was their favorite color? Style? Summon an image of each of your parents as you would like to remember them from childhood. Then choose a fabric to represent that image.
   Take a few minutes to re-experience visual, tactile, auditory, or olfactory memories (sights, sounds, textures, and smells) associated with each of the items to follow, and continue to select fabrics and place them in your bag.
3. Friends from childhood
4. Relatives and siblings
5. A childhood home (imagine your room)
6. First day of school (what did you wear?)

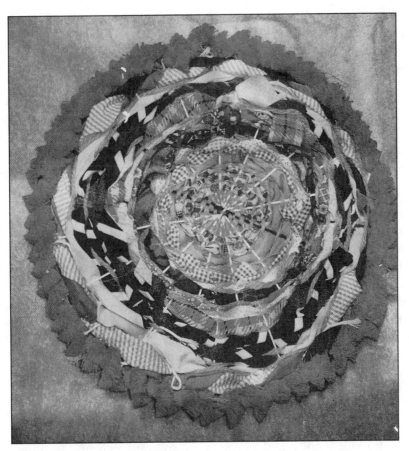

Figure 7-2. Fabric of life.

7. Communion, bar mitzvah, or joining a church
8. First date
9. First school dance
10. First boyfriend or girlfriend
11. Graduation
12. First job (or significant ones)
13. Marriage
14. First house or apartment
15. Death of loved one(s)
16. Important travels
17. Awards or promotions at work
18. Adult friends
19. Birth of children and their significant others
20. Marriage, graduation, or jobs of children
21. Birth of grandchildren

22. Organizations or committees
23. Adult hobbies or leisure activities
24. Other important events or milestones

Planning takes at least a 1-hour session and should be discussed before the session ends. Memories can be verbalized and elaborated. If desired, a small scrap of fabric can be taped to the paper and labeled after each item planned, so the group member will not forget which was chosen for which at the next session. Be sure to put names on paper bags. Planning paper can be folded and placed inside.

Procedure for Weaving: Begin with the ball of yarn that represents you. Tie the end to the center and weave it under and over each warp thread, clockwise around the circle for five or six rows. This yarn will touch and become a part of all the other materials you have chosen. How much of each other material you use depends on how large a part its associated element played in your life. Begin with childhood and work chronologically, adding chosen materials and weaving them over and under with the yarn, around and around the circle. From time to time, rake the yarn toward the center with your fingers to push it together. End when you have used up all the materials selected. Wind the yarn (or add ribbon or trim) around and around the wire circle to cover it, and tie in a loop knot at the end to hang it on the wall. (See Figure 7-2 for example.)

Discussion should be encouraged during the weaving process, and the therapist will help patients as needed. Feelings about the project at the end are especially important. The doing process often evokes many hidden feelings that need to be expressed and explored. Is the review of life positive or negative? Which parts are positive or negative? What is missing? Patients should be encouraged to keep their own projects and to reflect on the significance of them, and not to use them as gifts, at least for a while. Remember, a life review is only the beginning of the task of evaluation and integration which Jung and Erikson have suggested is necessary for contentment in old age.

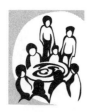

<h1 style="text-align:center">Developmental
Activity Example 7-4
The Doctor's Dilemma</h1>

This activity refers to Kohlberg's fourth and fifth stages of moral development. The group's discussion is intended to cast doubt upon a strict "law and order" kind of reasoning about morality, and to encourage empathy with more than one participant in a given situation.

Directions: First I will read you a story which has several characters who do not agree with one another. Listen carefully to the story and then, as a group, decide who is right, who is wrong, and what should be done about the situation.

Story: Jenny was a healthy 24-year-old woman who went into the hospital unexpectedly to have her appendix removed. It was 8:00 p.m. and Dr. Strothers had just completed a long, tiring day of surgery. Jenny's sister Carol brought her to the hospital in terrible pain; it was evident that she needed to be operated on at once. The emergency room nurse, Eva, interviewed Jenny and prepared her for surgery. Eva wrote down on her report that Jenny had her last meal 1 hour ago, which put her at considerable risk of choking when given general anesthesia. However, the doctor did not read the report carefully. He operated anyway, and the patient choked to death on the table.

Carol was in shock; she suspected negligence and sued the doctor for 1 million dollars. Although Jenny was not married and had no children, Carol missed her sister and felt that those who mistreated her sister should pay. But mostly, she could really use the money. She and her husband had just bought a house and had defaulted on the past few payments. Five hundred thousand dollars would just about pay off their mortgage, and prevent them from losing their home.

Eva, the nurse who prepared the report, was secretly in love with the doctor. Out of love, she offered to alter the report, changing the "1" hour since last meal to a "9." This would clear Dr. Strothers of any blame for Jenny's death. Eva saw that Dr. Strothers was a caring and brilliant young doctor, capable of saving many more lives if allowed to continue his practice. Of course, a verdict of guilty in the lawsuit would prevent him from ever practicing again. Eva was willing to give up nursing and take the blame for the man she loved. She hoped perhaps he would marry her if she did this, and after a brief jail sentence, they could live happily ever after.

Dr. Strothers was faced with a dilemma. Should he take the blame, plead guilty in the lawsuit, and give up his life's work? Should he accept Eva's offer to take the blame? Should he meet with Carol and offer to pay her $500,000 to withdraw the lawsuit? How should the story end? It is up to you.

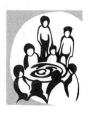

Developmental
Activity Example 7-5
Families of Clay

Margo Gross, MS, OTR/L, is acknowledged as the creator of this activity, which relates to Levinson's individuation in both the early adult and middle adult transitions.

Materials: A ball of soft clay, approximately 4 inches in diameter, a piece of cardboard or posterboard 18- x 24-inches for each member, clay modeling tools, water and paper towels for clean-up, markers, and small post-it notepads.

Directions: Divide your clay into sections for each member of your family, including yourself. Sculpt an abstract figure which represents how you feel about each person. Try to use non-concrete representations. Arrange the people on the board in such a way as to describe the relationships in your family. Label each member.

Discussion: Discuss how you saw your family system at ages 5, 15, 25, 35, etc. How would you like to see the relationships in your family placed, ideally? What happened to the structure when new members were introduced? Geographical moves? Marriage or divorce? Death?

Individuals beginning to separate from their family of origin can look at the structure and their place in it, from a distance. Assessing the aspects of learning derived from each parent, hidden messages, and alliances and conflicts between members is an important step in the individuation process. At mid-life, individuation takes on a qualitatively different process, as the role of parent to offspring ends, and becoming caretaker for one's own aging parents is more of a reality. Whether or not family ties remain close, individuation continues psychologically as one ages. One's perception of each family member alters as the individual becomes more fully integrated.

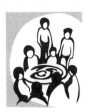

Developmental
Activity Example 7-6
Eulogy for Yourself

Margo Gross, MS, OTR/L, is acknowledged as the creator of this activity, which addresses Levinson's middle and late life transitions.

Materials: Pencil and paper for each member.

Directions: This exercise will help you see your life more clearly from the perspective of your imagined death. Write the eulogy that your best friend might read at your funeral. Include any major accomplishments, special family relationships, contributions to the community, and values or morals that you strongly uphold. What has been the significance of your life, and how might you be leaving the world a better place?

Within the group format, pass your eulogy to the person at your right, and take turns reading them out loud. Record your response as you hear about your life in retrospect.

Discussion: What periods of your life were the most/least fulfilling in terms of career, family relationships, involvement in community life? Where were the major turning points? What values did you act on consistently? How can you plan to complete any unfinished business in the time left before your death?

This exercise has direct implications for those individuals approaching mid-life, where the sense of aging becomes more acute due to the beginning of the physical and cognitive decline. Their sense of mortality is accentuated by the change in generational status, by the aging of parental figures, and by death or illness of friends or contemporaries.

Assessing the climb up the ladder of success and deciding whether earlier goals were attained or new goals need to be defined are aspects of this developmental period. The activity will reinforce the fact that each individual still has a period of life ahead to restructure a change to reach different or new goals.

For individuals in the late adult transition, the activity serves to assist in life review. It is a concrete way of seeing and hearing how the major themes and events in a life come together to unify the self.

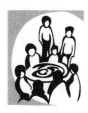

Developmental
Activity Example 7-7
Major Accomplishments

Margo Gross, MS, OTR/L, is acknowledged as the creator of this activity, which addresses Levinson's middle and late life transitions. Two 1-hour sessions are needed for this exercise.

Materials: 12- x 12-inch plywood boards for each member, sandpaper square, scissors, magazines, personal photographs if available, decoupage glue, water-based wood stain, rags, brushes, water and paper towels for clean-up, and permanent color markers.

Directions: Prepare the wood board by sanding the edges and corners, and also both surfaces of the wood until smooth to the touch. Wipe away the sawdust. Brush the stain onto all sides of the wood in the color of your choice. Use a small rag to wipe off excess stain and set aside to dry. From the magazines, choose pictures and words that describe your major accomplishments up to the present time. Arrange them in front of you as you process the first session. Write your name on the back of your board with a marker, and place your clippings in a plain envelope with your name.

Bring any photographs, actual newspaper clippings, or mementos you have found at home to the second session. Arrange the clippings and photos on the board in a pleasing manner. You may wish to overlap the pictures, which means applying several coats of decoupage glue to adhere each layer of the design. Be sure to smooth the pictures well to eliminate air bubbles underneath, which can cause wrinkling of the pictures as the glue dries. Apply a final coat of glue to finish the plaque, which gives the project a glossy shine. Be sure to apply decoupage glue to the edges to seal and protect the plaque. When dry, a tooth hook may be applied to the center of the back for hanging.

Discussion: Depending on the transitional period in which members of the activity group are involved, the pictures chosen will represent feelings about their accomplishments to date. Individuals in the middle adult transition will use this activity to re-evaluate the past and take stock of their progress. For late adult transitions, the plaque serves as a life review. Persons facing retirement, changes in financial status, or widowhood, may find the decoupage a concrete daily reminder of their self-worth, which may be shaky during such periods of adaptation. Categories of successes may be separated into family, career, or personal accomplishments. A discussion of how a future plaque might look will assist those in the process of designing a new life structure.

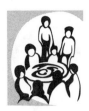

Developmental
Activity Example 7-8
Exploring Sex Roles

Margo Gross, MS, OTR/L, is acknowledged as the creator of this activity, which addresses Levinson's early adult transition.

Materials: Worksheets and pens for each member, large newsprint pad with easel, and magic marker.

Directions: This activity is designed to explore and clarify sex roles in our lives. Using the headings provided, fill in the incomplete sentences, trying not to censor any ideas that come to mind, even if the statements seem to be contradictory. After 10 to 15 minutes, ask the group to stop writing and look over their answers. On the newsprint pad, write down the men's and women's responses as they are shared.

Discussion: Which items on your list seem the most powerful or important to you? Which items are self-imposed? Which show family influences? Which items are similar for the men? For the women? Which items from the opposite sex surprised you the most? How might your roles be the same or different from roles of your parents? Which did you neglect, which did you emphasize? Which items are age specific for you right now?

Developmental
Activity Example 7-8
Exploring Sex Roles (continued)

Exploring Sex Roles Worksheet (Male)

If I were a woman, I could...

1.

2.

3.

4.

5.
Because I am a man, I must....

1.

2.

3.

4.

5.

Exploring Sex Roles Worksheet (Female)

If I were a man, I could...

1.

2.

3.

4.

5.
Because I am a woman, I must....

1.

2.

3.

4.

5.

From Cole, M. B. *Group Dynamics in Occupational Therapy, Second Edition.* © 1998 SLACK Incorporated.

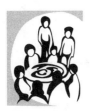

Developmental
Activity Example 7-9
Childhood Games and Occupational Choice

Margo Gross, MS, OTR/L, is acknowledged as the creator of this activity, which addresses one of the life tasks of Levinson's early and middle adult transitions.

Materials: Worksheets and pencils.

Directions: Children from a young age, until they are well into adolescence, spend much of their free time in some form of play. Make a list of 10 childhood games that you remember playing. Think about games you played alone, and ones you played informally with peers. Include both indoor and outdoor games, fantasy and make-believe, as well as group games and sports.

After you complete the list, analyze each game by placing next to it the symbols which best apply. Then apply these same symbols to your current occupation.

Discussion: What are the similarities and differences between your childhood play and current occupation? Consider whether your present occupation involves the characteristics of play that you enjoyed the most. Have you accepted or rejected aspects of yourself that you value and want to be a part of your life today?

Childhood Games and Occupational Choice (continued)

Childhood Games and Current Occupation Worksheet

Name:

Job title of current or most recent occupation:

List 10 childhood games you remember playing (before the age of 15):

1.

2.

3.

4.

5.

6.

7.

8.

9.

10.

After you complete the list, analyze each game by placing next to it the symbols which best apply:

M—Male oriented
F—Female oriented
U—Unstructured
S—Structured
A—Played alone
G—Played with others/groups
Ab—Abstract, fantasy oriented
C—Concrete, reality oriented
O—Objects or props necessary
M—Imagined or mentally created

Now apply these same symbols to your current occupation.

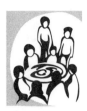

Developmental
Activity Example 7-10
Reminiscence

Life review has a place in almost every developmental theory addressing the older adult. Erikson, Jung, and Levinson all define some form of re-evaluation of the meaning of one's life as its end draws nearer. Reminiscence is a review of past experiences, with a goal of establishing a sense of integrity and satisfaction with oneself through the process of remembering. Drawing, writing, and storytelling are creative ways to assist members in recalling their specific experiences. Once written or drawn, members should share through discussion. Some suggested themes are:

- Specific years or events: The Great Depression, World War II, The 50s, The 60s.
- What were you doing when…Pearl Harbor was bombed? Franklin D. Roosevelt died?
- What was the most difficult period in your life?
- When did you get your first car? First house?
- Describe your first date. First job. First child.
- Describe your first encounter with death (relative, close friend).
- What was your proudest moment?
- Whom do you admire most in your family?
- What values would you choose to leave to your children? To society?
- Bring in favorite music/songs from the past and discuss their significance.

It should be noted that reminiscence does not restore memory for persons who have cognitive deficits. However, persons with mild or moderate dementia often retain remote memories, and discussing these in groups can help them re-establish a sense of normal social functioning.

Chapter 8

Sensory Motor Approaches

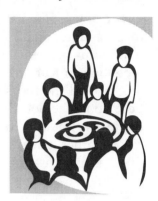

The sensory motor approaches are being used as a broad category which addresses sensory motor, perceptual, and cognitive problems due to brain dysfunction. Treatment in this frame, according to Trombly (1989), is aimed at promoting redevelopment of these abilities based on principles of neurophysiology. "When the treatment of these losses follows a developmental sequence and techniques reflect anatomical, functional, or behavioral reorganization in the central nervous system, the approach is called neurodevelopmental"(Trombly, 1989, p. 39). However, because the name "neurodevelopmental" is often associated with Bobath's approach (NDT) specifically, the title of this chapter has been changed to reflect a broader group of sensory motor approaches.

Focus

For occupational therapy, the primary use of this frame of reference has been with developmental disabilities affecting the central nervous system and those who have suffered trauma or disease to the central nervous system, such as stroke or traumatic brain injury. However, recent studies of the brain have linked neurophysiological abnormalities and central nervous system dysfunction to mental disorders as well. Applying neurodevelopmental principles of treatment with the geriatric population is increasing and shows promising results. Occupational therapy groups using this frame of reference should use activities that stimulate the senses, produce purposeful movement, promote cognition, and affect the central nervous system in a systematic way.

Basic Assumptions

This frame of reference encompasses many theorists (and techniques), among them Rood, Bobath, Brunnstrom, and Ayres, and proprioceptive neuromuscular facilitation (PNF). These approaches are not necessarily intended to be used with groups, however, the principles of treatment can be applied when planning group activities. Examples of occupational therapy group treatment approaches using these theories are reviewed, including the writings of King, Ross, and Levy. Central to all of these approaches is the assumption that rehabilitation of perceptual, sensory motor, and cognitive disorders follows a developmental sequence. All of the theorists agree on the importance of sensation in this process and the importance of repetition to learning. Disagreement centers around the focus of conscious attention. Rood, the Bobaths, and Ayres believe the focus should be on the goal of movement, rather than the movement itself. There is also disagreement about the role of primitive reflexes. Brunnstrom fosters the conscious use of reflexes to elicit movement in the disabled adult, while the Bobath approach actively inhibits reflexes (Trombly, 1979).

Rood

Margaret Rood's work preceded most of the other theorists covered in this chapter, and her ideas seem to have inspired many of the concepts of sensory integration developed later. Rood was the first to focus on the importance of reflexes. She states, "Motor patterns are developed from fundamental reflex patterns present at birth which are utilized and gradually modified through sensory stimuli until the highest control is gained on the conscious cortical level. It seemed to me then, that if it were possible to apply the proper sensory stimuli to the appropriate sensory receptor as it is utilized in normal sequential development, it might be possible to elicit motor responses reflexly and by following neurophysiological principles, establish proper motor engrams" (1954). Rood's theory has four basic components:

1. Sensory input is required for normalization of tone and evocation of desired muscular responses

2. Sensory motor control is developmentally based
3. Movement is purposeful
4. Repetition of movement is necessary for learning

Most occupational therapists recognize Rood's techniques of facilitation and inhibition. Light stroking, brushing, icing, and joint compression are used to facilitate movement. Joint approximation (light compression), neutral warmth, pressure on tendon insertion, and slow rhythmical movement are used to inhibit unwanted movement. Rood recommended the facilitation of normal movement in a developmental sequence. First, phasic reciprocal contraction, such as flexion to extension and back, are practiced repeatedly until learned. Next, stabilization through co-contraction of major muscle groups is facilitated. A third phase combines these, practicing movement imposed on stabilization, and a final phase incorporates the development of skilled movement.

This early theorist identified eight ontogenetic motor patterns as follows:
1. Supine withdrawal
2. Segmental rolling
3. Pivot prone (prone extension)
4. Neck co-contraction
5. Supporting self on elbows
6. All fours movement patterns
7. Standing
8. Walking

This sequence gives occupational therapists some very specific guidelines for planning movement activities for patients with neurodevelopmental disorders. When planning group treatment, each patient's unique developmental level with respect to movement needs to be carefully considered. Movement groups can be set up at many levels, but should progress from earlier to later stages in the ontogenetic sequence. Patients should not be asked to perform movements at higher levels than they are capable. Positioning is a primary concern, especially at the lower levels. It may involve the extensive use of mats, bolsters, beach balls, or other specialized equipment.

Many games can be devised that involve pushing and pulling, throwing and catching, rolling and creeping to move the body from one place to another. These activities should be set up to incorporate the correct therapeutic movement sequences for each patient, while the patients are participating in goal-directed activities.

The Bobaths

Dr. and Mrs. Bobath are a neurologist and a physiotherapist from England who originated the therapeutic technique best known as "neurodevelopmental therapy," or NDT (Bobath, 1972). One of their most important contributions to theory is their focus on sensory motor learning. It is not movement itself, but the sensation of movement that is learned and remembered. Much of the Bobaths' work was done on children with cerebral palsy and adult stroke patients. The techniques are widely known and used, but little researched, according to Trombly (1989). Following their focus on sensation, their handling of children with cerebral palsy and subsequently of adults with hemiplegia concentrated on repetition of correct motor responses. The assumption is that when patients experience normal movement, this results in correct sensory feedback to the central nervous system. NDT involves teaching the patient how correct movement feels (Trombly, 1989). To this end, great effort is made to inhibit primitive reflexes through "reflex inhibiting patterns"(RIPs) (Trombly, 1989, p. 113), and to elicit righting and equilibrium responses.

In NDT, sensory stimulation is regulated with great care. Weight bearing, placing and holding, tapping, and joint compres-

sion are used to activate normal movement and posture. However, these stimuli are withdrawn as soon as an abnormal response occurs. In hemiplegia, sensory deficits are interpreted as an indication of poor prognosis for regaining normal control of movement. Stress is avoided, since it is thought to promote abnormal tone and movement.

After stroke or head trauma, the sequence of relearning movement approximates normal development. Compensatory movement such as practicing dressing or feeding is discouraged because it results in increased spasticity and inactivity of the involved side. Recovery from stroke and trauma generally involves a flaccid stage followed by a spastic stage. Many specific exercises and handling are suggested in each of these stages following the developmental process. These involve positioning, weight bearing, holding and placing, balance reactions, and protective extension, among others. Trombly (1989) suggests a good source of both individual and group activities based on the Bobath NDT approach is Egger's *Occupational Therapy in the Treatment of Adult Hemiplegia* (1983).

Brunnstrom

Unlike the other theorists so far, Signe Brunnstrom took an opposite view of the use of reflexes. Her basic assumption was that as normal development progresses, spinal cord and brainstem reflexes become modified and their components rearranged into purposeful movement through the central nervous system. Therefore, reflexes can and should be used to elicit movement where none exists as part of a normal sequence (Trombly, 1989). Both proprioceptive (resistive) and exteroceptive (tactile) stimuli are used to elicit reflexes, and the patient is encouraged to think about the movement that results and try to gain control of that movement.

The Brunnstrom approach seeks to elicit associated reactions and synergies. Resistive stimuli are believed to achieve both reflexive movement on the non-involved side, for example, and similar synergistic movement on the involved side. A synergy is defined as the total flexion or extension movement of a joint or limb.

Six stages of recovery are defined by Brunnstrom for the upper and lower extremity. Generally these are:

1. Flaccidity, no voluntary movement
2. Synergies or minimal voluntary movement
3. Synergies performed voluntarily
4. Some deviation from synergy
5. Independent or isolated movement
6. Individual joint movement nearly normal with minimal spasticity

These are specifically defined, and interested students are encouraged to read about specific assessment and treatment techniques in Brunnstrom's *Movement Therapy in Hemiplegia* (1970).

Proprioceptive Neuromuscular Facilitation

The PNF approach, developed by neurophysiologist Herman Kabat, PhD, MD, uses proprioceptor stimulation to hasten the response and recovery of neuromuscular mechanisms. The theory has been developing since the early 1940s, and has had many esteemed contributors, including Sherrington, Gessell, and Pavlov. Diagonal and spiraling patterns of movement were identified to parallel functional movement such as that used in sports.

PNF literature states 11 basic principles (Trombly, 1989):

1. All human beings have potentials that are not fully developed.
2. Normal motor development proceeds in a cervico-caudal and proximodistal direction.
3. Early motor learning is dominated by reflex activity. Mature motor behavior is reinforced or supported by postural reflex mechanisms.
4. The growth of motor behavior has cyclic trends as evidenced by shifts between flexor and extensor dominance.
5. Goal-directed activity is made up of reversing movements.
6. Normal movement and posture are dependent upon "synergism" and a balanced interaction of antagonists.
7. Developing motor behavior is expressed in an orderly sequence of total patterns of movement and posture.
8. Normal motor development has an orderly sequence but lacks a step-by-step quality. Overlapping occurs.
9. Improvement of motor ability is dependent upon motor learning.
10. Frequency of stimulation and repetition of activity are used to promote retention of motor learning and the development of strength and endurance.
11. Goal-directed activities, coupled with techniques of facilitation, are used to hasten learning of total patterns of walking and of self-care activities.

The PNF techniques involve two diagonal patterns of movement for every major part of the body: head, neck, trunk, and extremities. These patterns combine the simplest movements: abduction, adduction, internal/external rotation, and crossing the midline. The patterns are unilateral and bilateral, symmetrical and asymmetrical, and total body movements. All functional movements are related to these patterns, which are learned and relearned through repetition. The techniques are similar to Brunnstrom in that they encourage the patient to think about the movement and assist the therapist, often using auditory commands: "Look up! Swing down! Help me move you!" (Trombly, 1989). These techniques are specifically described in Trombly (1989), and the interested student is referred to this text for a more in-depth description.

Groups using the principles of PNF as well as other neurodevelopmental theories may be designed with patients who have achieved a fair degree of voluntary movement. Exercise groups, movement to music, and simple games are best suited to these patients, many of whom are likely to have language and cognitive problems as well.

Ayres

A. Jean Ayres is best known for her contributions to the theory of sensory integration. This approach assumes that the central nervous system organizes and integrates sensory stimuli to produce an adaptive response. Ayres refers to the normal developmental sequence in her study of the use of sensory input. She suggests four levels of the sensory integrative process.

Primary Level

At this level, Ayres identifies the three basic sensory systems as vestibular, proprioceptive, and tactile. Visual and auditory are acknowledged but not thought to play a major integrative role in this early stage. Touch is cited as the basis for the infant's first emotional bond with mother. The processing of these initial touch sensations is seen to be responsible for establishing a basic sense of security.

The proprioceptive and vestibular senses offer another kind of basic security: gravitational security. These help the child develop balance for standing and walking and prevents the fear of falling. This level includes the eye movements, posture, balance, muscle tone, and gravitational security all resulting from the vestibular and proprioceptive integration. Sucking, eat-

ing, the mother-child bond, and tactile comfort are seen as the result of integration of tactile sensations.

Second Level

At this level, the three basic senses are integrated into a body percept, coordination of the two sides of the body, motor planning, attention span, activity level, and emotional stability. Sensory information from vestibular, proprioceptive, and tactile receptors are used to form percepts, or maps of the body which are stored in the brain. With this mechanism, one is constantly aware of where his body is and what it is doing. This percept has information about right and left sides of the body, which allow the two sides to work bilaterally to accomplish tasks. The percept also allows a person to plan motor actions (i.e., catching a ball or feeding himself). The organization of sensory input by the brain is also reflected in the ability to focus attention and adjust the level or pace of activity. Hyperactivity and hypoactivity and the inability to attend are thus explained by poor integration at the secondary level of sensory integration.

Third Level

Speech and language, eye-hand coordination, visual perception, and purposeful activity are possible at this level due to the impact of auditory and visual sensations. According to Ayres, the vestibular and auditory systems are intimately related. The vestibular system, as stated above, is responsible for the ability to attend to what is heard. Language comprehension likewise begins with the child's touching, moving, lifting, and otherwise interacting with the objects in his environment. Only through this experience can he begin to appreciate the unique properties of an object and know its name. Visual perception is also seen as an end product of earlier sensory integration: how big something is, how far away it is, and what its relationship is to other parts of the environment are all experienced first by reaching and touching. The visual experience is thus intimately related to the tactile and vestibular systems as well. With an understanding of what he hears and what he sees, the child's actions with respect to the environment can be purposeful. Visual sensation directs the child's hand to reach out to pet the kitten. He alters his posture to keep his balance as the kitten moves under his touch. The child hears the kitten purr and repeats the action. Visual, auditory, tactile, and vestibular systems all work together to help the child explore and learn about his environment.

Fourth Level

The fourth and final level of sensory integration includes the following end products: the ability to organize and concentrate, self-esteem, control and confidence, academic learning ability, capacity for abstract thought and reasoning, and development of dominance and hemispheric specialization. From Ayres' point of view, it does little good for occupational therapists to attempt to directly teach these skills when the earlier stages of integration are not adequately developed.

Skilled voluntary fine motor hand movement, for example, cannot be taught to the disabled child by giving practice exercises. Ayres describes the development of hand movement as a sequence of many steps:

1. Control of neck and eye movements
2. Trunk stability and balance
3. Scapular and shoulder stability and movement
4. Elbow motion
5. Gross grasp
6. Wrist positioning and movement
7. Release of grasp

8. Forearm supination and pronation
9. Individual finger manipulation

Overlapping this sequence is the coordination of visual and sensory motor mechanisms. Movements begin as spinal reflexes and are modified and refined to achieve a behavioral goal. In this way, reflex movement becomes voluntary. Regarding the role of sensation in this process, Ayres (1979) states two basic assumptions:

1. "Reflex movements (which) are the precursor to and the foundation of voluntary movement...are elicited by sensory stimuli."
2. "Ongoing motor learning and behavior are strongly influenced by if not dependent on incoming sensation."

She further reflects that although reflex movement can be elicited by direct stimulation, voluntary movement must be purposeful. A great deal has been written about sensory integrative function, and the reader is referred to A. Jean Ayres' *The Development of Sensory Integrative Theory and Practice* and *Sensory Integration and the Child* for a more in-depth discussion (Figure 8-1). An updated version of sensory integration theory by Fisher and Bundy is entitled *Sensory Integration: Theory and Practice* (1991).

Group Approaches

King

While most of the research of Ayres and her associates applies to children, several occupational therapists have written about the treatment of mentally ill adults using neurodevelopmental and sensory integrative techniques. The best known of these is Lorna Jean King, who pioneered the use of sensory integration approaches with chronic schizophrenic adults.

Lorna Jean King has noted the lack of sensory integration in both schizophrenic and autistic patients by observing the

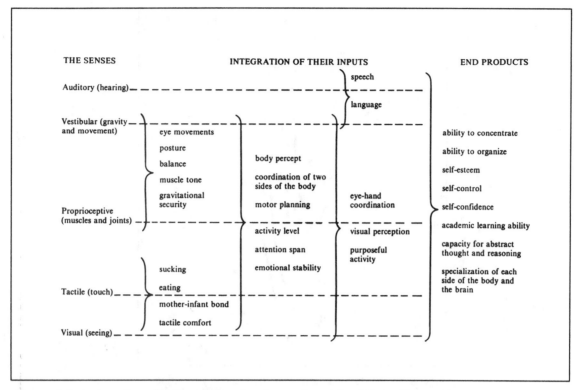

THE SENSES

Auditory (hearing)

Vestibular (gravity and movement)

Proprioceptive (muscles and joints)

Tactile (touch)

Visual (seeing)

INTEGRATION OF THEIR INPUTS

speech

language

eye movements
posture
balance
muscle tone
gravitational security

body percept
coordination of two sides of the body
motor planning

activity level
attention span
emotional stability

eye-hand coordination

visual perception
purposeful activity

sucking
eating
mother-infant bond
tactile comfort

END PRODUCTS

ability to concentrate
ability to organize
self-esteem
self-control
self-confidence
academic learning ability
capacity for abstract thought and reasoning
specialization of each side of the body and the brain

Figure 8-1. A. Jean Ayres sensory integration theory. Copyright 1979 by Western Psychological Services. Reprinted from *Sensory Integration and the Child* by permission of the publisher, Western Psychological Services, 12031 Wilshire Blvd., Los Angeles, CA 90025.

kinds of sensory stimulation they seek from the environment. For example, she evaluates a retarded and autistic adolescent by observing his preference for vibratory input (plays with a hand-held vibrator), proprioceptive input (constant self-hugging), and calming vestibular input (distractible and disruptive behavior is reduced by slow swinging and rocking) (Larrington, 1987).

Paul Schilder noted as early as the 1930s that schizophrenic patients are markedly underreactive to vestibular stimulation as measured by postrotary nystagmus (rapid eye movements) (King, 1974). King linked the vestibular system abnormalities with the postural and movement limitations (pacing, adduction, and internal rotation) observed in the chronic process schizophrenic patient, more currently called the negative symptom schizophrenic (Figure 8-2). Process schizophrenia is a subtype of

schizophrenia, a mental disorder which develops insidiously from childhood and is not the result of a severe or recognizable stress. Process schizophrenics do not respond readily to medical or behavioral treatment, and so tend to be chronically institutionalized.

King refers to numerous studies of the neurological deficits in schizophrenia (and also autism) which link faulty vestibular and proprioceptive processing to schizophrenic symptoms. Some of these symptoms include perceptual deficits, feelings of fatigue and slow movement, postural insecurity (fear of falling), concrete thinking, and lack of emotional response. King's hypothesis is that some schizophrenic patients have "defective proprioceptive feedback mechanisms, the vestibular component in particular being underreactive in its role in the sensory motor integration" (King, 1974, p. 534).

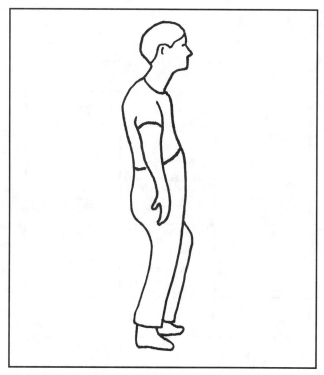

Figure 8-2. Postural abnormalities due to faulty propriocep-tive feedback in the person with process schizophrenia (flex-ion, adduction, internal rotation).

Considering today's emphasis on the biochemical etiology of all mental illness (including schizophrenia), King's postula-tions of the circular role of movement in altering biochemical states as well as bio-chemistry affecting movement remains timely. Movement and sensation are known to produce chemical changes just as taking medication produces changes in brain chemistry. Furthermore, King states that "This model...applies not only to eti-ology but also to treatment. Although we cannot be sure which chemicals to alter, or in what direction, we can intervene in the motor behavior of the individual with the knowledge that there will be affects upon the thought processes and upon biochem-istry" (1974, p. 534). In later publications, King notes the role of activities in coping with stress. A strenuous action, or "fight or flight" response to stress (Gal and Lazarus, 1975), was found to be responsi-ble for the rapid metabolism of stress hor-mones, thus preventing secondary dam-age to the system. This suggests that stren-uous or heavy work activity can serve to normalize the neurotransmitter balance which has been deranged by stress (King, 1978, 1988).

The treatment techniques King utilizes in treating groups of chronic schizo-phrenic patients are adaptations of the techniques Ayres used with children. They are gross motor movement activities aimed at normalizing patterns of excessive flexion, adduction and internal rotation, and increasing range of motion. Vestibular and tactile stimulation are provided through the use of the standard props—hammocks, scooter boards, balls, and blankets. Heavy work patterns suggested by Rood in King (1974) resisted use of tonic muscle groups, and co-contraction patterns are also incorporated. Other equipment King has added are para-chutes, balloons, and beanbag chairs.

King suggests two criteria for the selection of activities:

1. Attention must not be centered upon the motor process, but rather on the object or outcome
2. The activity must be pleasurable and evoke smiles, laughter, and a feeling of fun

Patients should not have to think about what they are doing or how they move; the goal is to elicit spontaneous movement and affect. Vestibular and proprioceptive processing occur at the brainstem level and produce automatic responses, not cortical (voluntary) responses. Therefore, if a ball is thrown to a patient and his hands extend spontaneously to catch it, we can assume that this automatic action reflects adaptive vestibular processing at the brainstem level. The goal of group activities using this frame of reference is to stimulate the sensory processing systems so that they will function more adaptively. As occupational therapists, we see spontaneous and purposeful motor responses as evidence that we are reaching that goal.

Ross

Mildred Ross further developed the use of sensory integrative theory and techniques with the chronic population. She extended the use of the sensory integration approach to the elderly, the neurologically impaired, the Alzheimer's patient, the mentally retarded, and the long-term chronic patient of any age with disabilities that prevent adequate functioning in the community (Ross, 1997). Ross developed her group techniques over more than 15 years of clinical experience. Her group sessions occur in five stages, which move developmentally from alerting activities involving tactile, kinesthetic, and proprioceptive input to graded opportunities for organized cognitive thought and behavior. The following is a summary of Ross' five-stage groups.

Stage I

Stage I acknowledges the presence of each member to every other member of the group. Introductions or saying names can easily accomplish this. The purpose of the session is established by the therapist or group members in Stage I and this orients members to the session. Explanations should be kept brief and on a level the members can understand. The attention of members should be captured in Stage I.

Stage II

Stage II provides maximum exertion in movement. A variety of gross motor movement is suggested here, incorporating all three planes: horizontal, vertical, and sagittal. Exercise, dance patterns, or games may be adapted for this stage. Pleasure, communication, and interaction or "cohesiveness" are possible goals. The effect of this stage is to stimulate or excite.

Stage III

Stage III emphasizes perceptual-motor skills. Activities may be chosen that require less vigorous movement and more judgment and focus action to accomplish a purposeful task. Making a fruit salad or drawing a picture are examples. The activities should be short-term and able to be finished in 30 minutes or less. This stage should have the effect of calming and focusing.

Stage IV

Stage IV is the time for cognitive stimulation. A discussion of the previous stages, memory games, or poetry reading are suggested by Ross. "This is the opportunity for cortical controls to be demonstrated through organized behavior such as impulse control or creative expression. It is the highest point for display of attentiveness and group cohesiveness" (Ross, 1997). The length of this stage may be changed depending on the activity chosen and the level and interest of the group. Music or current events discussion may take a major portion of the time, while a short inspiring poem may take less than 5 minutes. Preparation for closure should be kept in mind in selecting activities for this stage.

Stage V

Stage V provides resolution and termination. A way to say goodbye, when to meet next, or suggestions of what to do next time might serve as endings. When the therapist feels that the group was good, it may be appropriate to verbalize this in summarizing. Statements of satisfaction with the group by the therapist and patients can achieve a sense of peacefulness at its end.

Role of the Therapist

Using Ross' stages, the therapist plans and leads the activity, guided by knowledge of the principles of sensory motor integration and activity analysis, but taking her cues from the group as well. The occupational therapist must be quite skilled to lead this kind of group effectively, keeping control while gently encouraging members to get involved. The stages provide a clear structure around which to plan appropriate activities. In her book, *Integrative Group Therapy,* Ross offers excellent guidelines for "considering when an activity should be introduced and how it should be presented" (1997).

Levy

Linda Levy (1974) provides another example of the use of the sensory motor frames of reference. Levy uses Piaget's sensory motor stage as her guide. Piaget asserts that in normal development, a child progresses through a series of stages which culminate in a mature understanding of reality (Piaget, 1954). Adult psychotic patients, Levy states, mirror the characteristics of these stages. Mosey called this process the recapitulation of ontogeny (i.e., remission from psychosis is a replay of the original developmental process).

Several disorganized patients, Levy reports, have reverted to Piaget's earliest stage of learning, the sensory motor stage (learning through movement). Four of the six stages that Piaget conceptualizes can serve as guidelines for occupational therapy groups (Figure 8-3). The following is a summary of Levy's four-stage movement groups.

Stage 1 (Birth to 1 Month)

In the beginning, the infant depends on reflex movement. Functional assimilation means the infant uses his available movements to perform a function (e.g., sucking the breast). Generalizing assimilation occurs when the infant uses the same movement in new situations (i.e., sucking a bottle or pacifier).

The occupational therapist can make contact with even the most regressed patient through movement. At Stage 1, using kinesthetic cues (touching and moving body parts), the therapist can use the patient's available schemata (e.g., rocking) to begin to explore new situations (e.g., swaying, swinging). Almost any gross motor pattern displayed by the patient can be extended and generalized to new situations with the occupational therapist's guidance.

Stage 2 (1 to 4 Months)

Here the infant is interested in new movement patterns and tends to repeat those movements that bring pleasurable responses. The occupational therapist can imitate the patient's movement patterns and help the patient establish a consistent sequence of movement, such as rocking, walking, or running. This introduces a time sequence. Repetitive movement patterns can be applied to simplified sports,

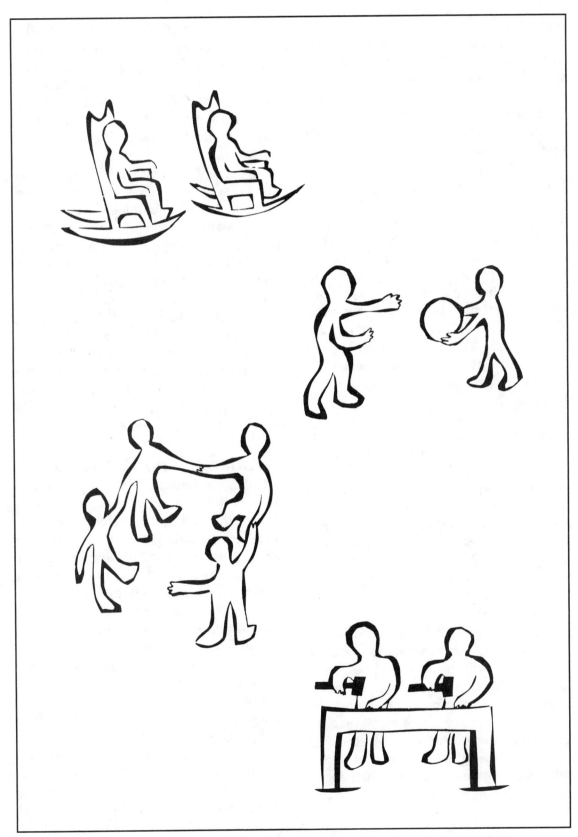

Figure 8-3. Guidelines for movement activities (Piaget's sensory motor stages from Levy, 1974).

such as balloon volleyball, shuffleboard, basketball, or games of catch. Movements that are habitual and reflexive in Stage 2 should be associated with a consistent result (e.g., the ball is caught and returned, the basketball goes through the hoop and bounces). The causal effect of movement is thus conveyed.

Stage 3 (4 to 10 Months)

The infant looks for the effect of his actions on the external environment. For example, he may kick and discover that he makes his cradle rock. In Stage 3, imitative exercise is appropriate, so the patient practices matching his movements to that of a model. Simple dance patterns and sequences are useful in groups at this stage, as long as they incorporate familiar movements. This stage is a precursor to the patient learning new skills through imitation.

Stage 4 (9 to 12 Months)

The infant can imitate model behaviors. When the mother pushes the teddy bear's stomach, it squeaks, so the infant tries it too. He imitates the action even if it does not have the same effect. When new learning becomes possible, the patient can apply his new skills to the more traditional task activities available in the occupational therapy clinic.

The sensory motor stages described are thought to be necessary to precede mature cognition. The infant begins to elaborate on the basic dimensions of space, time, and causality and relates them to movements. In this approach, Levy uses the development of the infant as a guide for planning motor activities that stimulate growth in the adult with mental illness who does not demonstrate normal cognitive functioning.

Function and Dysfunction

In the sensory motor frames of reference, functioning is adequate when a person is able to learn and use all of the adaptive skills characteristic of her age. Since there is assumed to be a sequence of neurological and physiological development, dysfunction can be defined as a lag in development causing the patient to function below her age level. An adult is dysfunctional when neurological or physiological malfunctioning interferes with normal daily activity and a normal course of life development. This view of dysfunction in any illness encourages the identification of a physical cause. Even mental illness, as King and Levy have discussed, can respond to a NDT approach which follows the guidelines of early development. In using movement and games, the patient's active participation is encouraged to produce an adaptive response in activities that are purposeful.

Change and Motivation

Change in sensory motor functioning is thought to be brought about through several methods. Physical activity can produce change through its effect on muscle tone, muscle strength, and range of motion. Physical activity has also been shown to produce chemical changes; this is how the "runner's high" has been explained. During occupational therapy activities, change in brain and body function can be brought about through sensory stimulation and repetition of movement.

It must be remembered in this frame that change occurs in a specific sequence, and progresses stage by stage up the hierarchy toward maturity. In an illness that has left patients without normal movement patterns and sensory processing skills, a baseline level must be established through careful sensory motor assessment. Then, through a repetition of the developmental sequence, sensory and motor components of activity can be utilized by the occupational therapist in such a way as to facilitate subcortical learning. Automatic movement and postural responses will precede more advanced cognitive responses. The changes we look for in the sensory motor frames can often be seen as spontaneous self-corrections, such as an increased state of alertness or a more functional body posture. These normalized neurological states can then serve as building blocks for working on more skilled purposeful movements and the use of language in interactions within groups.

As Ross points out, activities we offer patients can have powerful effects on the central nervous system. These effects can be both positive and negative. Activities should be carefully planned to approach the central nervous system in a way that it can accept and handle, and to do so in a way that facilitates positive change. The occupational therapist does this through control and limitation of sensory input (Ross, 1997).

Motivation comes in the form of accepting the challenge to be a more active participant in life. Patients, after illness or injury, may be motivated to go back to work and to do things the way they used to. The lack of motivation comes when they expect too much change too fast, and therefore they feel they have failed. With long-term physical dysfunction, patients may be unable to modify their goals or accept new methods for meeting their needs. Chronic illness may leave patients without hope. When cognitive impairment accompanies the physical or emotional dysfunction, long-term goals may no longer be understood. The spontaneous urge to advance one's development must often be rekindled after illness. Interventions such as sensory stimulation and movement play can encourage the chronic patient to have more active participation with others and the environment. Once success or pleasure is experienced, patients may be more motivated.

Group Treatment

King, Ross, and Levy, already cited, have given some helpful guidelines on how to structure groups. Gross motor activities are the common element. While movement activities are used extensively with pediatrics and physical dysfunction populations, movement is too often overlooked as an effective media for psychosocial dysfunction and geriatrics. As occupational therapists, we need to expand our repertoire of tools to include more activities involving movement. Much of our training in physiology, neuroanatomy, and sensory motor integration prepares us well for doing so. Perhaps our level of comfort in using movement with our patients is not as high as it could be. Often occupational therapists need to be comfortable with their own ability to move and play before they are able to share this with patients.

Role of the Occupational Therapist

In the sensory motor frames, the occupational therapist is a directive leader. The therapist needs a fairly thorough knowledge of neurodevelopment, neurophysiology, and sensory integration in order to lead these groups competently. In most cases, patients we are working with are at low levels of functioning. Often verbal communication is at a minimum, and it is through imitation and role modeling that our patients perform activities therapeutically. The occupational therapist plans movement, sensory, or cognitive activities that match their level and are relatively sure to succeed. The concept of the "just right challenge" applies here. Activities should interest and challenge the patients, but should not be so complex as to overwhelm them. In movement groups as described by King, Ross, and Levy, the occupational therapist is the undeniable leader. She comes prepared with equipment and ideas and guides the group from start to finish, taking cues from patients as needed along the way.

Neurodevelopmentally based movement groups can be effective with some higher cognitive level populations as well. When this is done, care should be taken to explain the purpose thoroughly so that patients understand how the exercises and movements will help them.

Goals

Some of the goals mentioned by the various theorists may be summarized as follows.

1. Provide sensory stimulation and opportunities for adaptive response. The patient will develop skill in sensory motor performance and strengthen normal sensory motor integration.
2. Improve and maintain muscle tone, posture, and motor planning. The patient will demonstrate these successfully during participation in activities.
3. Motivate the patient to participate. The patient will respond to stimulation by imitating or initiating activity.
4. Facilitate the development of higher level cognitive skills through the integration and assimilation of lower level skills. The patient will demonstrate higher level skills through participation in activity.
5. Achieve a sense of mastery and well-being. The patient will demonstrate positive affective responses during participation in activity.

Specific goals for individual patients may be easily set and measured. All of the goals may be worked on appropriately through the use of group activities.

Examples of Activities

Movement activities of all types may be adapted in this frame of reference, from simple calisthenics to dance and sports to laying bricks and digging in the garden. When working with adult populations, the therapist must be careful not to make the activities seem too childish.

New Games

One particularly rich source of activities which are adaptable is the handbook of the New Games Foundation (Fluegelman, 1976). The New Games Foundation is an organization that originated at San Francisco State College in 1966 as a resistance to the Vietnam War. The group was against any type of competition, even in sports, so they designed games that provided opportunities for individuals to express aggressiveness without anyone winning or losing. The games were designed for all ages and levels of activity, and since 1974, every few years they publish yet another book of newly invented games; see Activity Examples 8-1 and 8-2.

Parachute Games

King suggests parachute play as effective for spontaneous range of motion and postural correction as well as vestibular-proprioceptive stimulation (Figure 8-4). A real parachute (with no strings) works best and can be obtained in surplus stores or sports equipment supply catalogs.

Parachute games (Activity Example 8-3) are rich in sensory motor integration potential. The basic movement involved requires reaching high above the head, an extension of the shoulders, elbows, and wrists to the full range of motion. The head tends to roll back as the patient looks

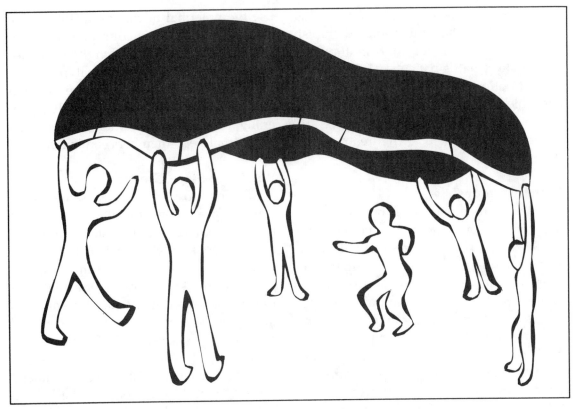

Figure 8-4. Parachute play.

at the effect of his movement, the parachute rising high in the air. Lowering the parachute to below the knee requires the patient to flex the spine forward at the waist and to extend the head forward, again following the movement of the parachute. The motion of the head and joints provides both proprioceptive and vestibular stimulation. Other movements may also be analyzed in this manner to aid in treatment planning to meet specific goals.

Bioenergetic Groups

These are groups aimed at the expression of feelings through movement. The major spokesman for this approach to movement is Alexander Lowen. Lowen's bioenergetic exercises were developed from his bioenergetic theory of personality, which is understood in terms of the body and its energetic processes (Lowen &

Lowen, 1977). More recently, Lowen's workshops have been offered as an extension of the myofascial release therapy workshops given by John Barnes, a physical therapist. Bioenergetic exercises can offer occupational therapists guidelines in the use of breathing and movement exercises to heighten emotional awareness and expression. Some of the bioenergetic exercises can release very powerful feelings, and should not be done without training. However, the basic concept is useful in planning expressive exercises in moderation. For further information about this approach, the reader is referred to Lowen's and Lowen's book *The Way to Vibrant Health* (1977).

The activity groups discussed in Activity Examples 8-4 and 8-5 are based on this concept, and have been used with adult psychiatric patients who are inhibited in the expression of feelings. In doing these activities, the occupational therapist should be careful not to overstimulate potentially volatile patients. The exercises should not be done with patients who are excitable or at risk for violent behavior. These neurophysiological techniques are especially well suited to the treatment of depression.

Exercise Groups

Exercise to music or dance activities has good potential as a therapeutic tool. Circle or group dancing is usually best suited to our purpose in occupational therapy. In physical disability areas where goals involve maintaining and increasing strength and range of motion, group activities that accomplish these goals are more enjoyable and motivating than individual exercise programs. A good example of this type of group is the "Range of Motion Dance," an exercise program for patients with rheumatoid arthritis developed by Diane Harlowe and Patricia Yu at St. Mary's Hospital Medical Center in Madison, Wisconsin (Van Deusen & Harlowe, 1987). This guided fantasy may be done with groups of patients seated in chairs. The exercises, while following the story, go systematically through the range of motion for nearly every joint in the body. Once the sequence of motions is learned, it can be repeated by the patients at home by listening to the story on an audiotape. Greenfield and Godinez have introduced a similar group for stroke patients, called "Self Range of Motion Exercises" (Greenfield & Godinez, 1989). They have defined eight skill levels for these exercises, ranging from complete dependence on the therapist leader to independence in performing the exercises.

In doing such groups, it is important to use the potential of the group to provide mutual support, encouragement, and feedback. Do not let the activity speak for itself; combine it with verbal reinforcement, progress checks, and education about how and why it is helping. It is generally the social and emotional aspects of a group that keep members coming back.

Ross' Five-Stage Groups

Mildred Ross gives us a sequence of specific guidelines for the selection of activities. Since the five-stage group is designed for severely impaired and chronic populations, movement and sensory stimulation are the key elements of activity. "A routine of organized sequences enhances the likelihood of an automatic habitual response" (Ross, 1997, p. 2). The purpose of the five separate, organized sequences is to motivate interaction with the environment. Sensory stimulation produces the heightened arousal and alertness to one's surroundings that maximizes the potential for adaptive responses. The outcome must be calm alertness that makes adults ready to move on, in an organized way, to the next activity of the day.

Table 8-1 may be useful in creating and modifying activities to help accommodate and manage the behaviors that emerge during the five-stage group.

Activity Examples 8-6 and 8-7 suggest specific organized sequences. In Ross' book *Integrative Group Therapy*, many other activity sequences are suggested. Another source of ideas for sensory integrative activities with adults is *Sensory Integration* by Vander Roest and Clements (1983). Because different populations have differences in their abilities to integrate sensory information, the examples given cover medium (Activity Example 8-6) and low (Activity Example 8-7) levels of sensory processing skill.

Table 8-1.
Adapting Ross' Five-Stage Groups: Alerting vs. Calming Sensory Stimuli

	Alerting	Calming
Environment	bright light, bright colors, high contrasts, loud sounds, rapid rhythms, uneven sounds	low light, pastel colors, similar hues, soft melodic sounds, slow even rhythms, closing one's eyes
Smell/Taste	pungent odors, cold/hot foods/liquids, crunchy, strong flavors	sweet or herbal smells, smooth textures, mild flavor, temperate foods
Touch/Movement	light touch, sudden touch, rapid movement, rotation or changing direction, jumping/hitting/clapping	steady moderate pressure, slow rhythmic movement, vibration, slowly rotating movement, holding on, hugging

Neurodevelopmental Therapy Groups with Handicapped Children

Sophie Levitt (1982) suggests therapeutic group work using a neurodevelopmental approach for children with cerebral palsy and motor delay. Both play groups and structured groups are seen as more effective than individual treatment for several reasons. The group often curtails rebellion and encourages cooperation. Children imitate other children and often instruct each other in doing what is required. Children seem to be able to concentrate longer with the stimulation of the group setting (1 to 1.5 hours as opposed to 20 minutes individually, Levitt reports) more than twice as long. Levitt emphasizes the interdisciplinary nature of these groups. Occupational and physical therapists, nurses, speech therapists, and teachers all contribute to planning and implementing the activity.

In groups with handicapped children, it is not useful to group by diagnosis. Children should be selected for the groups according to their functional problems. The basis of selection may be motor problems, such as poor grasp and release, poor balance, or recurring abnormal movement patterns or postures. The developmental or cognitive level of group members should be similar. Some children who are too severely involved to be aware of the group may not be appropriate. The selected group should be capable of working together and establishing a degree of group spirit. The specific activities should be selected according to the deficits of the members (Levitt, 1982).

It is evident that adults as well as children should be treated in groups of similar developmental level, and that the same principles for selection and planning apply. It would be encouraging to see more groups of physically disabled adults treated in a manner that encourages interaction and takes advantage of general group dynamics principles.

Music in Sensory Motor Groups

The use of music in therapy groups has been mentioned briefly. Music has qualities that can both relax and invigorate; it can energize a group, distract it, or put it to sleep. The choice of music should be made with care; instrumental rather than vocal may be less distracting. The patients' level of stimulation should be closely monitored, as Ross suggests. Music can change the mood of the group, but the key is to do it gradually. The music should match the mood of the patients to begin with, and then change little by little, accompanied by appropriate movement activities. It can arouse emotion easily because it has an effect on the body and the mind. Selection of music may depend to a great extent on what you want to accomplish with the patient. With depressed patients, the therapist may want to energize them by playing music with a lively beat. Patients susceptible to anxiety might benefit more from slow, mellow rhythms and ballads that soothe the nerves. In any case, occupational therapists usually use music in combination with movement activities, and it is the activity that should remain the focus with the music providing an appropriate background.

Group Leadership

Introduction

In sensory motor groups, the explanation of purpose should match the patients' ability to understand it. The level of cognition is the most important factor, and this varies widely in groups using sensory motor approaches.

The warm-up is essential, and takes on a somewhat different emphasis here. The warm-up should prepare the members for the activity not only psychologically, but physiologically as well. As Ross has stressed, "There is a systematic way to approach the central nervous system"(1997). If members are unable to screen out non-essential sensory stimulation, they may be overloaded very quickly. With patient populations that are at risk for this, such as stroke and head trauma patients, autistic and developmentally delayed patients, and the chronic mentally ill, the warm-up can offer limited and gradually increasing stimuli to test the group for an acceptable level of sensory stimulation.

Likewise, with the physically ill, the warm-up may be used as a testing experience to determine what level of physical exercise can be tolerated. Naturally the occupational therapist has evaluated the patient members prior to the group planning, so she should already be aware of the limits of safety. However, patients' conditions will vary on a daily (or hourly) basis and changes need to be taken into account. Based on the warm-up, the timeframe or the activity itself may have to be modified.

Activity

The activities used will vary widely depending on the patient population. Sensory motor or cognitive-perceptual tasks are most common. Activities will generally address some aspect of neurological or physical functioning and will facilitate some kind of adaptive response. Unlike previously described frames of reference, there may be several short-term activities planned during each session. The activities are organized and sequenced according to neurophysiological theory, so that simpler sensory motor activities can build up to advanced, more complex activities. Likewise, high stimulation activities are followed by slower, more calming ones, so that the central nervous system does not get overstimulated. Timing depends on the endurance and attention span of members, and sessions can be relatively short, 30 to 50 minutes. Materials that facilitate movement, like mats, balls, props, and pillows, are often used. Craft activities or work activities that incorporate gross motor actions are also useful.

Sharing and Processing

Sharing in movement groups occurs within the bounds of the activity. Patients can observe each other's movements; the cognitive or symbolic meaning of the movement is really not the point, and therefore not necessary to share. Processing involves expressing feelings about the group and, when possible, should be done verbally. Verbal processing can reveal hidden resistances and bring out other problems patients have while participating in the activity, which are important to note.

Generalizing and Application

The principles learned are associated with the effects of activity or movement of various kinds on the body and the emotions. The knowledge of the therapist may be shared with the group, when appropriate, to facilitate this learning. For example, a group of depressed patients may notice that after the physical expression of anger and hostility, they feel more energy. The lesson in this is that expression of feeling is natural and healthy. The application is to find ways to express feeling without hurting others or otherwise getting into trouble.

Application, even with lower functioning patients, may involve learning to repeat a desired adaptive response. When movement activities result in spontaneous laughter, for example, the pleasure of this response may motivate the patient to repeat the movement that produced it. The neurodevelopmental response to movement activities tends to be spontaneous and not planned. As patients integrate new movement patterns into their repertoire, they will use them spontaneously at times outside of the group. The goal is to stimulate the development of higher level skills and more adaptive functioning in the patient's everyday life.

Neither generalization nor application need to be separate phases of the sensory motor group. The verbal summary is sufficient to reinforce this learning.

Bibliography

Ayres, A. J. (1979). *Sensory integration and the child.* Los Angeles: Western Psychological Services.

Ayres, A. J. (1979). *The development of sensory integrative theory and practice.* Dubuque, IA: Kendall Hunt.

Bobath, B. (1972). The neurodevelopmental approach to treatment. In P. Pearson (Ed.), *Physical Therapy Services in Developmental Disabilities.* Springfield, IL: Charles Thomas.

Brunnstrom, S. (1970). *Movement therapy in hemiplegia.* New York: Harper & Row.

Eggers, O. (1983). *Occupational therapy in the treatment of adult hemiplegia.* London: William Heinemann Medical Books.

Fisher, A., & Bundy, A. (1991). *Sensory integration: Theory and practice.* Philadelphia: F. A. Davis.

Fluegelman, A. (1976). *New Games Foundation. The New Games book.* Garden City, NY: Doubleday.

Gal, R., & Lazarus, R. S. (1975). The role of activity in anticipating and confronting stressful situations. *Journal of Human Stress, 4,* 4-20.

Greenfield, J. M., & Godinez, M. (1989, April 20). Stroke clients learn independence by leading their own therapy group. *OT Week.*

King, L. J. (1974). A sensory-integrative approach to schizophrenia. *American Journal of Occupational Therapy, 28*(9), 529-536.

King, L. J. (1978). Toward a science of adaptive responses (Slagle lecture). *American Journal of Occupational Therapy, 32*(7), 429-437.

King, L. J. (1988). Occupational therapy and neuropsychiatry. In S. Robertson (Ed.), *Mental Health Focus.* Rockville, MD: American Occupational Therapy Association.

King, L. J. (1990). Moving the body to change the mind: Sensory integration therapy in psychiatry. *Occupational Therapy Pract, 1*(4), 12-22.

Levitt, S. (1982). *Treatment of cerebral palsy and motor delay.* Boston: Blackwell Scientific Publications.

Levy, L. L. (1974). Movement therapy for psychiatric patients. *American Journal of Occupational Therapy, 28*(6), 354-357.

Llorens, L. (1984). Theoretical conceptualizations of occupational therapy: 1960-1982. *OT in Mental Health, 2,* 1-14.

Lowen, A., & Lowen, L. (1977). *The way to vibrant health.* New York: Harper and Row.

Piaget, J. (1954). *The construction of reality in the child.* New York: Basic Books.

Rood, M. S. (1954). Neurophysiological reactions as a basis for physical therapy. *Phys Ther Rev, 34,* 444-449.

Ross, M. (1997). *1997 integrative group therapy: Mobilizing coping abilities with the five-stage group.* Baltimore, MD: American Occupational Therapy Association.

Trombly, C. (1989). *Occupational therapy for physical dysfunction* (3rd ed.). Baltimore, MD: Williams and Wilkins.

Vander Roest, L., & Clements, S. (1983). *Sensory integration.* Grand Rapids, MI: South Kent Mental Health Services.

Van Deusen, J., & Harlowe, D. (1987). The efficacy of the ROM dance program for adults with rheumatoid arthritis. *American Journal of Occupational Therapy, 41*(2), 90-95.

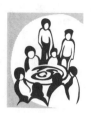

**Sensory Motor
Activity Example 8-1
Blob**

The Blob begins as a game of tag. When the person who is "it" catches someone, that person joins hands and becomes part of the Blob. Only the outside hand on either end of the Blob can snatch runaway players. Thus, the insidious Blob keeps growing, cornering stray runners and forcing them to join up. In large groups, the Blob may split itself into parts and organize raiding parties to round up the last few strays. Boundaries must be set for this game, so eventually everyone is caught. "The thrilling climax occurs when there's only one player left to put up a heroic last ditch stand on behalf of humanity" (Fluegelman, 1976, p. 107). The last survivor can start the next Blob as the game continues.

This game is obviously for people who are ambulatory, have good balance and coordination, and have enough cognitive understanding to be able to follow simple rules. Blob is a simple concept that can be fun even for those who do not grasp its deeper implications. Done inside a room with the elderly, a therapist can talk the group through any difficulties, or she can begin by being the Blob. It may be done slowly or quickly to adapt to patient ability, and it provides light exercise with an element of fun and challenge.

From Cole, M. B. *Group Dynamics in Occupational Therapy, Second Edition.* © 1998 SLACK Incorporated.

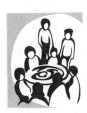

Sensory Motor
Activity Example 8-2
People to People

Here is a new game that is made for occupational therapy. It is especially good for integrating movement, motor planning, and cognition. Everyone chooses a partner and the game begins with a rhythmic clapping and snapping in unison (clap-clap-right hand, snap-snap-left hand). The caller names two body parts, one on the right snap, the other on the left snap (e.g., "elbow to ear"). On the next snap-snap the whole group repeats "elbow to ear" while simultaneously one partner places his elbow on the other partner's ear. The caller continues to name body parts, trying to challenge the group by naming obscure anatomical structures (esophagus to gastrocnemius) or forcing them to take awkward positions. When the caller gets tired of this, he may call out "people to people." Then everyone must change partners, and in the confusion, the caller grabs a partner, leaving another member to become the new caller.

Adaptations for this game are endless. At the very least, it is a great socialization ice breaker, sure to get everyone laughing. It is also an excellent way for occupational therapy students to study their anatomy. Patients can practice bilateral coordination (clapping and snapping), motor planning (touching parts with partner), body awareness (identifying parts), and cognition (naming and recognizing body parts). A fair amount of balance, coordination, and visual-motor integration are required to perform this activity successfully. Care should be taken with this and other games requiring touch that patients are not threatened by the close proximity to others.

The New Games followers suggest what occupational therapists already know—all the games can be adapted by changing the rules, or that new games can be invented to meet the special needs and goals of our patients.

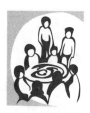

All the games begin with group members holding an edge of the parachute at even intervals. It will take a few tries to move the parachute up over heads and down to the knees in unison to "catch the air." When the group has accomplished this, members can take turns running under the chute and exchanging places with one another across the circle. Other variations of parachute play are as follows.

Popcorn—When the parachute is down, a few tennis balls can be tossed in the center. The group makes the balls "pop" into the air and catches them with the parachute.

Round the World—One ball is placed in the center of the parachute. The group is instructed to work together to make the ball roll around the edge of the parachute by moving it in unison.

Down the Drain—Two colored balls are placed in the parachute. One side (blue ball) tries to get the other side's ball (red ball) to drop through the hole in the middle of the parachute.

Secret Club—Billow the parachute by the unified above the head, below the knees motion of the group. Then on the count of three, group members bring the parachute edge down behind their backs and proceed to sit on the edge of the parachute. The air in the middle produces a "tent" in which the "secret club" can meet (but not for long or the air can get very stale!).

Shark—The members gather up the edge of the chute at just about waist level until a "calm sea" is produced. Then the "shark" ducks under and stalks the group with one finger pointing up touching the parachute from below, so that his movements may be observed from the top of the parachute. At an unexpected moment, the shark grabs the legs of an unsuspecting group member. The "victim" screams loudly as she is pulled under to become the next "shark." Two or three sharks at a time may be used in larger groups.

From Cole, M. B. *Group Dynamics in Occupational Therapy, Second Edition.* © 1998 SLACK Incorporated.

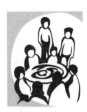

Sensory Motor
Activity Example 8-4
Expressing Anger with Movement

Materials: Exercise mats or thick carpeting and pillows.

Directions: Give directions for each step of the sequence and allow members to take the time they need for each step.

1. Lie down on your back on the mat and extend both legs. Kick your legs rhythmically and allow your energy to flow into this motion. Take a few minutes to do this, setting your own pace.
2. Stand up and form a circle. Kick alternately with the right, then the left leg into the center of the circle.
3. Clench your fists and as you kick into the center of the circle, say "No!" Louder!
4. What other words can we say? As members make suggestions, have the whole group try them. Try punching into the center of the circle and saying words or making sounds.
5. Rest a few minutes and concentrate on breathing. Walk slowly around the circle, then turn and walk the other way. The slow walking has a calming effect after the excitement of kicking and punching.
6. Lie down on stomach with pillow in front of you. Punch pillow with right and left fists in a rhythmic motion. Do this for a few minutes and set your own pace.
7. As you punch the pillow, say "No!" If you feel like kicking also, allow yourself to do this.
8. If you would like, give the pillow a name. (Therapists should do this with caution, so as not to arouse too much anger.)
9. After a few minutes, wind down and just breathe slowly, resting head on pillow.
10. Stand up again when rested. Shrug shoulders in a backward roll and loosen tension in the neck area.
11. As patients shrug, say "Get off my back!" Louder!
12. Sit in a circle and massage muscles in back of neck. Each person massages the back of the person in front of him or her.

This exercise must be processed so that patients are not left with unresolved angry feelings. One goal is awareness of anger so that its appropriate expression can be discussed. An other goal is eliciting normal movement patterns subcortically. The careful planning and adaptation of this type of activity can utilize the concepts of Rood, NDT, PNF, Brunnstrom, or sensory integration.

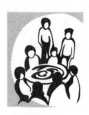

Sensory Motor
Activity Example 8-5
Acting Out Feelings

Materials: Twenty index cards with feeling words, paper, pencils, and stopwatch. Words for cards are: lonely, disgusted, excited, pleased, annoyed, infuriated, friendly, jealous, miserable, crabby, ecstatic, impatient, giddy, silly, moody, spacy, frightened, terrified, hopeless, hurt. Other feeling words may be added or substituted.

Directions: Each member draws a card and takes 30 seconds to act out the feeling on the card. Someone should be designated as timekeeper. Players may make sounds, but no words are allowed. Players can walk back and forth in front of the group, sit, stand, lie down, and make gestures and facial expressions. The entire 30 seconds should be used. Nonverbal interaction with other members may be allowed as long as no one is hurt.

Members do not shout out their guesses; this is not charades. When time is up, group members write down what they think the feeling is. As each "mini-drama" ends, members read out their feeling words and discuss why they thought so. After a brief discussion, the player shows the group the card. Members continue to draw cards and act out feelings until they are all used.

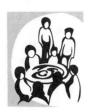

**Sensory Motor
Activity Example 8-6
Ross Five-Stage Group for
Medium/Verbal Members**

Materials: Six to eight patients, blackboard and chalk (or newsprint pad and large marker), and a basketball. Arrange chairs in a circle.

Directions: Stage I (5 minutes)—The therapist introduces self and states "We are all going to exercise our muscles and our brains so we can share ideas and learn from each other. To begin, I'd like each of you to take a turn coming up to the board and writing your name." The chalk is handed to the first volunteer, who sits back done when finished. The group will read each name aloud as it is written. Note that everyone is needed to complete the circle; gather any late or distracted members.

Stage II (10 to 15 minutes)—An agitated group is organized by asking members to pass the basketball from one to another with both hands while sitting. Members may then stand and bounce the ball to each other across the circle. Members take turns walking around the outside of the circle bouncing the basketball; then the members stand in a circle, facing right, an arm's length apart from each other. They must pass the basketball between their legs to the person behind them. The whole group jogs around the outside of the circle of chairs for maximum exertion. Members face left, arm's length apart, and pass the basketball backwards over their heads to the person behind them. The group can create its own movement sequences by requiring the ball to be passed without hands, or from member to member in a predetermined pattern.

Stage III (15 minutes)—Members move chairs back a few feet before sitting down, thus expanding the circle. A large, empty wastebasket is placed in the center. Members take turns bouncing the basketball once and trying to get it in the "basket." The group can be split into "teams," keeping score on the board. If teams are uneven, reshuffling should occur. Blocking may be done if skill permits for "offensive and defensive play." Members of teams sit alternately and attempt to block winning plays with arm movements. Different colored bandanas may be tied around the members' necks or heads to signify the different teams.

End group with a series of stretches (e.g., pantomime throwing a free point, reaching for the hoop, and blocking). Finally, pantomime congratulating each other on a winning game. Check level of excitement; use a calming strategy from Table 8-1 if needed.

Stage IV (15 minutes)—Discussion of favorite sports can follow. Each member takes a turn remembering an experience involving a sport. What athletics do members know? Admire? Dislike? What do they remember about Winter or Summer Olympics? What about leisure or solitary sports, such as swimming, fishing, or bicycling? The goal of the discussion is to learn about each other and from each other about different sports. Encourage members to ask each other questions or respond to one another's comments.

From Cole, M. B. *Group Dynamics in Occupational Therapy, Second Edition.* © 1998 SLACK Incorporated.

If discussion is somewhat beyond the group, substitute taking turns with the chalk and drawing a piece of sports equipment on the board. Have the group guess what it is or what sport uses the equipment. Examples include: fishing line with hook, swimming pool, boxing glove, golf club, baseball bat, tennis racquet, pair of skis. Congratulate the group for sharing their knowledge and experience with each other.

Stage V—To summarize, the therapist asks members to remember parts of the session. "What things did we do today? Which did you like best? What did you learn about each other?" End with a firm handshake and say goodbye by name as each member leaves.

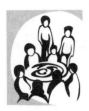

Sensory Motor
Activity Example 8-7
Ross Five-Stage Group for
Low/Nonverbal Members

Materials: Hand lotion, candle, balloons, party favor blowers, card table, cards with different colors, 10 to 12 pairs of matching objects, tray, and bag.

Directions: Stage I—Patients sit in a circle. The therapist greets each member by name and asks everyone to hold out their hands. A dot of herbal-smelling hand lotion is squeezed into their palms; the therapist demonstrates rubbing it into the hands. Ask members to notice how it smells. A vanilla or spice-scented candle is then passed from member to member, and sniffing is encouraged.

Stage II—Every member chooses a colored, blown-up, 6-inch diameter balloon to hold between their hands. "Don't let go…don't drop it…hold onto it." The therapist then asks members to imitate: holding it out in front, above the head, swinging to the left and the right (shoulder height), gently throwing and catching it, and touching the balloon to knees, ankles, floor, lap, chin, and each shoulder.

Put on music, such as a waltz tempo (e.g., Strauss) or a song that suits the members' age group. Ask the group to stand and imitate movements to the music: swinging the balloon back and forth, up and down, and around in a circle.

Batting balloons in the air begins as another song is played. Members try to keep all the balloons in the air until the music ends. Observe behavior and modify as needed.

Stage III—All balloons are collected except one. The therapist passes this balloon with her elbows and asks a member to begin passing it around the circle with no hands. This can be done sitting or standing. If it is someone's birthday, ask the members to sing "Happy Birthday" (many persons who no longer speak can still sing). Party blowers are passed out and everyone practices blowing by imitating the therapist. A small table is set up and balloons are placed on the table. Members attempt to knock all the balloons off the table using the party blowers (again, no hands). Pick them all up and do it again. Passing a single balloon from one side of the table to the other can follow.

Stage IV—Cards with different colors are passed to each member. Colored cards matching these are placed down on the table. Members take turns choosing a card from the table until they find one that matches.

The therapist makes a board or tray with 10 or 12 common objects. Matching objects are placed in a bag. Members draw an object, guessing what it is by touch if they can, and pointing to the matching object on the tray. The they look at the object to see if they guessed correctly.

Stage V—Play a short waltz tape and ask members to stand and join hands for a group sway.

Chapter 9

A Model of Human Occupation Approach

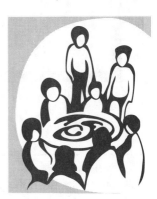

The model of human occupation (MOHO) emerged around 1980 as a further definition of the theory of occupational behavior developed by Mary Reilly (1962). The central idea of occupational behavior theory is that engagement in activity or occupation in itself will produce and maintain health. Human achievement and daily occupation are identified as the focal point for the development of the MOHO (Kielhofner, 1988). White (1959) is credited with introducing the concept of the human need for competence and achievement. Kielhofner, Burke, and Igi (1980) expanded on these concepts and combined them with general systems theory. They describe the human being as an open system, define the various parts of the system (volitional, habituation, and performance subsystems), and describe how it interacts with other systems (culture, tasks, social norms, human and non-human environment). The MOHO can be viewed as a superstructure that organizes concepts and expresses them in terms that can be readily applied to assessment and treatment.

Focus

Human occupation is a broad concept which is common to all mankind. As a therapeutic approach, it is holistic and universally applicable across ages, cultures, and disabilities. MOHO views the person as a system, which has the capacity to reorganize itself or be reorganized. "Humans self-organize through occupational behavior" (Kielhofner, 1995, p. 20). While the person's identity, or essence, remains the same, this capacity to change and adapt is equally important. The thrust of therapy in MOHO is to restore order to the system, both internally (person) and externally (fitting into one's environment). Injury or illness can bring about unwelcome change that is very disorderly. The function of occupational therapy is to facilitate an adaptive reorganization so that order can be restored.

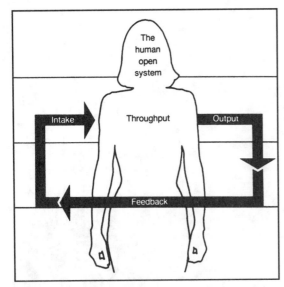

Figure 9-1a. The human open system. Reprinted with permission from Kielhofner, G. (Ed.). (1985). *The model of human occupation.* Baltimore, MD: Williams and Wilkins.

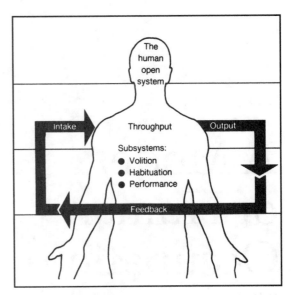

Figure 9-1b. The three subsystems. Reprinted with permission from Kielhofner, G. (Ed.). (1985). *The model of human occupation.* Baltimore, MD: Williams and Wilkins.

Basic Assumptions

The Human Open System

The basic assumption in applying systems theory to human functioning is that man is an open system that can change and develop through interaction with the environment. The human open system is described as a cyclical process involving output, feedback, input, and throughput (Kielhofner & Burke, 1985). The human being gives output to the environment, receives feedback in the form of input from the environment, and experiences throughput, a process of change and adaptation of the person resulting from the feedback given (Figures 9-1a and 9-1b). The system is divided into parts for the purpose of examining (assessment) and influencing (treatment) its processes.

The Three Internal Subsystems

Following systems theory, throughput occurs within the three internal subsystems—volitional, habituation, and perfor-

mance—which comprise the internal organization of the human system. These subsystems are consolidated and heterarchical, that is, they are interdependent with one another, contributing equally to the human system as a whole. The volitional subsystem maintains a belief in oneself and one's values, and exerts influence in choosing one's occupations and initiating occupational behavior. The habituation subsystem organizes and maintains occupational behavior in routines and role patterns (habit maps and role scripts). The mind-brain-body performance subsystem provides skills and motor capacities to carry out occupational behavior. The three subsystems work together in an integrated fashion to maintain the balance of work, play, and self-care activities.

The Volitional Subsystem

The volitional process involves anticipation, experiencing, choosing, and interpreting occupational behavior (Kielhofner,

Please note: Although this chapter is based on Kielhofner (1995) and subsequent workshops, these earlier illustrations (Figures 9-1a & b) are preferred for their simplicity in introducing basic MOHO concepts to the beginning student.

1995, p. 41). This system serves to direct and energize the other subsystems toward desired goals. However, this motivating force is highly influenced by the other subsystems (state of fatigue, habitual patterns) as well as external circumstances. Choices for occupation can be immediate (activities for today) or long-term (career choices, committed relationships). The three main components of this subsystem are:

1. Personal causation
2. Values
3. Interests

Personal causation refers to a belief in oneself, and is related to feelings of competence. A healthy individual is thought to possess needed skills, and to believe himself to be capable of using these skills to have a desired effect on the environment. A person who believes in himself expects to succeed through the use of his own abilities. A person who lacks a sense of personal causation may feel that what happens is controlled by fate or external circumstance. Such a person feels helpless to cope with the functional problems resulting from illness and disability.

Values in the MOHO refer to the meaningfulness of activities. Individuals are thought to spend time doing activities that have meaning and are thought to be good or morally right. For example, if a student thinks that having a college degree is good, she may work very hard at reading, writing, and studying, activities that will help her achieve that goal. Patients often find themselves unable to perform activities that they consider to be important or meaningful, such as going back to work. A reprioritizing of values might be a treatment goal. Using this model, patients can find alternate ways to perform a work role that are within their capabilities.

Interests in this model are defined as tendencies to find certain occupations attractive and pleasurable. If a person enjoys a particular activity, he may be inclined to participate in it frequently or for longer periods of time. Interests relate to work, play, and self-care activities, and are not limited to recreational endeavors. Occupational choices are highly influenced by the activities one finds attractive. A healthy individual uses his interests to guide present action and to plan his use of time. A person lacking in interests may need help in exploring his environment and in finding pleasure in activities.

In summary, the volitional subsystem guides the occupational behavior of the individual in ways that are meaningful and pleasurable, and are likely to have a desired effect on the environment.

The Habituation Subsystem

The concept of "habit training" dates back to the practice of Eleanor Clarke Slagle, reflected by the writings of Adolph Meyer. He describes the "systematic engagement of interest and concern about the actual use of time and work (as) an obligation and a necessity" in the treatment of chronic illness (Meyer, 1982, p. 81). The organization of activities throughout the day is the concern of the habituation subsystem, as conceptualized by the MOHO. Roles and habits are its components.

Habits are routine or typical ways in which a person performs tasks. Their familiarity provides a sense of stability and well-being that comes with predictability. For example, a morning routine may involve getting up at 7:00 a.m., bathing, dressing, and eating breakfast. Habits can decrease the effort required to perform tasks by making them so routine that they are almost automatic. Consider the effort needed to find one's way to a new place of work. After driving the same route for several days, one recognizes familiar landmarks and the trip requires much less conscious thought. This routine allows the individual to save his energy for the more challenging activities of the day.

However, research has shown that habits are not just mindless repetitions of behavior. Rather, they operate as habit maps, or guidelines, which must be improvised to accommodate each new circumstance. Habit maps include thoughts and perceptions as well as action sequences. Young (1988) views habits as internalized intuitive knowledge, which gives us our bearings (orients us), and allows us to anticipate the next step in familiar temporal, physical, and social surroundings. According to Young, habits that are shared by a social group are called "customs" and are the carriers of culture. They are the rules for living which keep us in harmony with our social environment (1988).

Illness often results in a breakdown of normal routines. Occupational therapy may be needed to relearn and reorganize one's habits after illness. Being in a familiar surrounding may provide a way for persons to maintain order in the face of illness or disability. MOHO stresses the importance of a familiar and safe habitat, and the necessity of assessing one's habitual ways of doing things. Often the initial intervention in occupational therapy is to reinforce familiar routines and existing skills.

A role is a position or status within a social group, along with its accompanying obligations and expectations. Some typical roles are worker, parent, family member, student, and volunteer. Functional individuals generally play a variety of life roles, and find it necessary to achieve a balance of these if they are to maintain order in their lives. The roles we play have an organizing effect on how we use time. The worker role and the family member role, for example, each require the performance of defined tasks which must be balanced and planned for if the day is to flow smoothly.

According to Kielhofner (1995), every role has a role script. Role scripts are structures that guide comprehension of social expectations and construction of performance actions (p. 72). Similar to habitual behavior, "role behavior is often preconscious, operating with a vague awareness of what is happening and of what one is doing" (p. 72). The role of a parent in the family, for example, suggests various tasks concerned with providing food and shelter, maintaining the household, and providing instruction, authority, and guidance for the children. The parent role also constrains behavior, because parents are expected to set an example for their children and to refrain from activities (e.g., gambling, alcohol abuse) that would be detrimental to the family unit. Some role scripts are more flexible than others. As circumstances change, role expectations may require rethinking, and their scripts adapted.

Our patients may lack social roles or may find it difficult to meet the obligations and expectations of their roles. The focus of therapy may be the development of new roles and/or the planning and modification of activities required within chosen roles. For treatment purposes, grouping patients who wish to continue in similar roles, such as returning to work or maintaining a home, allows persons with disabilities to share ideas and provide mutual support for adapting their role scripts to accommodate physical, emotional, or cognitive limitations.

The Performance Subsystem

This subsystem has been relabeled the "mind-brain-body" performance subsystem, which includes all of the constituents and skills required to perform purposeful activities. Constituents, or foundation abilities, include musculoskeletal, neurological, cardiopulmonary, and cognitive images. Three types of skills are identified:

1. Perceptual-motor
2. Process
3. Communication/interaction skills

A person's performance is directly linked to the output of the human open system. The volitional and habituation subsystems can only perform to the extent that existing capacities and skills will allow. Therefore, a lack of skills can prevent the needed organization of roles and habits, the pursuit of interests, and the accomplishment of valued goals. In this area, occupational therapy may treat deficit areas using other frames of reference, such as biomechanical or sensory integration, in a fragmented fashion. Authors of the updated MOHO theory caution against this "reductionistic" practice. The application of physiological, psychological, or biomechanical theory should always be in service to the more basic human need to engage in meaningful occupations.

Interaction with the Environment

The three subsystems discussed above are part of the throughput process of the human open system. Output, feedback, and input define the system's interaction with the environment. Since the health and adaptation of the individual is dependent on this interaction, the environment represents a vital part of the MOHO. MOHO first defines the influences of the environment on occupational behavior as affords (opportunities for performance) and presses (expectations or requirements of performance). Second, environments themselves are defined as physical or social, and finally, occupational behavior settings are defined.

Every environment offers the opportunity for a prescribed range of behaviors. The behavior that is selected depends upon the interaction of the person (intentions, habits, and skills), and the objects and circumstances of the surroundings.

Each environment affords opportunities within a range of possibilities. For example, a university environment offers multiple opportunities for academic and technical learning. Classrooms, laboratories, libraries or study areas, and office hours for dialogue with professors all suggest different modes of learning. Environmental press is the expectation of performance or behavior placed on an individual by a given environment (Barris, 1985). For example, a health club environment requires the individual to dress in a defined manner and to demonstrate a certain level of physical skill. Individuals generally seek out environments that fit their interests and their level of skill. Individuals who are disabled may find themselves in environments that do not match their competence level, and may need the services of an occupational therapist to help them change either their skill level or their environment.

Environments are described in both physical and social contexts. Physical environments operate according to the laws of science. They may be natural (untouched by humans) or fabricated (buildings, automobiles, roads, airports). Objects within these environments may also be man-made (clothes, dishes) or may occur naturally (trees, seashells). These environments are organized according to various purposes, and their contents and arrangement greatly influence human occupational behavior.

Social environments consist of social groups and occupational forms. Social groups, which assemble and meet regularly, define and assign occupational roles to individuals within them (a family, a corporation). An occupational form, according to Nelson (1988), is "the preexisting structure that elicits, guides, or structures subsequent human performance" (p. 633). For example, dinner is an occupational form that is accepted across cultures. Each culture has its unique ways of obtaining and preparing food, as well as acceptable ways of consuming it. Kielhofner defines occupational forms as "rule-bound sequences of action which are at once coherent, oriented to a purpose, sustained in collective knowledge, culturally recognizable, and named"(1995, p. 102). Many rules apply to the term "dinner." It implies a certain time of day, usually the early evening in American culture, and a time sequence (beverage, appetizer, salad, main course, bread and butter, dessert). It consists of foods from different groups (proteins, fruits and vegetables, breads and grains, dairy), cooked, chopped, diced, or otherwise combined in culturally prescribed ways. It is coherent in that a number of separate tasks are involved, such as shopping (gathering ingredients), cooking according to certain recipes, using certain tools (plates, glasses, utensils), and interacting in socially acceptable ways (blessing the food before eating, polite dinner conversation). The obvious purpose of dinner is to sustain life by supplying food to the body, but its purpose is also social, such as a time for a man and woman to get to know one another (dinner date) or for the family to communicate and be together (family dinner). This example demonstrates both the immediate/physical and the symbolic/cultural nature of occupational forms.

Occupational behavior settings combine the physical and social environments in ways recognizable to most people. These include homes, neighborhoods, schools, workplaces, and gathering or recreational sites. These are settings that should be evaluated by occupational therapists when planning and facilitating patient adaptation. Habitat refers to features within these settings that are familiar, and which suggest, guide, and sustain purposeful occupational behavior.

A general outline for organizing data about the human open system is found in Table 9-1. For definitions and elaboration of all these terms the reader is referred to Kielhofner's *A Model of Human Occupation* (1995).

Function and Dysfunction

When the human open system is functioning optimally, order exists within the system. This means that the individual competently performs everyday tasks of daily life in a routine and satisfying way (Rogers, 1982). This "order" produces and maintains a state of health in the individual. If a person can describe a typical day at work or home, identify a number of social roles he performs, and express satisfaction with these, then he is seen to be healthy.

Dysfunction is disorder, a lack of order in one's life which can be seen in dysfunctional daily routines, a lack of social roles, and/or dissatisfaction with any aspect of the person's life structure. When disorder exists, the occupational therapist evaluates the patient to determine what parts of the system are not operating properly. Barris, Kielhofner, and Watts (1983) suggest several specific kinds of disorder, including open system dysfunction, disruption in intrinsic motivation, poor decision-making capacity, role dysfunction, temporal dysfunction, disorder of environmental interactions, and disorder of performance components.

MOHO has specified three levels of occupational functioning (Reilly, 1974):
1. Exploration
2. Competence
3. Achievement

These have also been called levels of arousal and accomplishment (Kaplan, 1986; Kielhofner, 1988). Exploration is the lowest level and involves curious investigation of oneself and one's potential for action in conjunction with the properties

Table 9-1.
Components of the Model of Human Occupation

INTERNAL	(Examples)	EXTERNAL	(Examples)
Volitional		**Natural Environment**	Mountains, beach
Personal Causation	Knowledge of capacity (I can ski)	**Fabricated Environment**	House, airport, car, factory, supermarket
	Sense of efficacy (I can learn in college)	**Objects**	Clothes, dishes, machines, tools
Choices for Occupation	Activity choice (I need to buy milk)	**Social Environment**	
	Occupational choice (I want to be a doctor)	**Social Groups**	Family, corporation
Values	Personal convictions (be kind to others)	**Occupational Forms**	Driving a car, skiing, shopping, working
	Sense of obligation (always return what you borrow)	**Occupational Behavior**	
Interests	Attraction (loves reading, conversing)	**Settings:**	Homes
	Preference (enjoys the outdoors)		Neighborhoods
Habituation			Schools
Habits	Routines (getting dressed for work)		Workplaces
	Habit maps (operate a computer, adapt for different uses)		Gathering or recreational sites
Roles	Internalized roles (teacher, spouse, parent, friend) Role scripts (teaching = papers, preparing/giving lectures, etc.)		
Performance Subsystem (mind, brain, body)	Constituencies: musculoskeletal, neurological, cardiopulmonary, cognitive images	Skills: motor, process, communication, interaction	

of the environment. Competence involves striving to meet the demands of a situation through the development of skills and their organization. Achievement includes striving for excellence and the successful performance of roles.

Concurrent levels of occupational dysfunction are also described as inefficacy, incompetence, and helplessness. Inefficacy, the least dysfunctional level, implies a reduction of motivation.

There are dozens of assessment tools originating from this frame of reference, which can help occupational therapists to specify which parts of the system are disordered or malfunctioning. The state of order or disorder is easily observed in the patient's occupational behavior.

Change and Motivation

Change in the MOHO involves the restoration of order in the person's internal and external life structure. In recovering from illness, this often means restructuring a person's daily routines and re-establishing role performance. For example, Angie's roles were secretary, wife, and mother of a 5-year-old son. When at age 35 she was hospitalized for depression following a bitter divorce, all of her roles became inactive. The occupational therapist collaborated with Angie in restructuring her life so that she could resume her roles as worker and mother. Angie was able to volunteer while in the hospital to help maintain her secretarial skills. She arranged to have dinner with her son each evening and to take him on an outing one day on the weekend. In restoring these roles, Angie was able to organize her already existing skills into a normal daily routine. She showered and dressed each morning, went to her volunteer job each day, and met her son at a relative's house for dinner each evening. At night, she returned to the hospital.

The preceding therapy program addressed the components of the habituation and performance subsystems. Grieving over the loss of her role as spouse was dealt with in counseling and resulted in the addition of several activities to allow Angie to make new social contacts, like joining a tennis club and playing three times a week, and attending weekly meetings of a church social club.

The therapeutic work is not what activity is chosen, but in getting Angie moving toward the regular performance of desired occupational behaviors. Normal, everyday activities are the media used, and the patient herself makes the choices of activity, with the help and guidance of the occupational therapist.

Motivation in this frame of reference is attributed to an innate urge to explore and master the environment. Many writers have been credited with the elaboration of this concept, which is said to have a biological basis (Kielhofner, 1988). The best known of these is R. H. White (1960) who contributed the ideas of competence, adaptation, and motivation. Motivation speaks to the meaningfulness of activities. The meaning in occupation is derived not only from the individual, but from the context of her social and cultural environment. Part of the occupational therapist's job is not only to restore individual task

performance, but also to identify and restore meaningful roles in society.

A major value of the MOHO lies in its holistic view of the individual and its helpfulness in organizing data about patients' specific dysfunctions. Many examples exist in the literature of the application of the MOHO in identifying patterns of occupational dysfunction.

Group Treatment

Most of the literature on the MOHO does not address group treatment specifically. However, several aspects of its superstructure are helpful in program planning. A balanced occupational therapy program is assured, for example, when one incorporates group activities addressing the areas of self-care, work, and leisure. Another concept was to organize a program by using the three levels of occupational functioning. Kathy Kaplan (1986, 1988) writes about a group program for short-term psychiatry using group activities at the levels of exploration, competence, and achievement.

Exploration level groups incorporate simple activities to help the most severely disorganized patients to develop basic process skills (planning and problem-solving), perceptual motor skills, and communication/interaction skills. The occupational therapist selects the activities and organizes the environment. The group is structured in four stages:

1. Orientation and introductions
2. Warm-up activities
3. Selected activities
4. Wrap-up

Kaplan calls this type of group a "directive group." An exercise group is another example of an explorative level group.

At the competence level, it is assumed that the patients have basic skills but may need to integrate them into habit patterns: "These groups are designed to help patients identify goals, interests, and needs for meaning and action" (Kaplan, 1986, p. 476). Some examples of groups at this level are task groups and activity planning groups.

Groups at the achievement level are designed to help patients integrate skills into daily life roles (Kaplan, 1986). Examples of achievement level groups are assertiveness training and leisure awareness. For more information on the directive group the reader is also referred to Kaplan's *Directive Group Therapy* (1988).

Group Structure and Limitations

Within the components of the three subsystems, the most useful concept for organizing groups is roles. Roles will define the discharge goals for patients and will dictate the kinds of skills that will need to be restored or strengthened. Therefore, in MOHO, it is best to disregard diagnosis and focus on the social roles persons intend to return to or find. Grouping persons according to their need to maintain a home, care for children, socialize, participate in recreational activities, or engage in gainful employment allows them to learn from and support each other in adapting their routines, role scripts, and environments to accommodate physical or mental limitations.

It has been stated that the use of the MOHO is not limited by age or diagnosis. Functional levels are organized by levels of arousal and achievement and by the components of the three subsystems that are functioning within the human open system. The focus of occupational therapy in the MOHO is on roles and their associated activities and tasks, and not on emotions or process.

Role of the Therapist

The therapist in the MOHO plays the role of an adviser and collaborator. She counsels the patients in the various aspects of occupational functioning. Kaplan's "directive group" is so named because of the "active and supportive way in which the group leaders elicit adaptive behaviors and structure the environment to assure maximum participation of all the members" (Kaplan, 1986, p. 477). This role of leader as "director" is necessary for groups that have severely disorganized occupational behavior. However, even at this level, the occupational therapist encourages the active participation of the patients. The occupational therapist continues at higher levels to facilitate, not direct. Thus, the patient's sense of control and personal efficacy is reinforced by the occupational therapist as she continues to acquire new skills and make personal choices.

Goals

Goals are not discussed as a separate issue in the MOHO. The goal is to restore order in daily functioning, both internal and external. Therefore, the goal of group treatment may be seen as finding and engaging in meaningful occupations and meaningful roles in society. Group treatment goals are concerned with performance of normal daily occupations: work, daily living tasks, and play. They may involve any or all of the three subsystems. In the volitional subsystem, exploration of values and rekindling the urge to explore and master the environment may be goals. Habit formation or the acquisition of new roles may be goals in the habituation subsystem. Learning and practicing the skills necessary to perform the tasks of one's chosen or valued roles can be goals in the performance subsystem.

Examples of Activities

An updated criterion for placing patients in groups, according to Janice Burke, co-founder of MOHO, is to group them according to their anticipated social roles (1997, personal communication). Common roles, such as homemaker, caregiver, worker, or student, all suggest clusters of skills and tasks that may be selected for group activities. The MOHO stresses the use of the patient's normal daily activities as the modalities of choice. Groups designed around common roles, as Burke has suggested, can incorporate specific tasks or skills that need to be practiced or adapted. The more common media used in therapeutic groups include cooking, money management, home maintenance skills, parenting skills, leisure planning, and work skills. The patient's own interests guide activity selection and the focus is on the real problems of everyday living. Some kinds of activities necessitate longer sessions. The environment is important in providing feedback to the patient and challenging him to further exploration.

Part of the activity planning should address the intended roles and social environments the members will seek out or return to after recovery. Skills and tasks will seem meaningless unless they are connected to meaningful roles that reconnect them with their social groups and help them fulfill a useful purpose. This connection with society and with culture is what sets MOHO groups apart from groups in other frames of reference.

Some occupational therapy group activities used in a program based on MOHO are described in Activity Examples 9-1 through 9-4.

Group Leadership

In this frame of reference, the activity or occupation itself is considered health-producing, and the need to take great pains to share it or understand its process is deemphasized. In keeping with the greater emphasis on activities, two steps in the seven-step process have been eliminated: sharing and processing. There are longer and more frequent group meetings, and activities tend to be longer or ongoing, so that discussions of general principles and application are not necessary during every session. However, the introduction and summary should be done without fail, and should serve the purposes outlined in Chapter 1.

Introduction

Greetings and description of the purpose are done thoroughly at the outset of each activity. A warm-up is optional and can be used to set the mood or energize patients if appropriate. The expectations may be general and somewhat tentative as the members will have input and make choices as the group progresses. The timeframe often varies according to the activity and therefore should be started at the beginning of each session.

Activity

The thrust of all MOHO group activities should be moving patients toward meaningful roles in their own social environments. Persons with similar roles or intended roles are grouped together, so that their task choices are likely to be similar also. At the exploratory level, the activities selected for groups are generally designed to help patients develop specific skills. Patients who need to work on these skills are grouped together. For example, those who need to develop routines for self-care might do a series of skill-building sessions such as maintaining finger- and toenails, doing laundry, selecting appropriate clothing, applying make-up/shaving, care of teeth, and care of hair and skin.

At the competence level, choices are encouraged so that patients can apply their skills and organize them into habit patterns (Kaplan, 1986). Patients may be encouraged to set their own goals within the group context. For example, the title of the group may be "Time Management," and within that theme, patients may plan their own individual time schedules with tasks that are meaningful for them in their own social/cultural contexts.

Achievement level groups focus on life roles such as work support, leisure planning, and values clarification.

Generalizing and Application

The meaning of the activity is discussed with the group as outlined in Chapter 1. This is done after the activity is completed and focuses on how the activity relates to the life roles of the members. Similarities and differences among group members are de-emphasized. For example, in the vocational readiness group described earlier, the skills learned in doing a leather craft project may be generalized to a patient's actual job. Concentration, efficient use of tools, work neatness, and finishing on time are skills necessary for both. This kind of discussion leads directly into application. A group discussion in the vocational readiness group will necessarily focus on individual application of skills, as patients' vocational plans differ widely. Feedback from the occupational therapist on results of the vocational rating scale should also be presented in the group. The group focus is useful to confirm the therapist's observations and give a stronger message to patients. For example, a member may have done very careful work and showed considerable manual skills, but he may have taken excessive time to do so. The reality of the workplace is not only to do quality work, but also to meet deadlines. The group discussion may help the patient see the necessity to compromise and perhaps curb his perfectionistic tendencies.

Summary

The summary should review the purpose and goals of the group and determine what the group accomplished. Focus on individual achievements and strengths should be confirmed. The skills learned may be general or different for each member, and their application should be reinforced in the summary. Future plans, goal achievement, and life roles to which occupational therapy activities apply may be discussed by each member as part of the summary.

Bibliography

Barris, R. (1985). Occupation as interaction with the environment. In G. Kielhofner (Ed.), *A Model of Human Occupation: Theory and Application.* Baltimore, MD: Williams and Wilkins.

Barris, R., Kielhofner, G., & Watts, J. (1983). *Psychosocial occupational therapy: Practice in a pluralistic arena.* Laurel, MD: Ramsco.

Kaplan, K. (1986). The directive group: Short-term treatment for psychiatric patients with a minimal level of functioning. *American Journal of Occupational Therapy, 40*(7), 474-481.

Kaplan, K. (1988). *Directive group therapy.* Thorofare, NJ: SLACK Incorporated.

Katz, N. (1988). Interest checklist: A factor analytical study. *OT in Mental Health, 1,* 45-55.

Kielhofner, G., (Ed.). (1985). *A model of human occupation: Theory and application.* Baltimore, MD: Williams and Wilkins.

Kielhofner, G. (1978). General systems theory: Implications for theory and action in occupational therapy. *American Journal of Occupational Therapy, 32*(10), 637-645.

Kielhofner, G. (1988). Model of human occupation. In S. Robinson (Ed.), *Mental Health Focus.* Rockville, MD: American Occupational Therapy Association.

Kielhofner, G. (1995). *A model of human occupation* (2nd ed.). Baltimore, MD: Williams and Wilkins.

Kielhofner, G., & Burke, J. (1985). Components and determinants of occupation. In G. Kielhofner (Ed.), *A Model of Human Occupation.* Baltimore, MD: Williams and Wilkins.

Kielhofner, G., Burke, J., & Igi, C. (1980). A model of human occupation, part 4. *American Journal of Occupational Therapy, 34*(12), 572-581.

Kielhofner, G., Henry, A., & Walens, D. (1989). *A user's guide to the occupational performance history interview.* Rockville, MD: American Occupational

Therapy Association.

Lindquist J., Mack, W., & Parham, L. D. (1982). A synthesis of occupational behavior and sensory integration concepts in theory and practice, part 2: Clinical applications. *American Journal of Occupational Therapy, 36*(7), 433-437.

Mack, W., Lindquist, J., & Parham, L. D. (1982). A synthesis of occupational behavior and sensory integration concepts in theory and practice, part 1: Theoretical foundations. *American Journal of Occupational Therapy, 36*(6), 365-374.

Meyer, A. (1982). The philosophy of occupational therapy. *Occupational Therapy in Mental Health, 2*(3), 79-89. Reprinted from (1922). *Archives of Occupational Therapy, 1*, 1-10.

Nelson, D. (1988). Occupation: Form & performance. *American Journal of Occupational Therapy, 42*, 633-641.

Reilly, M. (1962). Occupational therapy can be one of the great ideas of 20th century medicine. *American Journal of Occupational Therapy, 16*, 1-9.

Reilly, M. (1974). An explanation of play. In M. Reilly (Ed.), *Play as Exploratory Learning: Studies of Curiosity Behavior* (pp. 117-155). Beverly Hills, CA: Sage Publications.

Rogers, J. (1982). Order and disorder in medicine and occupational therapy. *American Journal of Occupational Therapy, 36*(1), 29-35.

White, R. H. (1959). Motivation reconsidered: The concept of competence. *Psychological Review, 66*, 126-134.

White, R. H. (1960). *Competence and the psychosexual stages of development*. Nebraska Symposium on Motivation. Lincoln, NE: University of Nebraska.

Young, M. (1988). *The metronomic society*. Cambridge, MA: Harvard University Press.

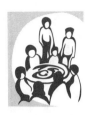

MOHO
Activity Example 9-1
The Special Events Group

This group is designed for exploratory level patients (chronic mentally ill) whose social relations and daily routines are severely disordered. The purpose is to increase orientation, to expand their level of awareness to the world outside themselves, and to work on time planning and social skills. The focus is on events in people's lives, such as holidays, birthdays, welcoming, and goodbyes, and how to celebrate them. The group is organized by the month, and begins with a planning session at the beginning of each month. The group meets for 2-hour sessions.

Materials: Posterboard with lines drawn up like a monthly calendar. Other materials are colored markers, colored paper, scissors, glue, blank cards and envelopes, cake mixes and frosting ingredients, large sheet cake pan, cake decorating kit, two large punch bowls, ingredients for punch, cake knife, serving ladle, paper supplies for parties, birthday candles, coffee maker, cream and sugar, and access to a kitchen for baking.

Directions: For a typical month, October.

Week 1—Organize monthly calendar (Figure 9-2).

Write name of month and numbers. Therapist begins by writing "1" on the day the month begins. Identify season and decorate calendar with designs appropriate for the season: pumpkins, cornstalks, leaves. Identify holidays for that month and write on calendar or decorate with appropriate symbols. Survey all patients and staff on ward to find out whose birthday is in October and write on calendar. Identify one day for the whole ward to celebrate October birthdays and Halloween and write on calendar.

Post the calendar in a prominent place on the ward. Other events, such as discharge dates and arrival or departure of staff, may also be added.

Plan what tasks need to be done for the celebration (e.g., make cards, bake cake, shop for supplies, think about masks or costumes for Halloween theme) and decide when to do each.

Week 2—Make cards. Identify birthday people and write names on index cards. Each member makes one card. If there are not enough birthdays, make some for Halloween, too. Each patient designs the card and writes the name and message inside. Stencils and markers, colored paper shapes, scissors, and glue should be available for the less "artistic."

Patients then circulate around the ward gathering signatures for the cards. A shopping list is made for needed refreshment items, eggs and milk for cake, ingredients for punch, etc. (The therapist does the actual shopping.)

Week 3—Bake cake and decorate. Group meets in kitchen. Needed items should be set out on table ahead of time (e.g., bowls, mixing spoons, measuring cups and spoons, eggs, confectioners' sugar, cake decorating supplies, etc.). The large sheet cake pan holds two complete cake mixes, so the recipe should be doubled (assuming a ward size of 20 or more).

The group divides into work teams and roles to accomplish this.

October						
S	**M**	**T**	**W**	**Th**	**F**	**S**

Figure 9-2. Special events group monthly calendar.

- Cake bakers—Recipe reader, measurer, mixer, timer
- Frosting makers—Recipe reader, measurer, mixer
- Designers—Choose motif or theme, border design, colors, and message

Supply frosting makers with desired food colors. Trace motif design on paper (jack o'lantern) and cut out. Write out message on paper and check spelling of "Happy Birthday" and "Happy Halloween."

Members learn to use decorating kit to decorate cake, frost in white, do border, trace motif, and write message. All may help with this "fun" part, and all help clean up (Figure 9-3).

When finished, the entire cake is frozen to be used the next week. The ward is informed of the date and the exact time and place are decided at a ward community meeting. Permission of staff is necessary.

Week 4—Celebration. Preparation time is 1 hour. Take cake out of freezer 2 hours ahead. Cover a large table with a sheet in the party room. Set up chairs in a large circle. Set out punch bowls and make punch. Make coffee in coffee maker, set out cream and sugar. Set out plates, forks, cake knife, cake, cups, ladle, spoons, and napkins. Bring the cards. Put the birthday candles on the cake. Bring matches or a lighter. When everything is ready, gather patients and staff.

Party—Estimate time is 30 minutes Give a toast. Members serve everyone punch, but do not drink it right away, save it for the toast. The whole group is asked to take turns proposing toasts or sharing wishes with honored members. Members lead group in singing "Happy Birthday." Candles are lit. Birthday people must come forward and blow out candles. Group members serve cake to all. Members serve themselves last. Informal socializing occurs while cake is being served. People help themselves to more punch or coffee.

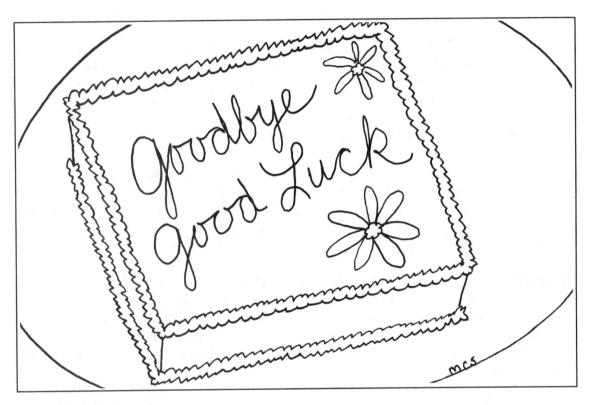

Figure 9-3. Cake decoration.

Clean up and discussion—Estimated time is 30 minutes. All members help clean up. When finished, group gathers in a meeting room to discuss and evaluate what roles members played, give feedback, verbalize what skills were learned, and discuss how to apply skills.

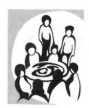

Vocational Readiness Group

This group uses craft or office activities to explore interests and practice work-related skills. The group runs for 4 weeks and has been used with competence level acute psychiatric patients and substance abuse patients. Appropriate members are those whose goal is to take on a work role after discharge. Group meets in 2-hour sessions. The goals of the group involve all three MOHO subsystems.

1. Volitional—Patients identify and explore their interests by selecting to do craft or office tasks.
2. Habituation—Patients gain and/or maintain good work habits, such as punctuality and following directions, in anticipation of regaining the worker role.
3. Performance—Patients practice basic work skills such as concentration, organization of time and materials, quality of workmanship, and task follow-through. Specific skills like typing and woodworking may also be learned and practiced.

Materials: Two typewriters, access to a copy machine, file cabinet with files and labels, typing tutorial manual, typing paper, workbench with vise, electric drill, band saw, pine boards, plywood, wood patterns, sandpaper, painting supplies, leather work supplies, belt blanks and key fob blanks, buckles, rivets, stamping tools, punch, mallets, bowls of water, sponges, and written directions for making several projects at several different levels of complexity.

Directions: Week 1—Evaluation and project choice. Members begin by doing a Work Activity Checklist. The basis for this is Noomi Katz's adaptation of Matsutsuyu's Interest Checklist (Katz, 1988.) For this group, the checklist has been modified to include work-related activities. The scale has been designed to include five work categories as follows.

Vocational Readiness Group (continued)

1. Office Work
Typing
Using computers
Filing
Answering phones
Using calculator
Accounting and math
Writing letters
Opening mail
Making appointments
Supervising employees

2. Building and Construction
Electrical wiring
Pipe fitting
Assembling parts
Working on cars
Woodworking
Refinishing furniture
Installing carpeting
Landscaping
Gardening
House painting

3. Communications/Teaching
Writing articles
Making posters
Painting signs
Broadcasting news
Introducing people
Reading books
Giving lectures
Giving exams
Taking notes
Teaching children

4. Sales/Service
Showing houses
Selling clothing
Doing make-up
Serving food
Styling hair
Giving sales pitches
Giving fashion shows
Travel planning
Dining with clients
Planning conferences

5. Home Maintenance
Washing dishes
Mopping floors
Cooking
Wallpapering
Arranging furniture
Grocery shopping
Menu planning
Doing laundry
Mixing drinks
Washing windows

From Cole, M. B. *Group Dynamics in Occupational Therapy, Second Edition.* © 1998 SLACK Incorporated.

MOHO
Activity Example 9-2
Vocational Readiness Group (continued)

Work Activity Checklist

Activity	INTEREST			PAST PERFORMANCE			FUTURE	
	Some	Casual	None	Usual	Some	Never	Yes	No
Typing	❑	❑	❑	❑	❑	❑	❑	❑
Electrical wiring	❑	❑	❑	❑	❑	❑	❑	❑
Writing articles	❑	❑	❑	❑	❑	❑	❑	❑
Showing houses	❑	❑	❑	❑	❑	❑	❑	❑
Washing dishes	❑	❑	❑	❑	❑	❑	❑	❑
Using computers	❑	❑	❑	❑	❑	❑	❑	❑
Pipe fitting	❑	❑	❑	❑	❑	❑	❑	❑
Making posters	❑	❑	❑	❑	❑	❑	❑	❑
Selling clothing	❑	❑	❑	❑	❑	❑	❑	❑
Mopping floors	❑	❑	❑	❑	❑	❑	❑	❑
Filing	❑	❑	❑	❑	❑	❑	❑	❑
Assembling parts	❑	❑	❑	❑	❑	❑	❑	❑
Painting signs	❑	❑	❑	❑	❑	❑	❑	❑
Doing make-up	❑	❑	❑	❑	❑	❑	❑	❑
Cooking	❑	❑	❑	❑	❑	❑	❑	❑
Answering phones	❑	❑	❑	❑	❑	❑	❑	❑
Working on cars	❑	❑	❑	❑	❑	❑	❑	❑
Broadcasting news	❑	❑	❑	❑	❑	❑	❑	❑
Serving food	❑	❑	❑	❑	❑	❑	❑	❑
Wallpapering	❑	❑	❑	❑	❑	❑	❑	❑
Using calculator	❑	❑	❑	❑	❑	❑	❑	❑
Woodworking	❑	❑	❑	❑	❑	❑	❑	❑
Introducing people	❑	❑	❑	❑	❑	❑	❑	❑
Styling hair	❑	❑	❑	❑	❑	❑	❑	❑
Arranging furniture	❑	❑	❑	❑	❑	❑	❑	❑
Accounting and math	❑	❑	❑	❑	❑	❑	❑	❑
Refinishing furniture	❑	❑	❑	❑	❑	❑	❑	❑
Reading books	❑	❑	❑	❑	❑	❑	❑	❑
Giving sales pitches	❑	❑	❑	❑	❑	❑	❑	❑
Grocery shopping	❑	❑	❑	❑	❑	❑	❑	❑
Writing letters	❑	❑	❑	❑	❑	❑	❑	❑
Installing carpeting	❑	❑	❑	❑	❑	❑	❑	❑
Giving lectures	❑	❑	❑	❑	❑	❑	❑	❑
Giving fashion shows	❑	❑	❑	❑	❑	❑	❑	❑
Menu planning	❑	❑	❑	❑	❑	❑	❑	❑
Opening mail	❑	❑	❑	❑	❑	❑	❑	❑
Landscaping	❑	❑	❑	❑	❑	❑	❑	❑
Giving exams	❑	❑	❑	❑	❑	❑	❑	❑
Travel planning	❑	❑	❑	❑	❑	❑	❑	❑
Doing laundry	❑	❑	❑	❑	❑	❑	❑	❑
Making appointments	❑	❑	❑	❑	❑	❑	❑	❑
Gardening	❑	❑	❑	❑	❑	❑	❑	❑
Taking notes	❑	❑	❑	❑	❑	❑	❑	❑
Dining with clients	❑	❑	❑	❑	❑	❑	❑	❑
Mixing drinks	❑	❑	❑	❑	❑	❑	❑	❑
Supervising employees	❑	❑	❑	❑	❑	❑	❑	❑
House painting	❑	❑	❑	❑	❑	❑	❑	❑
Teaching children	❑	❑	❑	❑	❑	❑	❑	❑
Planning conferences	❑	❑	❑	❑	❑	❑	❑	❑
Washing windows	❑	❑	❑	❑	❑	❑	❑	❑

From Cole, M. B. *Group Dynamics in Occupational Therapy, Second Edition.* © 1998 SLACK Incorporated.

The checklist is discussed with regard to interests, past work history, and satisfaction with current work skills. The expectations for the group are then shared. Members are expected to:

- Arrive on time or give prior notification of absence
- Appear well-groomed and dressed in clean work clothes
- Follow directions for project/task
- Respond positively to supervision
- Effectively deal with frustration
- Ask for help when needed
- Work independently
- Learn necessary skills
- Follow through on task (meet deadlines); strive for quality of workmanship

Several starter projects should be ready with written directions for each patient. Members may choose projects based on their interests and skills, and get started for the remaining time. Examples of starter craft projects are leather key fobs with stamped initials and border, wood wall plaque made from precut 6- x 8-inch pine board with picture to decoupage, or a wood trivet made from a kit. Examples of starter work projects are typing a short letter or sorting tiles by color. Starter projects are intended to teach basic skills and allow the therapist to evaluate patients' manual and cognitive abilities.

Weeks 2 through 4—Patients complete projects as assigned by the therapist. Each patient works independently on a different project. At the end of each session, members are evaluated with the Work Behavior Rating Scale and results are discussed with the patients.

Work Behavior Rating Scale

Name	Dates				
Arrives on time (gives prior notice of valid absence)					
Appropriate appearance (well-groomed, clean work clothing)					
Follows directions					
Responds positively to supervision					
Effectively deals with frustration					
Asks for help when needed					
Works independently					
Learns necessary skills					
Follows through on tasks (meets deadlines)					

Scale: 1=Independent and correct
          2=Requires some assistance
          3=Requires much assistance
          4=Is dependent or unmotivated

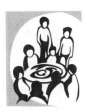

MOHO
Activity Example 9-3
The Perfect Parent

This activity is designed for mothers who have arthritis, or other physical illness involving chronic pain or limitation, who wish to continue being good parents to their young children.

Materials: Worksheets and pencils.

Directions: Have members begin by giving their names, and then the names and ages of children living with them. "The purpose of today's activity is to identify some specific concerns involving your ability to care for your children as you deal with the chronic pain and limitations of arthritis." Hand out worksheets and pencils, and give 15 minutes to complete. Areas to consider for parental tasks are: meal preparation, dressing, shopping, family events, school-related activities, sports, cultural and social activities, developing special talents or interests, and nurturing/emotional support.

Discussion: The group shares areas of concern from their individual worksheets. Priorities may be discussed, and ideas for coping with conflicts may be shared.

The Perfect Parent (continued)

The Perfect Parent Worksheet

Write name and age of each child:

List and describe five tasks you must perform for your children before 9:00 a.m. on a typical school day.

1.

2.

3.

4.

5.

List five tasks your children would appreciate your doing for them before they return home from school.

1.

2.

3.

4.

5.

List five tasks you must do for your children after 5:00 p.m. on a typical school day.

1.

2.

3.

4.

5.

   Go back over the above lists and place a * next to those tasks that present potential problems for you in terms of physical exertion or endurance, time constraints, or conflicting obligations.

The Perfect Parent (continued)

The Perfect Parent Schedule Worksheet

Directions: Write the tasks listed on the preceding page in the column "Things I Want to Do for My Children" at the appropriate times. Then, in the next column, schedule in your own needs for rest, exercise, socialization, and other obligations. Put a * next to possible conflicts between these.

Typical School Day	Things I Want to Do for My Children	Things I Need to Do for Myself
6:00 a.m.		
7:00 a.m.		
8:00 a.m.		
9:00 a.m.		
10:00 a.m.		
11:00 a.m.		
12:00 p.m.		
1:00 p.m.		
2:00 p.m.		
3:00 p.m.		
4:00 p.m.		
5:00 p.m.		
6:00 p.m.		
7:00 p.m.		
8:00 p.m.		
9:00 p.m.		
10:00 p.m.		
11:00 p.m. or later		

Conflict areas:

Coping strategies:

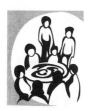

MOHO
Activity Example 9-4
Forming Good Habits

This activity is designed for persons whose daily structure have been disrupted by illness or injury. It starts at the beginning again, with self-care, and assists with building a supportive environment. This activity may require two or three sessions to complete, depending on attention span of members. Contact with family member of caregiver is needed for follow-up.

Materials: 3- x 5-inch cards with pictures of: toothbrush, toothpaste, glass, shower or bathtub, bathmat, soap, washcloth, towel, razor, shaving cream, cosmetics, nail file, nail clippers, hand lotion, hairbrush, comb, shampoo, conditioner, and a variety of clothing items appropriate to season and age of members. A second set of cards contains pictures of: dishes, utensils, breakfast items, kitchen sink/dishwasher, sponge, broom, dustpan, and trashcan. Duplicate cards should be made for each member. Pictures may be cut out of magazines as needed for this activity. Posterboards, glue or tape, and broad black markers are needed for the second part of this activity.

Directions: Members introduce themselves and discuss familiar morning routines they can remember having in the past. Cards for bathing, dental care, shaving, hair care, and make-up are distributed, and members asked to select those items used in the morning and place them in sequence in front of them on the table. Items may be sorted into categories and each given separately, depending on the skill level of group members. Dressing and breakfast cards are given in a likewise manner.

Discussion: How can members learn good morning habits? What is the best sequence of tasks for each individual? What is your home environment like? Where can you keep the items pictured on the cards so that you can find them easily each day?

Follow-Up: Posterboards are distributed with labels at the top of each: Grooming and Bathing, Dressing, Eating Breakfast, and Cleaning Up. Each member selects appropriate cards and pastes or tapes them to the posterboard in the desired sequence. Members take the posterboards home with them and obtain assistance in gathering the items pictured and finding appropriate storage for the items. The posters serve as reminders until sequences are repeated often enough to form good daily habits of self-care.

SECTION THREE
Planning an Occupational Therapy Group

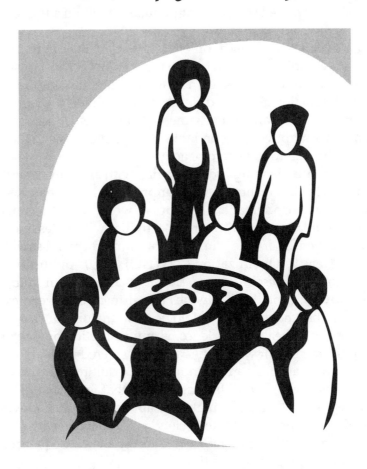

Chapter 10: Writing a Group Treatment Protocol

Chapter 11: A Group Laboratory Experience

Introduction to Section Three

The final step in the learning process of occupational therapy group treatment is applying our knowledge to patient populations. Chapters 10 and 11 take the form of guided learning experiences. Chapter 10, *Writing a Group Treatment Protocol*, gives guidelines for thinking about the needs of a patient population within a frame of reference and generating a written group plan.

One of the keys to successful application of theory lies in the understanding of patient dysfunction. It has been pointed out that the parts of function and dysfunction that are addressed changes in each frame of reference. In addition, it is important to remember that function and dysfunction are very different from diagnosis. Diagnosis is a medical term which identifies illness and guides medical treatment. Occupational therapy's emphasis on a patient's adaptive function looks beyond diagnosis to the consequence of illness and disease with regard to everyday activities.

In Chapter 10, the group planning process begins with an analysis of the patient population to be treated. This is a reality-oriented approach which looks at some of the typical treatment settings where occupational therapists work. As the occupational therapist assesses the patient population for which group activities will be designed, she must look carefully at the consequences of illness in terms of impairments, disabilities, and handicaps. The World Health Organization's (WHO) 1980 publication *International Classification of Impairments, Disabilities and Handicaps* is a helpful guide to our understanding of patient dysfunction. WHO defines impairment in the context of health as a loss or abnormality of psychological, physiological, or anatomical structure or function. Disability, in the context of health experience, is any restriction or lack of ability to perform an activity in the manner or within the range considered normal for a human being. A handicap is a disadvantage for a given individual, resulting from an impairment or a disability, that limits or prevents fulfillment of a role that is normal (depending on age, sex, and cultural factors) for that individual. A disability is considered within the context of the person, while a handicap relates to society or compliance with social norms. This distinction helps the occupational therapist to address the consequences of illness that can be best affected through group activities.

Chapter 11, *A Group Laboratory Experience*, offers a group membership experience as a context for learning about group dynamics. This chapter follows the guidelines of Chapter 10 and provides an example of the analysis of the needs of a student population. "Developing Your Professional Self" is an example of a group protocol which can be beneficial for students' professional development as they approach the clinical training phase of their education. In the 5 years we have been doing these groups for second semester juniors, the feedback from students has been excellent. In addition to learning and applying the principles of group dynamics, students have found the feedback for themselves invaluable for their own professional growth.

These two experiences should facilitate the application of theory in practice. The process of this text has gone from concrete (the format), to abstract (the frames), and then back to concrete (the plan). This is not unlike the clinical reasoning process itself, which swings back and forth between the empirical and the hypothetical as the therapy process progresses. A good group plan involves the empirical collection of data about patients' impairments, disabilities, and handicaps; the formation of a hypothesis about what kind of group activity might be helpful; and method for evaluation of treatment outcome after implementation (empirical again). The laboratory experience for students demonstrates this process.

Finally, as part of the practical application of theory to the group planning process, the student is encouraged to think about how the original seven-step format changes with each frame of reference. As a learning guide, a chart comparing group leadership in the seven frames of reference is presented in Appendix E.

Bibliography

World Health Organization. (1980). *International classification of impairments, disabilities and handicaps*. Geneva, Switzerland: Author.

Chapter 10

Writing a Group Treatment Protocol

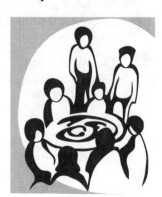

The group protocol is an extensive and detailed outline of a group to be planned by the occupational therapist for a specific patient population. This exercise is intended to prepare therapists to plan effective programs to meet the needs of patients in a wide variety of diagnostic categories and using a variety of frames of reference. Five steps have been outlined to clarify our clinical thinking about groups:

1. Identifying a patient population
2. Selecting a frame of reference
3. Selecting what aspect of treatment to address
4. Writing a group treatment outline
5. Planning individual sessions

Identifying Your Patient Population

For the purposes of learning, the student should choose one of the following treatment settings where occupational therapists typically treat patients. This will be the patient population around which you will plan your group. Use the Patient Population worksheet (Worksheet 10-1) to help you.

- Adolescent mental health inpatient (21 days)
- Adult substance abuse inpatient program (14 days)
- Stroke recovery unit (90 days)
- Chronic mental health inpatient (10 days)
- Unit for traumatic brain injured adults (90 days)
- Group home for adults with developmental disabilities
- Outpatient program for adults with physical disability (specify one type)
- Geriatrics, skilled nursing facility
- Cardiac recovery outpatient group
- Hand injury outpatient clinic
- Terminal illness outpatient group (AIDS, cancer)
- Senior center prevention/education
- Injury prevention in the workplace, health insurance seminar for employees
- Dementia home care, family/caregiver education

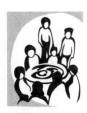

1. Population Choice
Choose a treatment setting from those listed on the previous page. If you like more than one, list pros and cons of each to help you decide.

First Choice _____

Pros	Cons
1.	1.
2.	2.
3.	3.

Second Choice _____

Pros	Cons
1.	1.
2.	2.
3.	3.

2. Population Definition
    a. Identify two centers nearby that treat this population.
    First Resource
    Center:

    Telephone number:

    Address:

    Contact person/therapist:

    Second Resource
    Center:

    Telephone number:

    Address:

    Contact person/therapist:

b. Describe patient characteristics typical of the center.

Age range:

Male/female (percentage of each):

Diagnostic categories and approximate percentages (list):

Patient's education level (average or range):

Patient's living arrangement when not hospitalized (list):

Occupation/work status (a few typical examples):

Socioeconomic status (average or range):

c. Predict rehabilitation potential.
Approximate level of functioning (high, medium, low):

Describe expectation of recovery or give approximate probabilities:
Full recovery
Partial recovery
Chronic disability
Gradual decline

Physical limitations:

Verbal ability/interaction potential:

Probable discharge plan (describe):
Independent
Home with assistance
Community placement
Institutional placement

d. Describe treatment setting.

Type of treatment setting (day treatment, inpatient, clinic, community):

Treatment setting's frame of reference (if known):

Settings should be chosen on the basis of interest, prior experience, or curiosity. The planning will incorporate a process of familiarization with the chosen population. Since most students do not have much experience, it is advisable to contact a local treatment center and arrange a visit. Fieldwork I experience or prior volunteer experience is also helpful. It is impossible to plan an effective group treatment experience without some knowledge of the population for which it is intended.

Another way to become more familiar with the population you choose is to do some reference reading. Many excellent books are available describing specific diagnostic categories, such as Alzheimer's disease, multiple sclerosis, drug abuse, eating disorders, and mental retardation. Reading case studies of people with these disorders is particularly helpful.

Writing a Group Treatment Protocol

Probably the most motivating way to choose a diagnostic category is personal experience. Many students have friends or relatives who may have a disorder that fits one of the listed categories. Writing a group protocol for a specific individual and others with the same disorder gives the student the advantage of greater personal understanding. It may be easier to imagine the impact of certain group activities and the barriers that may need to be addressed.

For those students who are unfamiliar with some of the diagnoses mentioned or implied in the list of populations, a short research assignment may be appropriate prior to attempting Worksheet 10-1. Once the patients in a given setting are defined with respect to diagnosis, one or two of the most common illnesses can be researched in medical textbooks.

How to Select a Frame of Reference

After you describe your patient population, the next decision to make is what frame of reference to use. There are several factors to consider in this decision. The preceding seven chapters can be consulted for a better understanding of the choices. While there are many frames of references in occupational therapy, for this assignment, try to stick with **one** of the seven included in this text and stick with options within that chapter. While personal beliefs usually have some influence over frame of reference selection, students should become competent in using all of them.

The major factor in the selection should be what is likely to work best for the patient. Sometimes the treatment setting has an identified frame of reference, and if so, the occupational therapist should find an occupational therapy frame of reference that is compatible with it. Some helpful factors to consider are: view of function and dysfunction, patient physical and cognitive level of function, change strategies, view of motivation, treatment timeframe, and treatment options. Use Worksheet 10-2 to summarize at least two choices of frames to be considered.

Factors to Consider

Definition of Function and Dysfunction

Each frame of reference has its unique point of view of disability. Looking at your patient population, compare their abilities and disabilities with the explanations of function and dysfunction given in each frame of reference. Which frame best explains the function and dysfunction you see in your patients? Why?

Patient Level of Functioning

Some frames of reference have a greater usefulness for higher functioning patients,

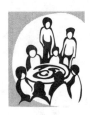

Worksheet 10-2
Selecting a Frame of Reference

Frame of reference selected (first choice): _____

Definition of function and dysfunction:

Patient level of functioning:

Change strategies:

Motivation:

Treatment timeframe:

Treatment options/modalities:

Selecting a Frame of Reference (continued)

Frame of reference selected (second choice): _____

Definition of function and dysfunction:

Patient level of functioning:

Change strategies:

Motivation:

Treatment timeframe:

Treatment options/modalities:

while some relate better to lower levels of functioning. Which frame offers treatment guidelines that have been effective for your patients' level of functioning? Summarize guidelines given to your patients.

Change Strategies

Another way the frames of reference differ is in their view of the change process. Some depend on the therapeutic relationship or on group interaction to facilitate change, while others rely more heavily on the components of tasks and activities or on the environment.

Think about what changes your patients need to make. Then look at the explanations given by the frames of reference on how change takes place. Which do you think might work the best for your patients? Why?

Motivation

How motivated are your patients? What forces do you think might motivate them to make positive changes? Each frame of reference explains motivation differently. The humanistic view is freedom from anxiety and self-actualization. The psychoanalytic, developmental, and sensory motor frames of reference and model of human occupation describe a drive toward mastery, but each defines something different to be mastered. The behavioral cognitive approaches look at various forms of reinforcement as the motivator. The goals of most of our occupational therapy groups are to help patients achieve a higher level of function or adaptation. However, it is not enough for the therapist to be motivated. We need to think about our patients' motivation as well. Which frame of reference best explains how our patients could be motivated? Why?

Treatment Timeframe

Some frames of reference work best for long-term treatment that encourages the development of relationships and insight, while others lend themselves to more immediate goals. For the purposes of this assignment, the treatment runs for six sessions of 1 hour each. But these could be spread out once a week for 6 weeks or condensed into two sessions a day for 3 days. If there is no center mentioned, what would be the most likely setting for the patient population you have chosen? Acute settings can be assumed to average 10 to 14 days. Substance abuse programs are generally 3 to 4 weeks of intensive inpatient treatment. Day treatment can go on for 1 year or more and chronic conditions can be treated for a lifetime. How long are your patients likely to be in treatment? Which frame of reference best fits the timeframe at your identified treatment center?

Treatment Options/Modalities

Each frame of reference has different guidelines for activity selection. Some have specific suggestions, while others are more flexible and able to be adapted. Some use creative modalities, movement, or sports activities, while others include learning skills through pencil and paper worksheets or group interaction exercises. Look at the activity examples suggested by the frame of reference and decide which would most interest you and your patients. Which frame of reference offers treatment options that would interest you? What are they? Which frame of reference offers treatment options or modalities that would interest your patients and/or best meet their needs? What are some options you might choose?

To further guide your selection of a frame of reference, the Leadership Style Guidelines in Chapter 1 may help you understand the implications for leadership and structure of groups. In addition,

Appendix E is designed to summarize the group guidelines in each of the seven approaches included in Section Two of this book.

Selecting What Aspect of Treatment to Address

All of the occupational performance areas and occupational components which make up the domain of concern of occupational therapy have been listed and organized in one convenient document. That document is called *Uniform Terminology for Occupational Therapy*, revised last in April 1994 by the American Occupational Therapy Association, along with a guide for its use by Dunn and colleagues (1994). The occupational performance areas listed are activities of daily living, work and productive activities, and play or leisure activities. Activities of daily living include: grooming, oral hygiene, bathing, toilet hygiene, dressing, feeding and eating, medication routine, socialization, functional communication, functional mobility, and sexual expression. Work and productive activities include home management, care of others, and educational and vocational activities. Play or leisure activities include both exploration and performance.

Performance components in Uniform Terminology are sensory motor components, cognitive integration and cognitive components, and psychosocial skills and psychological components.

A third section, performance contexts, includes temporal and environmental aspects. See Appendix D for the full Uniform Terminology document.

The best strategy is to go over Appendix D and decide what performance areas, components, and/or contexts your patients most need to work on or improve.

Most patients have more than one, and activities in occupational therapy can be designed to address several of these areas, components, or contexts. After looking over the document, list 10 performance areas, components, and/or contexts that your patient population may need to work on (Worksheet 10-3). In the next section, these identified aspects of treatment can help us to formulate goals for our group.

Group Treatment Plan Outline

Once the patient population is chosen and the frame of reference and aspects of treatment have been identified, the next step is to write a general outline. The outline should include all the factors inherent in designing a group. The general outline includes the following headings:
- Group title
- Author
- Frame of reference
- Purpose
- Group membership and size
- Group goals and rationale
- Outcome criteria
- Method
- Time and place of meeting
- Supplies and cost
- References

This outline is intended to include not only the ingredients of an effective group treatment protocol, but also factors which will be of interest to administrators. Often occupational therapists are asked to present a group protocol to administrators prior to implementation. Administrators will need to consider factors such as group size, space, scheduling, and cost. The plan you present must not only be therapeutically sound, but also cost-effective.

Group Title

The name of a group is often the patient's first impression of the role occupational therapy will play in treatment. Choose it with care. Not only should a title

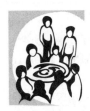

Worksheet 10-3
Performance Areas, Components,
and Contexts

List 10 performance areas, components, and/or contexts that your patient population may need to work on.

1.

2.

3.

4.

5.

6.

7.

8.

9.

10.

accurately reflect the goals and content of the group, but it should also attract the patient's interest. Some examples of good titles are: "Developing Self-Identity" (a group for substance abusing adolescents), "Art for Social Skills" (a group for persons with chronic mental illness), and "Re-entering Your Kitchen" (a group for post-operative cardiac patients).

Author

This includes your name and professional title: Jane Doe, OTS.

Frame of Reference

State the frame of reference you have decided to use to guide your approach to patients, organization of treatment groups, and selection of activities. A single sentence on why this frame of reference is appropriate will suffice: "The behavioral cognitive approach has been widely used with substance abuse patients, and it seems to help them change their own behavior by learning new ways of thinking about their lives."

Purpose

The purpose of the group is the group's general intent. Overall goals of the group should be stated, as well as the general nature of the activities to be used. This section should be short, preferably no longer than three sentences summarizing the overall scope of the group plan. For example, the purpose of a leisure planning group might be to assist patients whose disability requires a loss of the worker role, to identify and plan for leisure activities to meet their social and emotional needs. Patients will complete written exercises, participate in group discussions, and plan and carry out individual leisure activities as part of group requirements.

Group Membership and Size

The patient population for which your group is intended should be described in as much detail as possible. Not only general diagnostic factors, but factors such as age, functional level, gender, and role identity might be included. For purposes of referral, both inclusionary and exclusionary criteria should be described here. Inclusionary criteria describes characteristics that are appropriate for your group; exclusionary describes characteristics that are not appropriate. Some activities are appropriate for specific groups only, while others encompass a wide variety of characteristics. A target population should always be identified to give the group a focus. Broader applicability of the protocol should be described in a separate paragraph.

For the purposes of this assignment, the size of groups will be limited to three to eight members. It is generally not cost-effective to treat groups of less than three and not effective treatment for more than eight. The size of a group will depend on many factors, such as the degree of impairment, the need for individual attention, and the complexity of the tasks. Group membership may be open or closed. A closed group includes all the same patients at every session for the duration of the group. An open group allows members to be added or dropped from session to session. It is generally easier to plan for closed groups, since the membership is predictable and a sense of belonging is developed. Open groups are more practical for most treatment settings and are a necessity in acute settings where patients come and go rapidly. This assignment requires you to plan a closed group. This allows the student to plan specific sessions without having to adapt to unexpected changes in membership.

Group Goals and Rationale

The goals of a group are the specific treatment aims that are intended to be met by individuals participating in the group. No less than three and no more than eight goals should be stated. Less than three usually means that goals are too vague and therefore not useful in planning specific activities. More than eight gives the group too broad a focus. Ideally, there should be at least one specific goal for each individual session planned. However, since there is usually overlap (i.e., more than one goal met with any given activity), the exact number will vary.

Goals should be stated in measurable terms. They should state what the patient will do, that is, define, discuss, report, demonstrate. Vague terms like "learn," "understand," and "develop" should be avoided; "attend" and "participate" are generally not enough of a description to be meaningful.

Well-written goals are the backbone of any well-designed group. They will make the rest of the group easier to plan and the outcome easier to measure. For example, the goals of a money management group might be:

1. Recognize the need for a budget
2. List monthly income and expenses
3. Demonstrate ability to follow a budget for 1 week
4. Demonstrate specific banking skills
5. List anticipated needs and expenses
6. Practice comparative shopping techniques and skills to reduce impulse buying

Once these goals are identified, the activities used to reach the goals will logically follow. Perhaps each group session can focus on a different goal, or several sessions can include more than one goal. For example, goal number 4 can be addressed by giving each patient samples of a check register, check, deposit slip, and withdrawal slip. Simple addition and subtraction can be practiced and included when appropriate. Use of a banking machine or telephone banking can be taught and practiced. The outcome of this activity can be measured by examining the completed forms and watching the demonstrated procedures. Specific activities and measured outcomes should follow logically from each stated goal. Rationale for goal selection should relate goals to the chosen patient population and its inherent problems. This section should explain why the goals you selected are appropriate. Limitations of the group should be mentioned—for which patients are these goals inappropriate? For example, patients who will be institutionalized may not need the skills. Precautions that may need to be taken should also be mentioned in the rationale.

Adaptations that can be made to make the group useful to a wider variety of patients, perhaps in settings other than the target setting, should be mentioned here as well. For example, in the case of the money management group, the same goals can be applied to any group of patients with the goal of living independently.

Outcome Criteria

The desired results of the group should be stated in behavioral terms. By the end of the group, each patient should be able to show how he has progressed. The therapist needs to develop a measurable way to demonstrate the effectiveness of the group to the patient, the administrator, and to those responsible for payment of services. Specific procedures should be outlined, such as a pre- and post-questionnaire or a pre-post rating scale for each patient. An appropriate assessment tool can be identified, if one exists, or evaluation can be specific for the group offered. If verbal feedback is used, the therapist should specify where and how this information is to be recorded. A pre-post test, assessment, questionnaire, or documentation worksheet (e.g., Group Member Progress Rating) must accompany your group outline as a separate sheet.

Method

An outline of the media to be used and the kind of leadership offered are key elements here. Media can be as simple as structured discussions and as complex as learning to build a small engine. Most activities are fair game. However, complex media that require special training, such as biofeedback, systematic desensitization, bioenergetics, and psychodrama, should not be used. Therapeutic interventions which are the traditional roles of other disciplines, such as family therapy, unstructured verbal psychotherapy, or dietary planning, should also be avoided.

The kind of leadership offered depends upon the therapist's frame of reference. If a psychoeducational format is used, the therapist may include short lecturettes on skills to be learned. (The therapist's frame of reference will determine the type of introduction and explanation given to patients during each session.) The group protocol should reflect a consistent frame of reference. If a humanistic or an ego adaptive approach is used, more emphasis may be placed on group interaction. Cognitive groups for lower level patients require more structured environments with carefully planned therapist assistance.

Time and Place of Meeting

Several design elements should be described in this section. For the purposes of this assignment, the time will be limited to six sessions of 1 hour each. The scheduling of sessions will vary according to the treatment setting. Chronic settings will accommodate weekly sessions. Acute settings may require daily meetings. The length of sessions will vary with patient attention span and type of activity chosen.

The place of meeting should be chosen with specific requirements in mind. In an actual treatment setting, a room can be identified. For the purposes of this assignment, only the characteristics of the setting should be described. The following environmental factors could be included:

- Size of room
- Contents (tables, chairs, cabinets, sink, etc.)
- Lighting, windows
- Visual factors (bare walls or more home-like)
- Door opened or closed
- Noise factors (not next to gym or bathroom)
- Accessibility of medical assistance (special telephone equipment needed, kitchen for cooking activities)
- Availability of assistance from therapist
- Safety factors

This assignment will not limit any of these factors. A good room description will take into consideration the characteristics of the patient population chosen, as well as the activities to be included.

Supplies and Cost

The sum total of all materials and supplies and their total cost is listed here. It is recognized that copies of forms and paper and pencils or pens are generally available in most settings at no cost. Items other than these should be listed. If specific items such as videotapes or assessment materials are to be used, the name and address of the source of these should also be listed. This section will probably have to be done after specific sessions are outlined.

References

List all references that were used to create the material for the group sessions, including lecturettes, forms to be used as worksheets, and other copyrighted materials. References should use the format of the *Publication Manual of the American Psychological Association* (1994).

- Books—Author, date, title, place of publication, publisher.
- Articles—Author, date, title of article, journal name, volume, number, pages.
- Materials—Name of item, name and address of source (company, center, or hospital), telephone number, approximate cost.

Group Session Outline

A group session outline should be written for each of the six sessions of your group. Headings are as follows.

- Group title
- Session title
- Format (time sequence)
- Supplies
- Description

Session _____ of 6

The session number (this session) of total number of sessions planned indicates sequence. Your group sessions should be planned in logical order, from simple to complex, superficial to deep, general to specific, etc. In a closed group, the sessions should build on one another so that general group principles can be applied. It would make sense for the first session to be somewhat introductory, so that members begin to know not only the subject of the group, but each other as well. Subjects of a more personal nature should be saved for later in the sequence when members know one another better. The last session needs to deal with summary and termination of the group. The way you sequence the sessions will depend somewhat on your chosen population.

Group Title

This is the title of the group as a whole, for example, "Money Management."

Session Title

Like the group title, each session should be labeled with a word or phrase describing either the content or the goal for that session.

Format

This is a short outline stating what will happen when. For example, a session in "Balancing Your Checkbook" might have the following format.

Review last week—10 minutes
Introductory lecturette—10 minutes
Complete sample checkbook worksheet—10 minutes
Check answers with calculator—10 minutes
Discuss specific problems and summarize importance of balancing checkbook—20 minutes
Total—60 minutes

You need not include this last total figure, but make sure your timing fits the total time allotted for the group.

Supplies

This category includes a complete list of what is needed to complete the group. Do not assume patients will be carrying pens and pencils with them or will be wearing a watch. The supply list should include the correct number of each item needed. For a "Balancing Your Checkbook" session, supplies for a group of five patients would include the following:

5 worksheets (attach copy)
5 pencils
5 pocket calculators
1 large pad and 1 marker (for therapist to illustrate process)

Description

This is a step-by-step description of what will be included. The introduction should be fully described, including warm-up (if appropriate), explanation of purpose, expectations, and timeframe. If there are lecturettes, these must be outlined. If worksheets are to be written, a copy must be attached. Activities must be fully described including directions, choices, and timing. If the activity was selected from a text or prior experience, reference should be given. For the discussion part, a list of questions to be asked is included. The discussion questions should be divided into the following categories: *processing*, *generalizing*, and *application* (refer to Chapter 1 for a description of these phases of the group). Your discussions will vary depending on the frame of reference you are using. It is wise to be prepared with more questions than you will need. Also keep in mind the goals of the group when choosing discussion questions. An activity is generally more effective when the patients feel it has meaning for them. Relating each session's activity back to the original goals will help keep both patients and the therapist on track. A verbal summary at the end of each session is important. Include for each session some points to remember for the summary.

Instructions for Preparing Protocol

When you have written the entire protocol, you should type it into a computer. Each session should start a new page. When putting on the computer, use the exact headings in the order described. Capitalize the headings; use single spacing and 1-inch margins. It is not necessary to indent. Skip a line between each section or heading.

When rating sheets or worksheets are used, a copy should be attached to the outline or session to which it relates. Use the following forms to write your first draft of your Group Treatment Plan Protocol (Worksheet 10-4).

Note

James P. Klyczek is acknowledged here as the co-author of Chapter 10. Dr. Klyczek originated the concept of the group treatment plan assignment with the six session outlines in 1985 while teaching in the Occupational Therapy Program at SUNY Buffalo, New York. Currently, Dr. Klyczek is the Associate Dean of Graduate Studies and Academic Affairs and Dean of Health and Human Services, D'Youville College, Buffalo, New York.

Bibliography

American Psychological Association. (1994). *Publication manual of the American Psychological Association* (4th ed.). Washington, DC: Author.

American Occupational Therapy Association. (1994). *Uniform terminology for occupational therapy* (3rd ed.). Bethesda, MD: Author.

Dunn, W., et al. (1994). *Application of uniform terminology to practice*. Bethesda, MD: American Occupational Therapy Association.

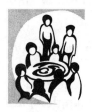

Worksheet 10-4
Group Treatment Plan Protocol

Group title:

Author:

Frame of reference:

Purpose:

Group membership and size:

Group goals:

1.

2.

3.

4.

5.

6.

7.

8.

Rationale (include limitations, adaptations, and precautions):

Outcome criteria (create a rating scale/format on a separate sheet to record progress of members). Describe how it will be used here:

Method:

Time and place of meeting:

Supplies and cost:

References:

Group Session Outline
Session 1 of 6

Group title:

Session title:

Format:

Supplies:

Description:

Group title:

Session title:

Format:

Supplies:

Description:

Group title:

Session title:

Format:

Supplies:

Description:

Group Session Outline
Session 4 of 6

Group title:

Session title:

Format:

Supplies:

Description:

Group Session Outline
Session 5 of 6

Group title:

Session title:

Format:

Supplies:

Description:

Group Session Outline
Session 6 of 6

Group title:

Session title:

Format:

Supplies:

Description:

A Group Laboratory Experience

The following is an example of a group protocol. It is a group designed as a laboratory experience for professional students. Ideally it is done in groups of eight students, with the instructor as leader. It addresses some of the most common professional issues for students and serves as a context for the discussion of the principles of group dynamics described in Chapter 2. The series of six sessions is planned in a sequence that moves toward greater intimacy as the group develops. The leadership is also intended to change from directive in the beginning toward a democratic, facilitative style at the end. The group leader models therapeutic interventions with various problem behaviors and fosters the exploration of here-and-now relationships. Members have the opportunity to take on various roles and to practice group interaction skills. Process illumination should be discussed as a part of each session, with a goal of learning and personal growth. Although this is a six-session sequence, it has been suggested by my students that three open sessions be interspersed.

An open session has no planned activity, and its purpose is to discuss the process of prior sessions. After Session 3 in my group, for example, there seemed to be little time to discuss the many issues and feelings resulting from giving and receiving feedback. An open group following this session would give the members a chance to discuss their concerns and to better understand their relationship to each other. Session 4 seemed to be too structured, and several of the groups felt the need to voice their urge to rebel against the structure and/or the directive leadership style. An open session following this one would allow for the discussion of group development and the significance of their rebellion in the context of group development theories. Another interesting addition to the sequence is a leaderless group. This forces the group members to take on leadership roles, and further illuminates the group process. This semester, many of the groups decided to end their group with a "termination" activity. One group brought in brunch, another had a pizza party, and another decided on a goodbye collage. With these additions, the group lab experience is expanded to 10 weekly sessions.

Group Treatment Plan Outline

Group title: "Developing Your Professional Self"

Author: Marilyn B. Cole, MS, OTR/L

Frame of reference: The frame of reference for this group is humanistic. The assumption is that members are motivated to know themselves better and to become competent professionals.

Purpose: This group is designed to help junior occupational therapy students to make the transition from a student role to a professional role. The six group activities are selected to deal with the most common areas of difficulty for students, such as being assertive, accepting feedback, and setting priorities in their lives.

Group membership and size: "Developing Your Professional Self" is designed for second semester junior occupational therapy students. Most of these students are between 20 and 22 years of age, although several are adults coming back to school. The majority are women who have lived independent of their families for at least 2 years, although there are several men and several students who commute from home. Having entered the junior year in an occupational therapy academic program, these students have all achieved and maintained a high academic average, and have survived at least one semester of difficult and challenging professional coursework. All have had at least one semester of clinical Fieldwork I experiences, allowing them a taste of what it is like to work with patients (a few hours per week). In choosing to become occupational therapists, these students have set a goal and are working to achieve it.

This will be a closed group of no more than eight members. The same members will be expected to attend all six sessions with no absences (Worksheet 11-1).

Group goals and rationale: The student will:
1. Discuss awareness of professional self in relation to clients and peers.
2. Demonstrate ability to problem solve, behave assertively, and set goals and priorities.
3. Identify strengths and weaknesses of self and others.
4. Express feelings directly and offer respectful feedback to others.
5. Accept feedback from others and use it constructively.
6. Clearly state professional values.
7. Demonstrate ability to interact effectively with peers.
8. Identify group behaviors and group process.

Students in the junior year are learning many of the skills necessary to treat patients. However, in order to use those skills effectively, the student needs to feel comfortable in the professional role. The "Developing Your Professional Self" group is designed to promote a needed self-awareness associated with professionalism. As a professional team member, future occupational therapists will need to interact effectively, behave assertively when necessary, share in group problem-solving, and learn constructively from other

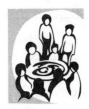

Worksheet 11-1
Contract for Group Membership

This contract should be reviewed and signed by each member of the group before beginning the first session.

I understand I am involved in a developmental process and therefore it is necessary to attend all sessions to benefit fully from the process. I realize that in order for me to be an effective member, it is important that I complete all assignments and arrive on time. I agree to participate as openly, honestly, and responsibly as I am able to, realizing that I am not under any group pressure to reveal personal data that I would regret sharing with the group. I agree to speak personally and make "I" statements as objectively and specifically as I can, trying not to generalize or talk in abstractions. I realize that no personal information about any group member should ever be discussed outside of the group.

Signed: _____

Date: _____

From Cole, M. B. *Group Dynamics in Occupational Therapy, Second Edition.* © 1998 SLACK Incorporated.

team members. Factors other than academic ones will influence professional effectiveness, such as warmth and empathy, flexibility and openness, ability to express feelings, and appropriate self-disclosure. The group format gives students an opportunity to explore and practice needed skills and attributes in preparation for their Fieldwork II experiences.

This group design, although planned for occupational therapy students, may also be useful for students in other disciplines. Adaptations would be minimal, simply substituting for "occupational therapy," nursing, physical therapy, social work, etc. The group and interpersonal skills needed by many health professionals are quite similar.

Outcome criteria:
1. The student will demonstrate interpersonal skills by verbal participation at least three times in each weekly session.
2. Students within the context of each session will discuss and demonstrate the skills required for self-disclosure, problem-solving, giving and receiving feedback, empathizing with or confronting others, behaving assertively, and setting goals and priorities.
3. The progress of each student may be rated twice on a 5-point scale, 1 being poor ability and 5 being excellent ability. The first rating should be before the first session, the second rating after the sixth session. This pre- and post-group rating will then show progress made by each student in each skill required. The Group Member Progress Rating chart (Worksheet 11-2) may be used to measure progress in each of these factors: self-disclosure, problem-solving, giving feedback, receiving feedback, empathizing with others, confronting others, behaving assertively, setting personal goals, and understanding dynamics.

Method: Structured group activities and discussions will occur each week. The activities will be graded from a superficial and safe level to a deeper level interpersonally. The activities will also be graded so as to encourage more group interaction and less dependence on the leader as each week progresses. Group development and interpersonal learning will be encouraged, and an understanding of the process of the group will be facilitated.

Time and place of meeting: The group will meet for 1 hour each week for 6 weeks. The rooms are selected to be free of noise distraction and to preserve the confidentiality of the group. A large table and nine chairs are preferable, so that members can work on group projects. On days when only discussion takes place, chairs may be arranged in a circle without the table. For the 1-hour meeting, it is important that no one leaves or comes late, and that there are no interruptions. The door should be closed, and a sign saying "Do Not Disturb, Group in Session" should be displayed outside.

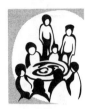

Worksheet 11-2
Group Member Progress Rating

Rating 1 (low) to 5 (high)	Session 1	Session 6 (or last)
Self-disclosure		
Problem-solving		
Giving feedback		
Receiving feedback		
Empathizing with others		
Confronting others		
Behaving assertively		
Setting personal goals		
Understanding dynamics		

Supplies and cost:

	Unit price	Total
9 sheets of white drawing paper 12 x 18 inches	donated	
16 assorted magazines	donated	
5 jars of glue	$1.50	$7.50
9 pairs of scissors	$2.50	$22.50
10 marking pens (set)	$2.50	$2.50
10 pencils (pack)	$1.50	$1.50
1 package 3- x 5-inch index cards	$1.25	$1.25
20 Xerox copies	$.10	$2.00
9 sheets typing paper	donated	
Total cost		$37.25

Reference: Rider, B., & Gramblin, C. (1987). *Activities card file.*

Group Session Outline
Session 1 of 6

Group title: "Developing Your Professional Self"

Session title: "Professional Self-Awareness Collage" (adapted from Rider & Gramblin, 1987)

Format:
> Warm-up—3 minutes
> Introduce group lab—2 minutes
> Instructions for activity—2 minutes
> Collage activity—20 minutes
> Sharing—10 minutes
> Discussion—20 minutes
> Summary—3 minutes

Supplies:
> 9 sheets white drawing paper 12 x 18 inches
> 5 jars of glue or 9 glue sticks
> 9 pairs of scissors
> 16 uncut magazines
> 10 marking pens, assorted colors

Description:
1. *Warm-up*—Ask each person in turn to give his or her name and something he or she likes and does not like about occupational therapy.
2. *Introduce activity* (group lab)—Group outline will be shared with the group.
3. *Instructions for activity*—The purpose of this activity is to help us think about ourselves as professionals. Give out bags and markers. "We will begin by signing our name at the top like this 'Jane Doe, OTS.'" Magazines, glue, and scissors are placed in center of table. "Look through the magazines and cut out pictures that represent qualities you have as a professional. We all have some characteristics that we will want to share and have others know about. These may be characteristics that will help us as professionals. Fold the drawing paper in half and paste the pictures representing these on the outside of the folder you have made. You may use both front and back covers.
  "We also have some characteristics we would rather not share. These may be a hindrance to our professional identity. Cut out pictures representing these and paste them on the inside of the folder you have made. When you are finished pasting the pictures, use markers to label each with the characteristic you intend it to represent. You have about 20 minutes to complete this task. We will discuss the collages when we are finished. This will be a good way to get to know each other better."
  Give warning when 5 minutes are left. After 5 minutes, collect all materials and place out of reach.
4. *Sharing*—Ask for a volunteer to start sharing the collages. Once started, go around

Group Session Outline
Session 1 of 6 (continued)

the group in order, forcing no one to share more than he or she wants.

5. *Discussion questions—*

   Processing:

   How did you feel about doing this?

   How many of us felt comfortable sharing the outside vs. the inside of the folder?

   Generalizing:

   How well do you know your professional self?

   What did you learn about yourself from doing this activity?

   What did you learn about others?

   How difficult was it to decide which parts of yourself are "professional"?

   Application:

   How will an activity like this help people build a professional identity?

6. *Summary—*Points to remember are to be taken from comments of members. Some might be:

- The "face" we show to the public is not what is really inside
- The outside represents what we wish to be, the inside what we fear we may be
- Students do not find it easy to think of themselves as professionals
- Some common characteristics are the wish to play a helping role and fondness and empathy for other people

Group Session Outline
Session 2 of 6

Group title: "Developing Your Professional Self"

Session title: "Difficult Decisions"

Format:
Warm-up—5 minutes
Introduce activity—5 minutes
Instructions for activity—5 minutes
Difficult decision writing—10 minutes
Discussion—30 minutes
Summary—5 minutes

Supplies:
8 3- x 5-inch index cards
8 pencils
Basket or box ("hat")

Description:
1. *Warm-up*—Ask members to give names and recall one characteristic about their professional self from last session.
2. *Introduce activity*—"Today we will discuss difficult professional decisions or problems. Each of you take an index card and a pencil and write on the card a professional problem or decision you have experienced in the past year. You may draw on Fieldwork I experiences, volunteer experiences, or situations in the classroom, as long as they concern some aspect of your chosen profession."
3. *Instructions for activity*—"You can write about a problem you had difficulty with or had trouble making a decision about. Give necessary background and detail, but you need not identify yourself. We will be putting the cards in a hat and drawing out someone else's problem to solve. You have 10 minutes to write your problem." Give 1 minute warning.
   Collect all cards after 10 minutes and shuffle them. Put them back in "hat" and ask each member to draw one out. If someone draws his own, he has the option of putting it back and drawing another. "Now think about the problem on the card you drew and get ready to share with the group how you would solve it. Take turns sharing solutions and discuss."
   For this activity, discussion will be during the sharing rather than afterward. Members have the option of identifying their problem and asking the group for additional help.
4. *Discussion questions*—
   Processing:
   What feelings are involved?
   How does it feel to need/ask for help? Receive help?

Group Session Outline
Session 2 of 6 (continued)

Generalizing:

Whose problem is it? Should it be?

What did you/others contribute?

What is the worst/best thing you could do?

If decision, what are pros and cons?

Whose decision is it?

Should it be?

What additional information is needed to decide/solve?

Application:

What can we learn from each other as professionals?

How can we help each other as professionals?

5. *Summary*—This activity usually produces much discussion and often members own up to their own problem. They have become a group of peers working together and trusting one another. A parallel should be drawn to the ideal in practice where no one should feel afraid to ask the help of their colleagues in facing a difficult problem.

Group Session Outline
Session 3 of 6

Group title: "Developing Your Professional Self"

Session title: "Giving and Receiving Feedback"

Format:
> Warm-up—5 minutes
> Introduce activity—5 minutes
> Instructions for activity—5 minutes
> Writing activity—15 minutes
> Discussion—25 minutes
> Summary—5 minutes

Supplies:
> 9 sheets of paper 8 1/2 x 11 inches
> 9 pens or pencils

Description:
1. *Warm-up*—Begin by asking members to say a few words about how they are feeling today.
2. *Introduce activity*—"Today we will be working on communication, self-awareness, and accepting feedback from others. Often the success of our professional interactions will depend on how well we understand our own feelings and express them to others. Even negative feelings can be expressed in positive terms. For example, if you are studying for a test, and your roommate is talking loudly on the phone, you might say to her: 'I know you're enjoying talking to your friend, but I'm having a hard time concentrating on my work. Would you mind calling your friend back later?'
   "Most people have an easier time giving positive feedback than negative. However, avoiding negative comments can cause all kinds of problems, especially when two people have to work together. This exercise is designed to practice giving positive and negative feedback to each other."
3. *Instructions for activity*—Pass out paper and pencils. "Fold paper in half. Put name on the outside folded half at the top. On the inside, write some ways you feel you need to grow professionally (skills needed, issues to deal with, etc.). Fold paper over so what you have written is not visible. Pass folded paper around circle—each person writes on the outside how he feels the person whose name is on the paper could grow professionally. To make this chore less difficult, you may also write one thing you admire about the person. Both positive and 'change needed' comments should be expressed constructively. Even if you do not know everyone that well, do the best you can."
   Give 15 minutes for this part—after that stop, even if not finished. Each reads own paper for a few minutes. Then members share the results with the group. If possible, each should read a few positive and growth comments to the group.

Group Session Outline
Session 3 of 6 (continued)

4. *Discussion questions—*
   Processing:
   How do you feel about the feedback you received?
   How did you feel about giving feedback to others?
   What problems did you encounter in doing this exercise?
   Generalizing:
   How do the comments about yourself compare with comments of others?
   What feedback from others do you agree/disagree with?
   What did you learn from doing this exercise?
   Application:
   Whom would you like feedback from in your professional role?
   How can you use feedback in everyday life?
   How can you become more comfortable in giving constructive feedback to others?
   To patients?
5. *Summary*—Ask members to summarize.

Group Session Outline
Session 4 of 6

Group title: "Developing Your Professional Self"

Session title: "Professional Values"

Format:
> Warm-up—5 minutes
> Introduce activity—5 minutes
> Instructions for activity—5 minutes
> Activity—15 minutes
> Discussion—25 minutes
> Summary—5 minutes

Supplies:
> 9 pencils
> 9 Values worksheets (Worksheet 11-3)

Description:
1. *Warm-up*—Begin by summarizing last week's activity. How are people left feeling about the group? Is there any unfinished business? (Any comments, either negative or positive, should be accepted by the leader without judgment and acknowledged.)
2. *Introduce activity*—"Knowing our professional values can help us set priorities and use our time at work and away from work more constructively. For example, if I want to balance my career with a meaningful relationship with my family, then I will be careful not to work overtime or make work-related commitments on weekends. Professional values should also guide our behavior at work. If you believe a good rapport with patients is important, you may take extra time with them to show your concern."
   Pass out Values worksheets and pencils. Follow instructions on top of sheet. Allow 15 minutes to complete. When finished, each member shares his responses with the group.
3. *Instructions for activity*—The discussion guidelines written on the sheet are to come up with a group consensus on values held in common.
   (Generalizing is done by the group.)
   One group member can be a recorder and allow group to collaborate on what professional values they can agree on. A separate Values worksheet may be used for note taking of group values.
4. *Discussion questions*—
   Processing:
   How did the group perform without leader intervention?
   How did you feel about doing the activity on your own?
   How did the structure affect your interaction?
   Application:
   How do values affect your interpersonal relationships?

Group Session Outline
Session 4 of 6 (continued)

What role do values play in your professional life?
How do values determine how you spend your time?

5. *Summary*—In summary, the recorder can read her notes back to the group and accept final revisions and/or comments.

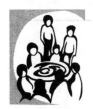

Worksheet 11-3
Values

Directions: Complete the following sentences in your own words. Then compare your responses to those of the other members of your group in order to generate a set of commonly held values in interpersonal relations. In the discussion, you have four tasks:
  1. To make yourself heard
  2. To hear others accurately
  3. To listen for themes
  4. To collaborate on the group consensus

A professional should:

A professional should not:

A supervisor:

A student:

A colleague:

A spouse or boyfriend/girlfriend:

I want to be remembered as a person who:

Our group:

Group Session Outline
Session 5 of 6

Group title: "Developing Your Professional Self"

Session title: "Assertiveness Role Play"

Format:
    Warm-up—5 minutes
    Introduce activity—2 minutes
    Instructions for activity—3 minutes
    Activity writing—10 minutes
    Sharing (role playing)—25 minutes
    Discussion—10 minutes
    Summary—5 minutes

Supplies:
    8 3- x 5-inch index cards
    8 pencils

Description:
1. *Warm-up*—Define assertive, passive, and aggressive and discuss the differences between these.
2. *Introduce activity*—"One of the most common problems students have in making the transition to professionals is not acting assertively. Lack of assertiveness can lead to difficulty even on fieldwork experiences, as many of you have already discovered. For example, one student on a Fieldwork I experience overheard a discussion by staff members who were setting up a family conference in the patient lounge at 2:00 p.m. This student was already scheduled to run an occupational therapy group in that room at 2:00 p.m. However, she did not say anything about it to the staff group. The student was left without a place to run group and became very frustrated. Afterward, when staff became aware of the problem, they wondered why the student did not speak up! They could have met in several other places. This situation could have been avoided if the student had behaved more assertively."
3. *Instructions for activity*—Pass out index cards and pencils. "You will now write down on the card a professional situation in which you would like to have responded more assertively but did not. You may either have been too passive or overly aggressive instead. On the front of the card, describe the situation: who, what, where, and when and whatever background information is necessary. On the back, state what your actual response was (if possible, give a quote) and state how you felt afterward."
4. *Sharing*—Each member shares the situation written on the front of the card. Then members decide as a group which situations they would like to role play. Group chooses first, second, and third choices, using group decision-making techniques to do this.
    Role play one to three situations as time allows:

Group Session Outline
Session 5 of 6 (continued)

- Allow protagonist to direct role play
- Protagonist chooses members of group to play significant characters
- Protagonist sets up room, props
- Role play situation as it really happened first, then discuss
- Reverse roles and play situation using assertive behavior as discussed by the group
- Allow a few alter egos to present feelings and/or alternate responses

5. *Discussion questions*—
   Processing:
   How did you feel about doing the role play?
   Which characters did you identify with?
   How do you feel about being assertive? Passive? Aggressive?
   What are you feeling about the protagonist's situation?
   Generalizing:
   What passive, assertive, and aggressive behaviors can you identify in the role play?
   What are the advantages of assertive behavior?
   Application:
   What did you learn about being assertive professionally?
   What steps do you personally need to take to be able to behave assertively in the professional setting? As a student? As an occupational therapist?

6. *Summary*—Summarize by reinforcing assertive behaviors, reviewing the role of feelings and habits, and thanking role players for their participation.

Group Session Outline
Session 6 of 6

Group title: "Developing Your Professional Self"

Session title: "Group Evaluation"

Format:
> Warm-up—5 minutes
> Introduce activity—5 minutes
> Instructions for activity—5 minutes
> Activity—15 minutes
> Discussion/Summary of all six sessions—20 minutes
> Summary—10 minutes

Supplies:
> 9 Group Evaluation worksheets (Worksheet 11-4)
> 9 pencils

Description:
1. *Warm-up*—Begin by stating that this will be the final group of the series and ask members to say how they feel about ending the group.
2. *Introduce activity*—"An important part of the termination of groups is to review all the sessions and summarize what has been valuable. As professionals, we will all need to evaluate our patient groups, so this will be good practice. The Group Evaluation worksheet has been designed to help you think specifically about this group and to apply some of what you have learned about group dynamics." Give out worksheets.

   "First, you are asked to identify the roles your fellow members played in the groups, and for this you will have to name names. In our discussion, these questions will serve as the basis of giving one another feedback about our participation. Next, we will look at the events of the group. These are emotionally charged situations which often emerge unexpectedly. In the context of activities, often it is the conflicts and problems groups encounter which become the turning points from which we learn the most. You are asked to identify three such events over the last five sessions.

   Norms are the "ground rules" of behavior in groups. You are asked to identify the implicit or implied norms over the course of the group. The stage of development is sometimes difficult to identify in the short time this group has been meeting. We will use Schutz's stages of inclusion, control, and affection as a guide (Chapter 2). Sometimes the characteristics of stages overlap and this can be confusing, so you are asked to justify your choice with behaviors you see or have seen in this group. Your feeling about the group may be an important clue about what stage the group has achieved.

   "Finally, you are asked to look at the group leadership. What style was used, and how has it changed over the course of the group? You have 15 minutes to complete the worksheet."

Group Session Outline
Session 6 of 6 (continued)

3. *Instructions for activity*—Members share their answers to some or all of the questions on the sheet, as time allows. After each question, ask the group to discuss their answers and come to a consensus. Be sure to leave the last 15 minutes to summarize.

4. *Discussion questions/Summary of all six sessions*—Take a few minutes to reflect on the past six sessions.

   Processing:

   What parts of the group experience are most memorable?

   Which experiences did you like best/least?

   How do you feel about your role in the group?

   Generalizing:

   What things did you learn from being a part of this group?

   Application:

   What parts of this group experience can you take with you and apply to future roles both personally and professionally?

5. *Summary*—End by summarizing results and asking each person to say in his or her own words what parts of this group experience he or she values and feels good about.

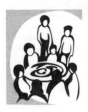

Worksheet 11-4
Group Evaluation

Directions: Answer the following questions about your group as it has developed from Session 1. Be sure to identify members by name.

Participation and Roles:
1. Who are the most outspoken participants?

2. Who are the least frequent participants?

3. Who talks to whom? What patterns have you observed? (Identify any subgroups that exist.)

4. Who keeps the ball rolling?

5. Who/what has blocked the group?

6. What rivalries have you observed during the group? Who has challenged the leadership?

Events: Name three interactions or situations that were high points or turning points for the group. Describe each situation briefly.
   1.

   2.

   3.

Norms:
   1. What behaviors are acceptable to the group today?

   2. What behaviors are not acceptable today?

   3. How have norms changed from the beginning of the group?

Group Evaluation (continued)

Stage of Development:
   1. What stage of development has this group achieved? Justify your answer.
      a. Inclusion
      b. Control
      c. Affection

   2. How do you feel about the group right now?
      a. It means a lot to me. I'm sorry it's ending.
      b. I feel good about the other members.
      c. I feel indifferent.
      d. It feels uncomfortable. I'm glad it's ending.
      e. I strongly dislike the group.

Leadership:
   1. What was the leader's style of leadership? Why?
      a. Directive
      b. Facilitator
      c. Leader as adviser

   2. How has the role of the leader changed over the course of the group?

Other Process Observations:

APPENDICES

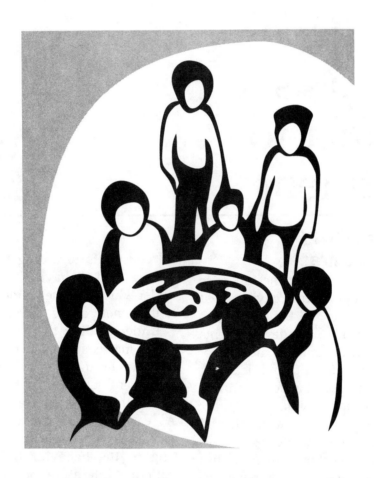

Appendix A: The Task-Oriented Group as a
Context for Treatment

Appendix B: The Concept and Use of Developmental Groups

Appendix C: Summary of Mosey's Adaptive Skills

Appendix D: Uniform Terminology for
Occupational Therapy, Third Edition

Appendix E: Comparison of Group Leadership
Guidelines in Seven Frames of Reference

The Task-Oriented Group as a Context for Treatment

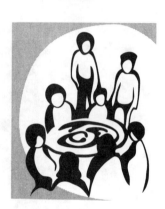

Gail S. Fidler, OTR

Abstract

Increasing recognition of the influence of man's social and cultural environment on behavior has extended the parameters of patient treatment. Such developments are manifested in the gradual melding of sociologic, psychoanalytic and learning theories and the emerging focus on ego functions and adaptive skills. This paper explores concepts of the task-oriented group within this context, offering a definition and delineation of purpose for its use in occupational therapy as a remedial-learning experience for the schizophrenic patient.

Returning the hospitalized psychiatric patient to an acceptable productive role in the community and appreciably reducing the rate of recidivism is a complex problem. Such concern has led to intensive studies of both psychotherapeutic procedures and organizational structures of the mental hospital. The impact of sociologic inquiry into the mental hospital has been to add another dimension to our theoretical constructs regarding both individual feeling and behavior, and conditions under which such behavior may be altered to the benefit of the patient.

Understanding the significance of the social matrix in which the patient functions has brought more sharply into focus factors influencing ego function in addition to the intrapsychic and intrapersonal. As early as 1931 Harry Stack Sullivan[1] spoke of the importance of the social setting to the behavior of schizophrenic patients. Literature of the past fifteen years is replete with the investigations and analyses of the import of environment on patient functioning.[2-4] This focus has inevitably led to theoretical and practical attempts to relate concepts of ego psychology to social theories of the environment.[5,6] Such linkage as well as the social scientist's interest in group phenomena has given impetus to increased exploration of the many facets of group process and group therapy.

Group Process and Group Psychotherapy

Group psychotherapy is firmly established as a method of treatment for mental illness. It has its foundation in psychodynamic personality theories and emerged in America essentially from a psychoanalytic frame of reference stressing personality change through exploration of intrapsychic and interpersonal pathology believed to be at the root of conflicts and problems.[7-10] The group has been seen as a setting in which the individual with the help of the therapist and through sharing with other members could explore and work through those unconscious conflicts and problems which inhibited personality change and growth. Such a frame of reference places primary importance on unconscious phenomena and explores "here-and-now" feelings and behavior as a means to arriving at an awareness and understanding of intrapsychic conflict. The role of the therapist is to facilitate such awareness and elicit the involvement and help of members in exposing and working through personal conflicts and problems.

The social scientist's interest in groups emanated from a sociologic orientation rather than from personality theories. This frame of reference stresses the impact of society and the group on individual behavior and seeks to explain behavior based on the nature of the society in which a man lives. This ideology is exemplified by Lewin[11] who theorized that behavior was determined by the situation in which it occurred as well as by personality factors. The sociologist's beginning involvement with groups was via his interest in organizational structure and this was reflected in an early focus on the use of the group to accomplish a task or to effect a change in management.[12] Such experimentation inevitably led to the development of theories regarding the use of such groups in teaching and learning.[13]

Theories and practice in the field of group dynamics have focused on the group as a dynamic force in facilitating learning and behavioral change. Emphasis on "the group" as the primary change-producing agent thus accentuates the importance of exploring the dynamic forces within the here-and-now group to both understand and facilitate such change. Group structure and membership roles become significant and individual feeling and behavior is viewed only as it contributes to or deters from cohesive structure and contributory roles.

As the group therapist, the psychiatrist and social scientist work collaboratively in an attempt to resolve some of the complex problems of the mentally ill, these two seemingly disparate theories have moved closer together. There are increasing efforts to integrate not only practice of group psychotherapy and group dynamics but also the more apparently divergent concepts of each. One has but to survey current literature to be impressed with the ubiquity of these efforts.

Experimental Studies

In *Social Psychology in Treating Mental Illness*[14] Fairweather describes an experimental approach combining the psychodynamic doctrine of patient treatment with theories of social psychiatry, sociology and the small group. This program focused around patient-led, small task-oriented groups for the chronic regressed schizophrenic. Such an approach, Dr. Fairweather points out, "called for an altered perception of the patient's role from that of a subordinate to that of a peer group member with responsibilities to himself and his group members, and away from that of a passive recipient within the limits of his abilities, despite existing psychopathology."[15] Tasks around which these autonomous patient-led groups were organized concerned the current and future living of each member. Thus task levels ranged according to the capacity of the patient from personal care and ward responsibility to responsibility for vocational planning and placement. These groups provided the opportunity for patients to explore and develop their capacities for independent function, creating patient roles within the hospital which were more consistent with those of the outside community.

This study made an important contribution to patient programming and treatment. Although it concerned itself entirely with problems of the chronic regressed schizophrenic, there is much that would seem to be directly applicable to other patient categories and most certainly to patient groups in rehabilitation settings.

Marshall Edelson's experimental study[16] at the University of Oklahoma was concerned with "making possible the meaningful integration of both group experience and individual psychotherapy in an intensive treatment program designed to accomplish fundamental alteration in characterological disorder rather than solely rapid relief of acute secondary symptomatology and restoration of an ability to function marginally in the community." This work combines ego psychology and group dynamics in a therapeutic community as the basis for intensive psychotherapy. The focus of this study is aptly stated by Dr. Edelson in these words: "The therapeutic community (and small group) is organized to provide opportunities for the appearance of the patient's characterological difficulties or way of life as these are expressed in activities and other aspects of group living and for the confrontation of the patient and the group with these difficulties and their consequences to the life of the (hospital) community."

A third innovative experiment was Robert Morton's use of the laboratory method with psychiatric patients.[17] This study describes the design and use of the group process laboratory training program for hospitalized mental patients. The laboratory is a structured, small group experience designed to bring about change by establishing conditions whereby participants are forced to test their assumptions regarding interpersonal and group relations. Not only is the application of the laboratory experience to hospitalized psychiatric patients a creative innovation, but it is even more provocative to learn that they were autonomous, staff-leaderless, patient groups. Morton agrees with Fairweather that cohesive decision-making groups with psychotics cannot be explored if a professional leader is present. It is their contention that even the most permissive therapist-leader reinforces dependency for the psychotic to a detrimental extent. This experiment provides some useful and creative postulates regarding small group experiences for psychiatric patients and should stimulate further research and study in the adaptation of this technique in treatment and rehabilitation programs.

It is interesting to note that in follow-up studies on the Morton experiment only two findings seemed to be suggestive.[18] Training laboratory patients were employed a mean of 5.92 months during the nine month follow-up period whereas the group therapy patients were employed 4.70 months. In the Fairweather study, patients participating in the small-group program were significantly better than the control group in community adjustment with regard to areas of employment, verbal communication with others and friendships.

These three experimental studies are examples of the way in which the small group is being used and adapted to meet treatment needs and essentially bridge the apparent gap between theories of individual psychodynamics and sociology.

The Task Group in Occupational Therapy

Development of task-oriented treatment groups approximately four years ago within the occupational therapy program at New York State Psychiatric Institute emanated from several not unrelated observations. First, the increasing conviction that as patients engaged in activities or created objects they expressed characterological difficulties and that attention to these problems as they emerged and were operant in the here-and-now seemed to be of benefit to the patient. Second, a seemingly evident relationship between problems evidenced by the patient in his activity experiences and difficulties he encountered in the workday world. Third, the nature of the occupational therapy setting which expects active involvement in doing, provides a microcosm of life-work situations which can be seen and explored as they occur rather than in retrospect. Fourth, recognition of the relationships between verbal skills and learning and our experience which indicated that learning and concomitant growth were enhanced when problems in doing were identified and explored. Finally, our belief that the shared, small group experience is conducive to the exploration and amelioration of some problems in ego function.

Groups were organized with approximately eight members selected on the basis of their particular difficulties in doing and being productive as well as their readiness and need for a small group experience. All patients admitted to these early groups were male schizophrenics and placement in a given group was determined by the level of ego function. Meetings were held three to four times a week for periods of one and one-half hours. Each group was responsible for choosing its own common task and arriving at a consensus regarding procedures for accomplishing that task.

Definition and Purpose

Task as it relates to such groups is defined as any activity or process directed toward creating or producing an end product or demonstrable service for the group as a whole and/or for persons outside of the group. Some examples of tasks chosen by these groups were: publishing a newspaper, cooking, building a playhouse for the children's' service, gardening, organizing a patient council, play reading and ward decoration and improvement.

The intent of the task-oriented group is to provide a shared working experience wherein the relationship between feeling, thinking and behavior, their impact on others and on task accomplishment and productivity can be viewed and explored. Alternate patterns of functioning can be considered and tested within the context of the here-and-now, to the end that such learning may induce ego growth and improve function. Task accomplishment is not the purpose of the group but hopefully the means by which purpose is realized. It is seen as the catalytic agent which elicits behavior and interaction, brings into focus both functional capacities and limitations, facilitates collaboration in working through problems and provides a concrete reality factor against which to measure learning and achievement. Furthermore, the task provides a frame of reference which helps to keep in focus what is relevant to explore and work through and what conflicts and issues belong more appropriately in other treatment settings. In such a group, issues and problems which directly effect the cohesiveness and/or task accomplishment are the appropriate agenda items.

Such groups are not unique in eliciting or diagnosing conflicts of the schizophrenic but it would seem that use of a common task within a small group setting does facilitate delineation of certain problems and their amelioration. Responsibility for selecting and accomplishing a task provides an opportunity for the group to explore problem-solving and decision-making skills, to have concrete evidence of their ability to function as well as to identify those expectations which give rise to conflict. The expectation that an activity needs to be chosen and implemented makes it necessary for the group to look at concepts regarding self and others that have impaired problem-solving skills and gives impetus to working toward their resolution.

The ability to perceive cause and effect relationships is a well-recognized problem of the schizophrenic and learning in this area requires consistent, repeated opportunities to see and have evidence of cause and effect. The task-oriented group with its focus on the relationship between feelings, thinking, behavior and task achievement thus creates excellent learning opportunities. Following through on a task procedure, the nature of doing or not doing, gives ample confirmation of cause and effect regarding behavior and function. When task responsibility must be shared and when the nature of one's doing is viewed in terms of its contribution to the group, such learning is further amplified.

Reality testing through consensual validation is an essential process in every group and is of particular value to the schizophrenic. In addition to the shared reality indigenous to group structure and interaction, a clearly delineated task with standard procedures and techniques provides a shared reality from which perceptions can be tested and shared. Shared participation in an activity, the necessary interdependence makes possible an objective, demonstrable assessment of one's capacities and limitations. One of the values of the task-oriented group is the consensual validation of the patients' capacity to grow and change as evidenced in the accomplishment of a task.

The need to work together as well as talk together about one's doing contributes to learning to conceptualize and verbalize more accurately and directly. Identification of problems in functioning, discussion of these as well as exploration of alternatives, combines feeling, behavior and cognition and provides the necessary components of learning and change. The shared decision-making, working experiences available in these groups and the opportunity to explore and work through problems that interfere with satisfactory function make integrated learning possible. If we are to teach new and better ways of functioning then we need to combine the patient's doing with his thinking and bring such relationships into awareness in order that he may integrate such learning.

Collaboration on a concrete, clearly defined task encourages more direct and clear communication and coupled with group support provides a safe area in which to practice such skills. In addition, experiences in working and sharing help the schizophrenic to begin to perceive and conceptualize his needs within the context of gratification potential with increasing awareness of his own potential for obtaining gratification rather that the expectation of rejection or frustration outside himself.

The task-oriented group with its focus on function related to here-and-now tasks and doing their corresponding responsibilities bear a closer resemblance to living in the outside community and provides learning which correlates more directly with those skills and expectations required in community adjustment.

It would seem useful at this time to make some distinction between these groups and verbal psychotherapy and delineate some values to the patient when both experiences are correlated. Within the task-oriented group setting, issues concerning feelings, perceptions and behavior are discussed and explored only insofar as they are shared by others and impede or contribute to the problem-solving and/or activity accomplishment of the group. Personal, intrapsychic and historical determinants are not emphasized but are reserved for investigation in psychotherapy. Many personal and interpersonal perceptions and responses are elicited but not dealt with in the group. Psychotherapy provides an opportunity to explore these in depth, interrelating the unconscious, the historical, the personal and interpersonal to the here-and-now. Likewise, the task-oriented group provides a life-like action and doing setting in which insights gained in psychotherapy can be tested and consolidated through performance. The extent to which the task-oriented group and psychotherapy is correlated, the degree which the purpose of each and their relationship is understood by both staff and patients, may well determine the extent to which treatment potential will be realized.

Leadership

The role of staff leader or therapist is an important determinant in the group. The function of the leader is to facilitate a process and milieu which will be conducive to the kind of learning and growth to which these groups are directed. The role of the leader is to make learning possible and not to assume responsibility for the group. Fulfillment of objectives will depend in good measure on the leader's concepts of the mental patient and himself, as well as his skill in group and interpersonal processes.

Confidence in the inherent capacity of the group to be constructively self-determining, in its ability to ultimately recognize problems and reach realistic solutions to these, is a basic requirement. The foundation for such an attitude is belief in the right of the patient to be self-determining and a trust sufficient to allow exercise of freedom in exploring and testing his capacities. The group needs to be perceived as a therapeutic agent in its own right and leadership not as giving treatment but rather as the agent which helps to maximize the therapeutic and learning potential of the group.

It would seem that we tend to see patients as more fragile and thus needing more guidance and direction than seems warranted, at least on the basis of our experience. Perhaps this view of the patient is sustained by our need to be needed and important to the patient and to be recognized as having expertise. Autocratic leadership confirms for the patient his dependent position and tends to reaffirm his concept of self as inept and inadequate, while hesitant, aloof permissiveness increases his sense of vagueness, unpredictability and limitlessness. Jay W. Fidler[19] defines the nature and extent of leader activity as it pertains to working with groups of psychotics, emphasizing the importance of active interventions based on sensitivity and understanding of the schizophrenic's particular problems with reality testing and other ego functions.

Such understanding and attitude sets however, are not the only basis of leadership skills for these groups. An intimate knowledge of and skill in problem-solving procedures is essential if the group is to be helped toward learning and developing such capacities. The extent to which problem-solving skills are an inherent part of the leader's way of thinking and functioning and his ability to make these appropriately apparent in identifying and dealing with issues will, by and large, determine the extent to which the group will be able to learn these processes and incorporate them into their functioning.

The extent and quality of the leader's receptivity to looking at himself and his relations to others, his freedom to participate in the learning and growth process, his ability to share perceptions and his openness to exploring all aspects of his functioning in the group, will either make learning and growth possible and a less threatening expectation for members, or confirm the many doubts and distortions they bring to the experience. The leader cannot expect from his group what he is not willing or able to do himself.

Problems of the Schizophrenic

Several aspects of the task-oriented group seem to bring into focus particular problems of the schizophrenic patient. First, decision-making is particularly difficult, especially the decision regarding task choice. There seems to be little question that groups expect the staff leader to make the choice for them. Some groups have insisted that this be done while others have behaved as though this was what they both wanted and expected. Groups have discussed their anxieties and conflicts about decision-making and these discussions suggest that problems in this area are related to dependency needs, fear of responsibility and the ultimate unacceptability of any decision they might make. It would seem that since they conceptualize themselves as worthless and "bad", any

decision they make as well as its implementation will be worthless and "bad" and reflect basic ineptness and inadequacy. It would also seem they expect authority (the parental figure) to find any decision they make unacceptable and inadequate. However, groups resent and may forcefully reject any task choice suggestion made by the leader. Ambivalence with regard to dependency, coupled with problems related to self-concept, compose one of the major conflictual areas which need to be worked through before meaningful growth can occur. Some of these findings would seem to support Fairweather's hypothesis that the dependency needs of the psychotic contraindicate staff leadership in task-oriented groups.

More recently we have been experimenting with a standard task for each beginning group in an effort to assess the extent to which decision-making problems may be altered or reduced when task choice is not an initial requirement. It is further hoped that such a procedure may lead to the development of a group diagnostic implement. However, the issue is not so much whether we deny or gratify the patient's dependency needs but rather how we can teach decision-making. It seems reasonable to conjecture that teaching such skills is a problem because of our limited understanding of the full nature of blocks to learning and thus our inability to identify and utilize techniques and procedures which facilitate learning.

Second, expectations of a shared group are frightening. It is as though fluid ego boundaries and difficulties in perceiving self as separate from others makes the closeness inherent in the small group an additional threat to identity. For some patients there is also the expectation that narcissistic needs will be frustrated and that sharing in a group will deny dependency needs. In addition, anticipation of shared doing seems to represent a threat to the schizophrenic's defenses and orientation. However, the structured, predictable aspects of the task and engagement with non-human objects increase opportunities for supportive consensual validation of observable abilities and facilitates identification of those perceptions which they share in common.

Third, great difficulty is experienced in problem-solving. Although some of the dilemmas operant in problem-solving are obviously related to dependency needs and authority relationships, difficulties which emerge in these groups suggest also that many patients have never learned even the basic procedures for identifying problems and exploring possible solutions, or have lost the ability to appropriately perceive and organize perceptions into logical concepts.

The combined thinking and doing, the cognitive perceptual skills at both the motor and verbal level inherent in the product of these groups, seem to bring clearly into focus disturbances and abilities in thinking and learning.

Fears associated with learning and related conflicts, disturbances in cognition and resultant dysfunction become readily evident. By the same token, the structure and focus of these groups make possible a sense of competence and learning less conflictual, the task providing evidence of movement toward achievement. Task activity furthermore creates opportunities to engage and relate in a more concrete way making it possible to be involved at a conceptual level commensurate with current capacities rather than consistently requiring a higher symbolic thinking order. The task also facilitates gradation of learning. As we become more knowledgeable about blocks to learning and their impact on function we should be able to articulate more meaningfully related

learning experiences and use more fully the potential of the task-oriented group.

Finally, two generalized responses have been evident in these groups. There are those who find expectations of doing, the intrinsic action, learning and responsibilities, very threatening. These patients place a high premium on talking about their problems and intellectualization is used as a way of avoiding the more hazardous and fearful doing of a task. These groups have great difficulty arriving at a choice of task and such a decision may be prolonged for an inordinate period of time. Other patients seem driven to an excessive emphasis on the task, to a flight into activity as a means for avoiding bringing problems into awareness and working them through. Furthermore there would seem to be a correlation between the leader's characteristic way of functioning, what he perceives as the more important "therapeutic set" and a group's sustained focus or movement toward a more equitable balance between these two responses.

One further observation would seem to be useful and this relates to the kind of task choices made by groups. There seems to be an identifiable relationship between the task selected by a group, the level and nature of their primary emotional needs and the conflicts surrounding those needs. Furthermore, task choice seems to reflect the group's progress or regression. Further study of this phenomenon should increase our understanding of need-gratifying processes and enhance our ability to make growth potential opportunities available to the patients.

Returning the schizophrenic patient to the community as a potentially productive, contributing member with an increased capacity to sustain such a role, is a multi-faceted, complex problem. The task-oriented group represents one of many attempts to reduce the problem. It seems that at least it provides a structure wherein dysfunction can be observed and explored. Hopefully these and other explorations will make it possible to ultimately articulate more clearly the essential factors of remedial processes. As we become increasingly able to inter-relate psychodynamic and sociologic concepts, as we enhance our knowledge of the cognitive process and its relationships to intrapsychic phenomena and overt behavior, our efforts may come closer to realizing the ultimate goal of satisfactory community living for our patients.

Acknowledgment

The author is indebted to Dr. Lothar Gidro-Frank and Dr. Eugene Friedberg for their interested support and to Miss Patricia Mayer, OTR, whose creative thinking and skillful leadership contributed so much to our learning.

References

1. Sullivan HS. Socio-psychiatric research: its implications for the schizophrenic problem and mental hygiene. *Am J Psychiat.* 1931;10.
2. Stanton AH, Schwartz MS. *The Mental Hospital.* New York: Basic Books; 1954.
3. Caudill W. *The Psychiatric Hospital as a Small Society.* Cambridge, Mass: Harvard University Press; 1958.
4. Jones M. *The Therapeutic Community: A New Treatment Method in Psychiatry.* New York: Basic Books; 1953.
5. Cummings J, Cummings E. *Ego and Milieu.* New York: Atherton Press; 1963.
6. Edelson M. *Ego Psychology, Group Dynamics and the Therapeutic Community.* New York: Grune & Stratton; 1964.
7. Slavison S. *Group Psychoanalytic Psychotherapy.* New York: International University Press; 1964.
8. Wolf A. The psychoanalysis of groups. *Am J Psychother.* 1949;3.
9. Bach G. *Intensive Group Psychotherapy.* New York: The Ronald Press; 1954.
10. Mullan H, Rosenbaum M. *Group Psychotherapy, Theory and Practice.* Glencoe Free Press; 1962.
11. Lewin K. *Dynamic Theory of Personality.* New York: McGraw Hill; 1945.
12. Schien E, Bennis W. *Personal and Organizational Change Through Group Methods.* New York: John Wiley & Sons; 1965:357-368.
13. Bradford L, Gibb J, Benne K. *T-Group Theory & Laboratory Method.* New York: John Wiley & Sons; 1964.
14. Fairweather GW. *Social Psychology in Treating Mental Illness.* New York: John Wiley & Sons; 1964.
15. Ibid, 14.
16. Ibid, 6.
17. Morton RB. The uses of the laboratory method in a psychiatric hospital. In: *Personal and Organizational Change Through Group Methods.*
18. Johnson DL, Hanson PG, Rothaus R, Morton RB, Lyle E, Moyer R. Follow up evaluation of human relation training for psychiatric patients. In: *Personal and Organizational Change Through Group Methods.*
19. Fidler JW. Group psychotherapy of psychotics. *Am J Orthopsychiat.* 1965;35(4).

The Concept and Use of Developmental Groups

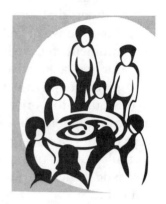

Anne Cronin Mosey, PhD, OTR

Developmental groups are task-oriented groups structured in such a manner as to stimulate the various types of nonfamilial groups usually encountered in the normal development process. Five types have been identified:

1. Parallel
2. Project
3. Egocentric-cooperative
4. Cooperative
5. Mature

The concept of developmental groups was formulated in an attempt to apply recapitulation of ontogeny in the treatment of patients who are deficient in their ability to interact effectively in small groups. In dealing with this area of dysfunction, consecutive participation in the various types of developmental groups provides a framework for planned change. Group experiences are graded so as to provide opportunities for acquisition of basic group interaction skills. It is suggested that learning occurs through reinforcement of behaviors or approximation of behaviors that are necessary for successful participation in a given type of developmental group and nonreinforcement of behaviors that are inconsistent with successful participation.

A subtle change in orientation seems to be taking place among practitioners and scientists. There is movement away from the medical model, with its focus on concepts of pathology, toward an organization of thinking and effort around the concepts of growth. Scientists have shown renewed interest in exploring the development of various mature human capacities (here referred to as skills) and identifying factors that promote or cause development of these skills. Practitioners are beginning to think in terms of lags, deficits, or deviations in the normal developmental process. Classical diagnostic categories are being discarded for a more functional delineation of areas of adequate development and areas in which there is need for continued or redirected development.[1]

Treatment that emphasizes the nurturing of growth rests upon three major postulates:

1. Deviations in development can be altered.[2]
2. Subskills fundamental to mature adaptive skills must be acquired in a sequential manner.[3]
3. Mature adaptive skills can be acquired through participation in situations that simulate those interactions between individual and environment believed to be responsible for the sequential development of a given adaptive skill.[4]

It is out of this orientation, of treatment as recapitulation of ontogeny, that the concept of "developmental groups" has been formulated. It is presented principally as a heuristic device for discussing one facet of patient care.

Description of Developmental Groups

Developmental groups are clinical simulations of the various types of nonfamilial groups usually encountered in the normal developmental process.[5] These groups and their community-based counterparts are described as task-oriented and primary. Task-oriented refers to members' active engagement in the accomplishment of a definable project or task.[6] "A primary group is a face-to-face organization of individuals who cooperate for certain common ends, who share some common ideas and patterns of behavior, who have confidence in and some degree of affection for each other, and who are aware of their similarities of bonds of association."[7] The family (in its ideal form) is one example of a primary group. However, there are many nonfamilial groups that have the above listed characteristics. It is this type of group that is of concern in this paper.

Five types of developmental groups have been identified: parallel, project, egocentric-cooperative, cooperative and mature.[8] In a clinical setting, they would be described as follows:

A parallel group is made up of an aggregate of patients who are involved in individual tasks with minimal necessity for interaction. Group members may act as sources of stimulation for one another or tentatively test the effect of their behavior on others. However, task accomplishment does not require interaction. The therapist provides assistance with tasks and takes responsibility for meeting the social-emotional needs of each member.

In a project group, members are involved in common, short-term tasks that require some interaction, cooperation, and competition. The task is paramount. Mutual interaction outside the task is not expected. The therapist provides or assists the group in selecting tasks that require interaction of two or more persons for completion. He or she responds to the social-emotional needs of group members.

Egocentric-cooperative groups are characterized by group members selecting, implementing, and executing relatively long-term tasks through joint interaction. The task remains central but satisfaction of some social-emotional needs of fellow group members is encouraged. There is emphasis on the reciprocal satisfaction that can be gained by responding to others' needs. The therapist gives support and guidance relative to the task and continues to satisfy a considerable portion of each member's emotional needs.

In a cooperative group, members are encouraged to identify and gratify each other's social-emotional needs in conjuction with task accomplishment. This type of group often includes only members of the same sex. The therapist acts primarily in the role of an advisor and may not be present at all group meetings.

A mature group is heterogeneous in composition and characterized by members taking those task and social-emotional roles that are required for adequate group functioning. Maintenance of a proper balance between productivity and personal need satisfaction is stressed. The therapist interacts as a coequal group member.

Division of developmental groups into five types is arbitrary—an attempt to provide demarcation points. It is more accurate to perceive these groups as being on a continuum. Thus, in the clinical setting, a given group may be best described as standing somewhere between two adjacent types of developmental groups.

When used in the treatment process, developmental groups are seen as agents of planned change. It is postulated that change occurs through the individual experiencing the consequence of his behavior in the group setting.[9] Developmental groups are so structured that adaptive behavior leads to a positive reinforcing stimulus while maladaptive behavior does not. A positive reinforcing stimulus is an event that causes need reduction. The need may be outer-directed as in the need for companionship, or inner-directed as in the need to be competent.[10]

Treatment of Group Interaction Skill Deficiency

The concept of developmental groups was formulated originally to delineate and describe a method of treating deficiency in group interaction skill. It grew out of the attempt to apply recapitulation of ontogeny in the treatment of patients who were deficient in their ability to interact effectively in small groups. Although developmental groups may be utilized in other areas (which will be briefly discussed later) they are seen as particularly useful in treatment of inadequate development of group interaction skill.

Group interaction skill is here considered to be an adaptive skill. It is defined, in its mature form, as the ability to partici-pate in a variety of groups in a manner that is satisfying for oneself and for one's fellow group members. It is postulated that this skill develops sequentially, each stage in its development being marked by acquisition of behavior that is required for adequate participation in the community-based counterpart of the five types of developmental groups. It is further postulated that group interaction skill is acquired through participation in these various types of groups in conjuction with the opportunity to experience the consequences of appropriate and inappropriate behavior.[11]

It is beyond the scope of this paper to give a detailed description of evaluative methods for group interaction skill. Ideally, the therapist and patient collaborate in identifying what stages of this skill the patient has successfully integrated. Pertinent information may be acquired by observation of the patient in a group situation and discussion with the patient about his participation in groups outside the clinical setting. Evaluation also involves identifying what behavior the patient needs to acquire for successful interaction in small groups and current behavior that is interfering with successful participation.

The therapist must determine when deficiency in group interaction skill will be dealt with in the treatment process. The criterion suggested for making this judgment is treatment is initiated when the patient shows evidence of having acquired those abilities or skills that are normally learned prior to involvement in nonfamilial groups. The first step in treatment is engagement of the patient in that type of developmental group that is compatible or nearly compatible with his current capacity for meaningful group interaction.

Briefly, the treatment process consists of providing positive reinforcers for behaviors or approximation of behaviors that are necessary for successful participation in a given type of developmental group and withholding positive reinforcers for behaviors that are inconsistent with successful participation. These predetermined consequences are believed to be the central factor in bringing about change. The developmental group provides the structure; it sets and defines classes of behavior that are to be learned. Participation in a developmental group in and of itself is not conducive to planned behavioral change. Participation must be concurrent with deliberate and controlled reinforcement.

There are several methods that the therapist may use to increase the probability of the patient emitting desirable behaviors so that they can be reinforced. The method or methods selected will be determined primarily by the other adaptive skills available to the patient and his fellow group members. The most primitive method is simply to wait until the patient exhibits an approximation of the behavior he needs to acquire. This behavior is differentially reinforced as it moves in the direction of becoming an affective behavior pattern. Other initiating methods are:

1. Encouraging imitation of the therapist or other group members
2. Suggesting specific patterns of behavior to the patient
3. Identifying the patient's ineffectual responses and encouraging him to experiment with other forms of behavior
4. Group discussion regarding the behavior of self and others with mutual encouragement for engaging in appropriate and effective group behavior
5. Experimentation with various behaviors through role-playing exercises.[12]

Pragmatically, the therapist uses those initiating methods that appear to be successful.

An effort is made in all developmental groups to engage the patients in helping each other to acquire group interaction skill. Patients are encouraged to give and withhold reinforcers on the basis of the behavior exhibited by fellow group members. In order for patients to function as ancillary therapists, they must be able to comprehend what behavior is appropriate for a given type of developmental group and have sufficient self-control to give and withhold reinforcing stimuli. If it is deemed appropriate, the initial phase of treatment may be devoted to helping group members take on this ancillary therapist role.

Treatment continues to take place within the context of a specific type of developmental group until the patient has acquired the ability to function effectively in that group. He is then ready to begin learning the behavior that is necessary for competent functioning in the next, sequentially more advanced, developmental group. Depending upon the particular clinical situation and the extent to which the patient's fellow group members have progressed in an analogous manner, the patient is either placed in a new group or his original group as a whole is altered in the direction of the next type of developmental group. Treatment continues as previously outlined.

The treatment of deficiency in group interaction skill is terminated when any of the following criteria are met:

1. The patient has attained the ability to function in the type of group that is typical for his age.
2. He is able to participate in the kinds of groups that he is likely to encounter in his community environment (given its culture and the patient's preferred lifestyle).
3. The patient appears to be able to con-

tinue the development of group inter-action skill outside the treatment situation.

Additional Comments

The concept of developmental groups was formulated in the attempt to apply recapitulation of ontogeny in the treatment of patients who were deficient in their ability to interact effectively in small groups. This concept may prove useful in three other areas. These areas are:

1. Treatment of deficiency in other adaptive skills
2. Meeting mental health needs
3. Describing the evolution of small groups

Many of the subskills that are fundamental to the development of mature, adaptive skills are acquired through interaction in the familial group. These are usually the most basic or primitive subskills. However, more advanced subskills are often learned in the context of nonfamilial groups. The familial group may, indeed, continue to play a strongly supportive role, but interaction in nonfamilial groups is essential for adequate learning. (Treatment of those subskills that are usually developed within the family group is outside the scope of this paper.) In regard to those subskills that are partially or completely acquired through interaction in nonfamilial groups, it is suggested that they can be learned most easily through participation in a group that is structurally similar to the type of group in which the subskills are normally acquired. The concept of developmental groups could be used as a guide for selecting and forming appropriate groups. The difference between using developmental groups in the treatment of group interaction skill deficiency and deficiency in other adaptive skills is one of focus. The therapist would be primarily concerned with regulating reinforcement of behavior specific to the skill being learned as opposed to concentrating on helping the patient to learn how to function in the group. These two foci are not mutually exclusive, but it may be useful to deal with them as such to clarify treatment goals and methods.

That area of patient care here identified as meeting mental health needs refers to patient-therapist-nonhuman object interactions that are directed toward satisfying the normal human needs of the patient and maintaining his ability and desire to function.[13] The majority of mental health needs are most successfully met in a small group situation. However, needs cannot be satisfied unless there is synchronization of the individual's capacity to function in a particular group and the demands inherent in the structure of that group. In attempting to meet mental health needs, it is suggested that the therapist structure groups along a developmental continuum and that patients be encouraged to become involved in the type of group that is compatible with their group interaction skill. When a developmental group is oriented to satisfying mental health needs, the therapist is not concerned with bringing about a predetermined change in the patient's behavior. Therefore, the process of providing and withholding reinforcement is minimally important. The purpose of the group is to give pleasure, to have fun, to enjoy.

Preliminary, and somewhat superficial, observation indicates that the concept of developmental groups could be a useful tool in describing the evolution of task-oriented groups. This observation is not restricted to patient groups. As a task-oriented group moves toward becoming an effective working unit, there appear to be sequential patterns of interaction that are similar in many respects to the five types of developmental groups. Further study of this phenomenon may provide useful information for those persons who are concerned with facilitating the maturation and productivity of task-oriented groups.

The concept of developmental groups has been presented as a heuristic device. It is meant to stimulate interest and to encourage discovery. Its usefulness will be confirmed or refuted as we learn more about the human growth process, this entity that we call illness or dysfunction, and the effectiveness of treatment founded on the principles of recapitulation of ontogeny.

References

1. A. Jean Ayres, "Perceptual Motor Dysfunction in Children," paper presented at the Ohio Occupational Therapy Association Conference, 1964; John Flavell, *The Developmental Psychology of Jean Piaget* (New York: D. Van Nostrand Company, 1963); Anne Mosey, *Occupational Therapy: Theory and Practice* (printed through support of R.S.A. Training Grant No. 543-T-65 by Pothier Brothers, Medford, MA 1968); Maya Pines, "Why Some 3-Year Olds Get A's-and Some Get C's", The New York Times Magazine , July 6, 1969; Kenneth Overly, "Developmental Theory and Occupational Therapy-Considerations for Research," paper presented at the American Occupational Therapy Association Convention, Portland, Oregon, 1968; Marguerite Sechehaye, *A New Psychotherapy in Schizophrenia* (New York: Grune and Stratton, 1965).

2. Overly, "Developmental Theory and Occupational Therapy...."

3. Flavell, *The Developmental Psychology of Jean Piaget*...

4. Ayres, "Perceptual Motor Dysfunction in Children"; Mosey, *Occupational Therapy*....

5. Mosey, *Occupational Therapy*....

6. Gail Fidler, "The Task-Oriented Group as a Context for Treatment", *American Journal of Occupational Therapy, 23*, (1969).

7. H. English and A. English, *A Comprehensive Dictionary of Psychological and Psychoanalytic Terms* (New York: David McKay Co., 1958).

8. Erik Erikson, *Childhood and Society* (New York: W.W. Norton and Co., 1950); Anna Freud, *Normality and Pathology in Childhood* (New York: International University Press, 1965); T. Parsons and R. Bales, *Family, Socialization and the Interaction Process* (Glencoe, IL: The Free Press, 1955); J. Pearce and S. Newton, *The Conditions of Human Growth* (New York: Citadel Press, 1963).

9. C. Ferster and M. Perrott, *Behavior Principles* (New York: Appleton-Century-Crofts, 1961); Gregory Kimble, *Hilgard and Margis' Conditioning and Learning* (New York: Appleton-Century-Crofts, 1961); B.F. Skinner, *Science and Human Behavior* (New York: The Macmillan Co., 1953); A. Smith and V. Tempone, "Psychiatric Occupational Therapy Within a Learning Theory Context", *American Journal of Occupational Therapy* (September-October 1968); Kenneth Spence, *Behavior Theory and Conditioning* (New Haven, CT: Yale University Press, 1956).

10. Spence, *Behavior Theory and Conditioning*...

11. Parsons and Bales, *Family, Socialization, and the Interaction Process*; George Mead, *Mind, Self and Society* (Chicago, IL: University of Chicago Press, 1934); Theodore Mills, *The Sociology of Small Groups* (Englewood Cliffs, NJ: Prentice-Hall, 1963).

12. Fidler, "The Task-Oriented Group...."

13. G. Fidler and J. Fidler, *Occupational Therapy: A Communication Process in Psychiatry* (New York: The Macmillan Company, 1963).

From Mosey, A. C. (1970). The concept and use of developmental groups. *American Journal of Occupational Therapy, XXIV*(4), 272-275. Copyright 1970 by the American Occupational Therapy Association. Reprinted with permission.

Summary of Mosey's Adaptive Skills

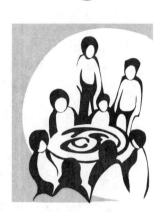

Sensory Integration Skill: The ability to receive, select, combine, and coordinate vestibular, proprioceptive, and tactile information for functional use.

1. The ability to integrate the tactile subsystems (birth-3 months).
2. The ability to integrate primitive postural reflexes (3-9 months).
3. Maturation of mature righting and equilibrium reactions (9-12 months).
4. The ability to integrate the two sides of the body, to be aware of body parts and their relationship, and to plan gross motor movements (1-2 yr).
5. The ability to plan fine motor movements (2-3 yr).

Cognitive Skill: The ability to perceive, represent, and organize sensory information for the purpose of thinking and problem-solving.

1. The ability to use inherent behavioral patterns for environmental interaction (birth-1 month).
2. The ability to interrelate visual, manual, auditory, and oral responses (1-4 months).

3. The ability to attend to the environmental consequence of actions with interest, to represent objects in an exoceptual manner, to experience objects, to act on the bases of egocentric causality, and to seriate events in which the self is involved (4-9 months).
4. The ability to establish a goal and intentionally carry out means, to recognize the independent existence of objects, to interpret signs, to imitate new behavior to apprehend the influence of space, and to perceive other objects as partially causal (9-12 months).
5. The ability to use trial-and-error problem-solving, to use tools, to perceive variability in spatial positions, to seriate events in which the self is not involved, and to perceive the causality of other objects (12-18 months).
6. The ability to represent objects in an image manner, to make believe, to infer a cause given its effect, to act on the bases of combined spatial relations, to attribute omnipotence to oth-

ers, and to perceive objects as permanent in time and place (18 months-2 yr).

7. The ability to represent objects in an endoceptual manner, to differentiate between thought and action, and to recognize the need for causal sources (2-5 yr).

8. The ability to represent objects in a denotative manner, to perceive the viewpoint of others, and to decenter (6-7 yr).

9. The ability to represent objects in a connotative manner, to use formal logic, and to work in the realm of the hypothetical (11-13 yr).

Dyadic Interaction Skill: The ability to participate in a variety of dyadic relationships.

1. The ability to enter into trusting familial relationships (8-10 months).

2. The ability to enter into association relationships (3-5 yr).

3. The ability to interact in an authority relationship (5-7 yr).

4. The ability to interact in a chum relationship (10-14 yr).

5. The ability to enter into a peer, authority relationship (15-17 yr).

6. The ability to enter into an intimate relationship (18-25 yr).

7. The ability to engage in a nurturing relationship (20-30 yr).

Group Interaction Skill: The ability to engage in a variety of primary groups.

1. The ability to participate in a parallel group (18 months-2 yr).

2. The ability to participate in a project group (2-4 yr).

3. The ability to participate in an ego-centric group (9-12 yr).

4. The ability to participate in a cooperative group (9-12 yr).

5. The ability to participate in a mature group (15-18 yr).

Self-Identity Skill: The ability to perceive the self as a relatively autonomous, holistic, and acceptable person who has permanence and continuity over time.

1. The ability to perceive the self as a worthy person (9-12 months).

2. The ability to perceive the assets and limitations of the self (11-15 yr).

3. The ability to perceive the self as self-directed (20-25 yr)

4. The ability to perceive the self as a productive, contributing member of a social system (30-35 yr).

5. The ability to perceive the self as having an autonomous identity (35-50 yr).

6. The ability to perceive the aging process of oneself and ultimate death as part of the life cycle (45-60 yr).

Sexual Identity Skill: The ability to perceive one's sexual nature as good and to participate in a relatively long-term sexual relationship that is oriented to the mutual satisfaction of sexual needs.

1. The ability to accept and act on the basis of one's pregenital sexual nature (4-5 yr).

2. The ability to accept sexual maturation as a positive growth experience (12-16 yr).

3. The ability to give and receive sexual gratification (18-25 yr).

4. The ability to enter into a sustained sexual relationship characterized by the mutual satisfaction of sexual needs (20-30 yr).

5. The ability to accept the sex-related physiological changes that occur as a natural part of the aging process (40-60 yr).

Reprinted with permission from Mosey, A. (1986). *Psychosocial components of occupational therapy* (pp. 416-418). New York: Raven Press.

Uniform Terminology for Occupational Therapy, Third Edition

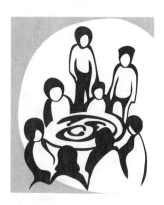

This is an official document of the American Occupational Therapy Association. This document is intended to provide a generic outline of the domain of concern of occupational therapy and is designed to create common terminology for the profession and to capture the essence of occupational therapy succinctly for others.

It is recognized that the phenomena that constitute the profession's domain of concern can be categorized, and labeled, in a number of different ways. This document is not meant to limit those in the field, formulating theories or frames of reference, who may wish to combine or refine particular constructs. It is also not meant to limit those who would like to conceptualize the profession's domain of concern in a different manner.

Introduction

The first edition of Uniform Terminology was approved and published in 1979 (AOTA, 1979). In 1989, the *Uniform Terminology for Occupational Therapy— Second Edition* (AOTA, 1989) was approved and published. The second document presented an organized structure for understanding the areas of practice for the profession of occupational therapy. The document outlined two domains. **PERFORMANCE AREAS** (activities of daily living [ADL], work and productive activities, and play or leisure) include activities that the occupational therapy practitioner emphasizes when determining functional abilities. **PERFORMANCE COMPONENTS** (sensorimotor, cognitive, psychosocial, and psychological aspects) are the elements of performance that occupational therapists assess and, when needed, in which they intervene for improved performance.

This third edition has been further expanded to reflect current practice and to incorporate contextual aspects of performance. Performance Areas, Performance Components, and Performance Contexts are the parameters of occupational therapy's domain of concern. Performance areas are broad categories of human activity that are typically part of daily life. They are activities of daily living, work and productive activities, and play or leisure activities. Performance components are fundamental human abilities that—to varying degrees and in differing combinations—are required for successful engagement in performance areas. These components are sensorimotor, cognitive, and psychosocial and psychological. Performance contexts are situations or factors that influence an individual's engagement in desired and/or required performance areas. Performance contexts consist of temporal aspects (chronological, developmental, life cycle, and disability status) and environmental aspects (physical, social, and cultural). There is an interactive relationship among performance areas, performance components, and performance contexts. Function in performance areas is the ultimate concern of occupational therapy, with performance components considered as they relate to participation in performance areas. Performance areas and performance components are always viewed within performance contexts. Performance contexts are taken into consideration when determining function and dysfunction relative to performance areas and performance components, and in planning intervention. For example, the occupational therapist does not evaluate strength (a performance component) in isolation. Strength is considered as it affects necessary or desired tasks (performance areas). If the individual is interested in homemaking, the occupational therapy practitioner would consider the interaction of strength with homemaking tasks. Strengthening could be addressed through kitchen activities, such as cooking and putting groceries away. In some cases, the practitioner would employ an adaptive approach and recommend that the family switch from heavy stoneware to lighter weight dishes, or use lighter weight pots on the stove to enable the individual to make dinner safely without becoming fatigued or compromising safety.

Occupational therapy assessment involves examining performance areas, performance components, and performance contexts. Intervention may be directed toward elements of performance areas (e.g., dressing, vocational exploration), performance components (e.g., endurance, problem solving), or the environmental aspects of performance contexts. In the last case, the physical and/or social environment may be altered or augmented to improve and/or maintain function. After identifying the performance areas the individual wishes or needs to address, the occupational therapist assesses the features of the environments in which the tasks will be performed. If an individual's job requires cooking in a restaurant as opposed to leisure cooking at home, the occupational therapy practitioner faces several challenges to enable the individual's success in different environments. Therefore, the third critical aspect of performance is the performance context, the features of the environment that affect the person's ability to engage in functional activities.

This document categorizes specific activities in each of the performance areas (ADL, work and productive activities, play or leisure). This categorization is based on what is considered "typical," and is not meant to imply that a particular individual characterizes personal activities in the same manner as someone else. Occupational therapy practitioners embrace individual differences, and so would document the unique pattern of the individual being served, rather than forcing the "typical" pattern on him or her and family. For example, because of experience or culture, a particular individual might think of home management as an ADL task rather than "work and productive activities" (current listing). Socialization might be considered part of play or leisure activity instead of its current listing as part of "activities of daily living," because of life experience or cultural heritage.

Examples of Use in Practice

Uniform Terminology—Third Edition defines occupational therapy's domain of concern, which includes performance areas, performance components, and performance contexts. While this document may be used by occupational therapy practitioners in a number of different areas (e.g., practice, documentation, charge systems, education, program development, marketing, research, disability classifications, and regulations), it focuses on the use of Uniform Terminology in practice. This document is not intended to define specific occupational therapy interventions. Examples of how performance areas, performance components, and performance contexts translate into practice are provided below.

- An individual who is injured on the job may have the potential to return to work and productive activities, which is a performance area. In order to achieve the outcome of returning to work and productive activities, the individual may need to address specific performance components such as strength, endurance, soft tissue integrity, time management, and the physical features of performance contexts, like structures and objects in his or her environment. The occupational therapy practitioner, in collaboration with the individual and other members of the vocational team, uses planned interventions to achieve the desired outcome. These interventions may include activities such as an exercise program, body mechanics instruction, and job site modifications, all of which may be provided in a work-hardening program.

- An elderly individual recovering from a cerebral vascular accident may wish to live in a community setting, which combines the performance areas of ADL with work and productive activities. In order to achieve the outcome of community living, the individual may need to address specific performance components, such as muscle tone, gross motor coordination, postural control, and self-management. It is also necessary to consider the sociocultural and physical features of performance contexts, such as support available from other persons, and adaptations of structures and objects within the environment. The occupational therapy practitioner, in cooperation with the team, utilizes planned interventions to achieve the desired outcome. Interventions may include neuromuscular facilitation, practice of object manipulation, and instruction in the use of adaptive equipment and home safety equipment. The practitioner and individual also pursue the selection and training of a personal assistant to ensure the completion of ADL tasks. These interventions may be provided in a comprehensive inpatient rehabilitation unit.

- A child with learning disabilities is required to perform educational activities within a public school setting. Engaging in educational activities is considered the performance area of work and productive activities for this child. To achieve the educational outcome of efficient and effective completion of written classroom work, the child may need to address specific performance components. These include sensory processing, perceptual skills, postural control, motor skills, and the physical features of performance contexts, such as objects (e.g., desk, chair) in the environment. In cooperation with the team, occupational therapy interventions may include activities like adapting the student's seating in the classroom to improve postural control and stability, and practicing motor control and coordination. This program could be developed by an occupational therapist and supported by school district personnel.

- The parents of an infant with cerebral palsy may ask to facilitate the child's involvement in the performance areas of activities of daily living and play. Subsequent to assessment, the therapist identifies specific performance components, such as sensory awareness and neuromuscular control. The practitioner also addresses the physical and cultural features of performance contexts. In collaboration with the parents, occupational therapy interventions may include activities such as seating and positioning for play, neuromuscular facilitation techniques to enable eating, facilitating parent skills in caring for and playing with their infant, and modifying the play space for accessibility. These interventions may be provided in a home-based occupational therapy program.

- An adult with schizophrenia may need and want to live independently in the community, which represents the performance areas of activities of

daily living, work and productive activities, and leisure activities. The specific performance categories may be medication routine, functional mobility, home management, vocational exploration, play or leisure performance, and social interaction. In order to achieve the outcome of living independently, the individual may need to address specific performance components such as topographical orientation, memory, categorization, problem solving, interests, social conduct, time management, and sociocultural features of performance contexts, such as social factors (e.g., influence of family and friends) and roles. The occupational therapy practitioner, in cooperation with the team, utilizes planned interventions to achieve the desired outcome. Interventions may include activities such as training in the use of public transportation, instruction in budgeting skills, selection of and participation in social activities, and instruction in social conduct. These interventions may be provided in a community-based mental health program.

- An individual with a history of substance abuse may need to reestablish family roles and responsibilities, which represent the performance areas of activities of daily living, work and productive activities, and leisure activities. In order to achieve the outcome of family participation, the individual may need to address the performance components of roles, values, social conduct, self-expression, coping skills, self-control, and the sociocultural features of performance contexts, such as custom, behavior, rules, and rituals. The occupational therapy practitioner, in cooperation with the team, utilizes planned intervention to achieve the desired outcomes. Interventions may include roles and values exercises, instruction in stress management techniques, identification of family roles and activities, and support to develop family leisure routines. These interventions may be provided in an inpatient acute care unit.

Person-Activity-Environment Fit

Person-activity-environment fit refers to the match among skills and abilities of the individual; the demands of the activity; and the characteristics of the physical, social, and cultural environments. It is the interaction among the performance areas, performance components, and performance contexts that is important and determines the success of the performance. When occupational therapy practitioners provide services, they attend to all of these aspects of performance and the interaction among them. They also attend to each individual's unique personal history. The personal history includes one's skills and abilities (performance components), the past performance of specific life tasks (performance areas), and experience within particular environments (performance contexts). In addition to personal history, anticipated life tasks and role demands influence performance.

When considering the person-activity-environment fit, variables such as novelty, importance, motivation, activity tolerance, and quality are salient. Situations range from those that are completely familiar, to those that are novel and have never been experienced. Both the novelty and familiarity within a situation contribute to the overall task performance. In each situation, there is an optimal level of novelty that engages the individual sufficiently and provides enough information to perform the task. When too little novelty is present, the individual may miss cues and opportunities to perform. When too much novelty is present, the individual may become confused and distracted, inhibiting effective task performance.

Humans determine that some stimuli and situations are more meaningful than others. Individuals perform tasks they deem important. It is critical to identify what the individual wants or needs to do when planning interventions.

The level of motivation an individual demonstrates to perform a particular task is determined by both internal and external factors. An individual's biobehavioral state (e.g., amount of rest, arousal, tension) contributes to the potential to be responsive. The features of the social and physical environments (e.g., persons in the room, noise level) provide information that is either adequate or inadequate to produce a motivated state.

Activity tolerance is the individual's ability to sustain a purposeful activity over time. Individuals must not only select, initiate, and terminate activities, but they must also attend to a task for the needed length of time to complete the task and accomplish their goals.

The quality of performance is measured by standards generated by both the individual and others in the social and cultural environments in which the performance occurs. Quality is a continuum of expectations set within particular activities and contexts.

Uniform Terminology for Occupational Therapy— Third Edition

"Occupational Therapy" is the use of purposeful activity or interventions to promote health and achieve functional

I. Performance Areas	II. Performance Components	III. Performance Contexts
A. Activities of Daily Living	A. Sensorimotor Components	A. Temporal Aspects
1. Grooming	1. Sensory	1. Chronological
2. Oral Hygiene	a. Sensory Awareness	2. Developmental
3. Bathing/Showering	b. Sensory Processing	3. Life Cycle
4. Toilet Hygiene	(1) Tactile	4. Disability Status
5. Personal Device Care	(2) Proprioceptive	
6. Dressing	(3) Vestibular	B. Environmental Aspects
7. Feeding and Eating	(4) Visual	1. Physical
8. Medication Routine	(5) Auditory	2. Social
9. Health Maintenance	(6) Gustatory	3. Cultural
10. Socialization	(7) Olfactory	
11. Functional Communication	c. Perceptual Processing	
12. Functional Mobility	(1) Stereognosis	
13. Community Mobility	(2) Kinesthesia	
14. Emergency Response	(3) Pain Response	
15. Sexual Expression	(4) Body Scheme	
	(5) Right-Left Discrimination	
B. Work and Productive Activities	(6) Form Constancy	
1. Home Management	(7) Position in Space	
a. Clothing Care	(8) Visual-Closure	
b. Cleaning	(9) Figure Ground	
c. Meal Preparation/Cleanup	(10) Depth Perception	
d. Shopping	(11) Spatial Relations	
e. Money Management	(12) Topographical Orientation	
f. Household Maintenance	2. Neuromusculoskeletal	
g. Safety Procedures	a. Reflex	
2. Care of Others	b. Range of Motion	
3. Educational Activities	c. Muscle Tone	
4. Vocational Activities	d. Strength	
a. Vocational Exploration	e. Endurance	
b. Job Acquisition	f. Postural Control	
c. Work or Job Performance	g. Postural Alignment	
d. Retirement Planning	h. Soft Tissue Integrity	
e. Volunteer Participation	3. Motor	
	a. Gross Coordination	
C. Play or Leisure Activities	b. Crossing the Midline	
1. Play or Leisure Exploration	c. Laterality	
2. Play or Leisure Performance	d. Bilateral Integration	
	e. Motor Control	
	f. Praxis	
	g. Fine Motor Coordination/Dexterity	
	h. Visual-Motor Integration	
	i. Oral-Motor Control	
	B. Cognitive Integration and Cognitive Components	
	1. Level of Arousal	
	2. Orientation	
	3. Recognition	
	4. Attention Span	
	5. Initiation of Activity	
	6. Termination of Activity	
	7. Memory	
	8. Sequencing	
	9. Categorization	
	10. Concept Formation	
	11. Spatial Operations	
	12. Problem Solving	
	13. Learning	
	14. Generalization	
	C. Psychosocial Skills and Psychological Components	
	1. Psychological	
	a. Values	
	b. Interests	
	c. Self-Concept	
	2. Social	
	a. Role Performance	
	b. Social Conduct	
	c. Interpersonal Skills	
	d. Self-Expression	
	3. Self-Management	
	a. Coping Skills	
	b. Time Management	
	c. Self-Control	

outcomes. "Achieving functional outcomes" means to develop, improve, or restore the highest possible level of independence of any individual who is limited by a physical injury or illness, a dysfunctional condition, a cognitive impairment, a psychosocial dysfunction, a mental illness, a developmental or learning disability, or an adverse environmental condition. Assessment means the use of skilled observation or evaluation by the administration and interpretation of standardized or nonstandardized tests and measurements to identify areas for occupational therapy services.

Occupational therapy services include, but are not limited to:

1. The assessment, treatment, and education of or consultation with the individual, family, or other persons

2. Interventions directed toward developing, improving, or restoring daily living skills; work readiness or work performance; play skills or leisure capacities; or enhancing educational performances skills

3. Providing for the development, improvement, or restoration of sensorimotor, oral-motor, perceptual or neuromuscular functioning; or emotional, motivational, cognitive, or psychosocial components of performance.

These services may require assessment of the need for and use of interventions such as the design, development, adaptation, application, or training in the use of assistive technology devices; the design, fabrication, or application of rehabilitative technology such as selected orthotic devices; training in the use of assistive technology, orthotic or prosthetic devices; the application of physical agent modalities as an adjunct to or in preparation for purposeful activity; the use of ergonomic principles; the adaptation of environments and processes to enhance functional performance; or the promotion of health and wellness (AOTA, 1993, p. 1117).

I. Performance Areas

Throughout this document, activities have been described as if individuals performed the tasks themselves. Occupational therapy also recognizes that individuals arrange for tasks to be done through others. The profession views independence as the ability to self-determine activity performance, regardless of who actually performs the activity.

A. *Activities of Daily Living*—Self-maintenance tasks.

1. *Grooming*—Obtaining and using supplies; removing body hair (use of razors, tweezers, lotions, etc.); applying and removing cosmetics; washing, drying, combing, styling, and brushing hair; caring for nails (hands and feet); caring for skin, ears, and eyes; and applying deodorant.

2. *Oral Hygiene*—Obtaining and using supplies; cleaning mouth; brushing and flossing teeth; or removing, cleaning, and reinserting dental orthotics and prosthetics.

3. *Bathing/Showering*—Obtaining and using supplies; soaping, rinsing, and drying all body parts; maintaining bathing position; transferring to and from bathing positions.

4. *Toilet Hygiene*—Obtaining and using supplies; clothing management; maintaining toileting position; transferring to and from toileting position; cleaning body; and caring for menstrual and continence needs (including catheters, colostomies, and suppository management).

5. *Personal Device Care*—Cleaning and maintaining personal care items, such as hearing aids, contact lenses, glasses, orthotics, prosthetics, adap-

tive equipment, and contraceptive and sexual devices.

6. *Dressing*—Selecting clothing and accessories appropriate for the time of day, weather, and occasion; obtaining clothing from storage area; dressing and undressing in a sequential fashion; fastening and adjusting clothing and shoes; and applying and removing personal devices, prostheses, or orthoses.

7. *Feeding and Eating*—Setting up food; selecting and using appropriate utensils and tableware; bringing food or drink to mouth; sucking, masticating, coughing, and swallowing; and management of alternative methods of nourishment.

8. *Medication Routine*—Obtaining medication, opening and closing containers, following prescribed schedules, taking correct quantities, reporting problems and adverse effects, and administering correct quantities using prescribed methods.

9. *Health Maintenance*—Developing and maintaining routines for illness prevention and wellness promotion, such as physical fitness, nutrition, and decreasing health risk behaviors.

10. *Socialization*—Accessing opportunities and interacting with other people in appropriate contextual and cultural ways to meet emotional and physical needs.

11. *Functional Communication*—Using equipment or systems to send and receive information, such as writing equipment, telephones, typewriters, communication boards, call lights, emergency systems, Braille writers, telecommunication devices for the deaf, and augmentative communication systems.

12. *Functional Mobility*—Moving from one position or place to another, such

as in-bed mobility, wheelchair mobility, transfers (wheelchair, bed, car, tub/shower, toilet, chair, floor); performing functional ambulation and transporting objects.

13. *Community Mobility*—Moving self in the community and using public or private transportation, such as driving, or accessing buses, taxi cabs, or other public transportation systems.

14. *Emergency Response*—Recognizing sudden, unexpected hazardous situations, and initiating action to reduce the threat to health and safety.

15. *Sexual Expression*—Engaging in desired sexual activities.

B. *Work and Productive Activities*—Purposeful activities for self-development, social contribution, and livelihood.

1. *Home Management*—Obtaining and maintaining personal and household possessions and environment.

   a. *Clothing Care*—Obtaining and using supplies; sorting, laundering (hand, machine, and dry clean); folding; ironing; storing; and mending.

   b. *Cleaning*—Obtaining and using supplies; picking up; putting away; vacuuming; sweeping and mopping floors; dusting; polishing; scrubbing; washing windows; cleaning mirrors; making beds; and removing trash and recyclables.

   c. *Meal Preparation/Cleanup*—Planning nutritious meals; preparing and serving food; opening and closing containers, cabinets, and drawers; using kitchen utensils and appliances; cleaning up and storing food safely.

   d. *Shopping*—Preparing shopping lists (grocery and other); selecting and purchasing items; selecting method of payment; and completing money transactions.

e. *Money Management*—Budgeting, paying bills, and using bank systems.

f. *Household Maintenance*—Maintaining home, yard, garden appliances, vehicles, and household items.

g. *Safety Procedures*—Knowing and performing preventive and emergency procedures to maintain a safe environment and prevent injuries.

2. *Care of Others*—Providing for children, spouse, parents, pets, or others, such as giving physical care, nurturing, communicating, and using age-appropriate activities.

3. *Educational Activities*—Participating in a learning environment through school, community, or work-sponsored activities, such as exploring educational interests, attending to instruction, managing assignments, and contributing to group experiences.

4. *Vocational Activities*—Participating in work-related activities.

a. *Vocational Exploration*—Determining aptitudes, developing interests and skills, and selecting appropriate vocational pursuits.

b. *Job Acquisition*—Identifying and selecting work opportunities, and completing application and interview processes.

c. *Work or Job Performance*—Performing job tasks in a timely and effective manner; incorporating necessary work behaviors.

d. *Retirement Planning*—Determining aptitudes, developing interests and skills, and identifying appropriate avocational pursuits.

e. *Volunteer Participation*—Performing unpaid activities for the benefit of selected individuals, groups, or causes.

C. *Play or Leisure Activities*—Intrinsically motivating activities for amusement, relaxation, spontaneous enjoyment, or self-expression.

1. *Play or Leisure Exploration*—Identifying interests, skills, opportunities, and appropriate play or leisure activities.

2. *Play or Leisure Performance*—Planning and participating in play or leisure activities; maintaining a balance of play or leisure activities with work and productive activities, and activities of daily living; obtaining, utilizing, and maintaining equipment and supplies.

II. Performance Components

A. *Sensorimotor Components*—The ability to receive input, process information, and produce output.

1. *Sensory*

a. *Sensory Awareness*—Receiving and differentiating sensory stimuli.

b. *Sensory Processing*—Interpreting sensory stimuli.

(1) *Tactile*—Interpreting light touch, pressure, temperature, pain, and vibration through skin contact/receptors.

(2) *Proprioceptive*—Interpreting stimuli originating in muscles, joints, and other internal tissues to give information about the position of one body part in relation to another.

(3) *Vestibular*—Interpreting stimuli from the inner ear receptors regarding head position and movement.

(4) *Visual*—Interpreting stimuli through the eyes, including peripheral vision and acuity, awareness of color and pattern.

(5) *Auditory*—Interpreting and localizing sounds, and discriminating background sounds.

(6) *Gustatory*—Interpreting tastes.

(7) *Olfactory*—Interpreting odors.

c. *Perceptual Processing*—Organizing sensory input into meaningful patterns.

(1) *Stereognosis*—Identifying objects through proprioception, cognition, and the sense of touch.

(2) *Kinesthesia*—Identifying the excursion and direction of joint movement.

(3) *Pain Response*—Interpreting noxious stimuli.

(4) *Body Scheme*—Acquiring an internal awareness of the body and the relationship of body parts to each other.

(5) *Right-Left Discrimination*—Differentiating one side of the body from the other.

(6) *Form Constancy*—Recognizing forms and objects as the same in various environments, positions, and sizes.

(7) *Position in Space*—Determining the spatial relationship of figures and objects to self or other forms and objects.

(8) *Visual-Closure*—Identifying forms or objects from incomplete presentations.

(9) *Figure Ground*—Differentiating between foreground and background forms and objects.

(10) *Depth Perception*—Determining the relative distance between objects, figures, or landmarks and the observer, and changes in planes of surfaces.

(11) *Spatial Relations*—Determining the position of objects relative to each other.

(12) *Topographical Orientation*—Determining the location of objects and settings and the route to the location.

2. *Neuromusculoskeletal*

a. *Reflex*—Eliciting an involuntary muscle response by sensory input.

b. *Range of Motion*—Moving body parts through an arc.

c. *Muscle Tone*—Demonstrating a degree of tension or resistance in a muscle at rest and in response to stretch.

d. *Strength*—Demonstrating a degree of muscle power when movement is resisted, as with objects or gravity.

e. *Endurance*—Sustaining cardiac, pulmonary, and musculoskeletal exertion over time.

f. *Postural Control*—Using righting and equilibrium adjustments to maintain balance during functional movements.

g. *Postural Alignment*—Maintaining biomechanical integrity among body parts.

h. *Soft Tissue Integrity*—Maintaining anatomical and physiological condition of interstitial tissue and skin.

3. *Motor*

a. *Gross Coordination*—Using large muscle groups for controlled, goal-directed movements.

b. *Crossing the Midline*—Moving limbs and eyes across the midsagittal plane of the body.

c. *Laterality*—Using a preferred unilateral body part for activities requiring a high level of skill.

d. *Bilateral Integration*—Coordinating both body sides during activity.

e. *Motor Control*—Using the body in functional and versatile movement patterns.

f. *Praxis*—Conceiving and planning a new motor act in response to an environmental demand.

g. *Fine Coordination/Dexterity*—Using small muscle groups for controlled movements, particularly in object manipulation.

h. *Visual-Motor Integration*—Coordinating the interaction of information from the eyes with body movement during activity.

i. *Oral-Motor Control*—Coordinating oropharyngeal musculature for controlled movements.

B. *Cognitive Integration and Cognitive Components*—The ability to use higher brain functions.

1. *Level of Arousal*—Demonstrating alertness and responsiveness to environmental stimuli.

2. *Orientation*—Identifying person, place, time, and situation.

3. *Recognition*—Identifying familiar faces, objects, and other previously presented materials.

4. *Attention Span*—Focusing on a task over time.

5. *Initiation of Activity*—Starting a physical or mental activity.

6. *Termination of Activity*—Stopping an activity at an appropriate time.

7. *Memory*—Recalling information after brief or long periods of time.

8. *Sequencing*—Placing information, concepts, and actions in order.

9. *Categorization*—Identifying similarities of and differences among pieces of environmental information.

10. *Concept Formation*—Organizing a variety of information to form thoughts and ideas.

11. *Spatial Operations*—Mentally manipulating the position of objects in various relationships.

12. *Problem Solving*—Recognizing a problem, defining a problem, identifying alternative plans, selecting a plan, organizing steps in a plan, implementing a plan, and evaluating the outcome.

13. *Learning*—Acquiring new concepts and behaviors.

14. *Generalization*—Applying previously learned concepts and behaviors to a variety of new situations.

C. *Psychosocial Skills and Psychological Components*—The ability to interact in society and to process emotions.

1. *Psychological*

a. *Values*—Identifying ideas or beliefs that are important to self and others.

b. *Interests*—Identifying mental or physical activities that create pleasure and maintain attention.

c. *Self-Concept*—Developing the value of the physical, emotional, and sexual self.

2. *Social*

a. *Role Performance*—Identifying, maintaining, and balancing functions one assumes or acquires in society (e.g., worker, student, parent, friend, religious participant).

b. *Social Conduct*—Interacting using manners, personal space, eye contact, gestures, active listening, and self-expression appropriate to one's environment.

c. *Interpersonal Skills*—Using verbal and nonverbal communication to interact in a variety of settings.

d. *Self-Expression*—Using a variety of styles and skills to express thoughts, feelings, and needs.

3. *Self-Management*

a. *Coping Skills*—Identifying and managing stress and related reactors.

b. *Time Management*—Planning and participating in a balance of self-care, work, leisure, and rest activities to promote satisfaction and health.

c. *Self-Control*—Modifying one's own behavior in response to environmental needs, demands, constraints, personal aspirations, and feedback from others.

III. Performance Contexts

Assessment of function in performance areas is greatly influenced by the contexts in which the individual must perform. Occupational therapy practitioners consider performance contexts when determining feasibility and appropriateness of interventions.

Occupational therapy practitioners may choose interventions based on an understanding of contexts, or may choose interventions directly aimed at altering the contexts to improve performance.

A. *Temporal Aspects*
1. *Chronological*—Individual's age.
2. *Developmental*—Stage or phase of maturation.
3. *Life Cycle*—Place in important life phases, such as career cycle, parenting cycle, or educational process.
4. *Disability Status*—Place in continuum of disability, such as acuteness of injury, chronicity of disability, or terminal nature of illness.

B. *Environmental Aspects*
1. *Physical*—Nonhuman aspects of contexts. Includes the accessibility to and performance within environments having natural terrain, plants, animals, buildings, furniture, objects, tools, or devices.
2. *Social*—Availability and expectations of significant individuals, such as spouse, friends, and caregivers. Also includes larger social groups which are influential in establishing norms, role expectations, and social routines.
3. *Cultural*—Customs, beliefs, activity patterns, behavior standards, and expectations accepted by the society of which the individual is a member. Includes political aspects, such as laws that affect access to resources and affirm personal rights. Also includes opportunities for education, employment, and economic support.

References

American Occupational Therapy Association. (1979). *Occupational therapy output reporting system and uniform terminology for reporting occupational therapy services*. Rockville, MD: Author.

American Occupational Therapy Association. (1989). Uniform terminology for occupational therapy (2nd ed.). *American Journal of Occupational Therapy, 43*, 808-815.

American Occupational Therapy Association. (1993). Definition of occupational therapy practice for state regulation (Policy 5.3.1). *American Journal of Occupational Therapy, 47*, 1117-1121.

Authors

The Terminology Task Force:
Winifred Dunn, PhD, OTR, FAOTA—Chairperson
Mary Foto, OTR, FAOTA
Jim Hinojosa, PhD, OTR, FAOTA
Barbara A. Boyt Schell, PhD, OTR/L, FAOTA
Linda Kohlman Thomson, MOT, OTR, OT(C), FAOTA
Sarah D. Hertfelder, MEd, MOT, OTR/L—Staff Liaison
for The Commission on Practice
Jim Hinojosa, PhD, OTR, FAOTA—Chairperson

Adopted by the Representative Assembly July 1994.

Note: This document replaces the following documents, all of which were rescinded by the 1994 Representative Assembly:

Occupational Therapy Product Output Reporting System (1979)

Uniform Terminology for Reporting Occupational Therapy Services—First Edition (1979)

Uniform Occupational Therapy Evaluation Checklist (1981)

Uniform Terminology for Occupational Therapy—Second Edition (1989)

Comparison of Group Leadership Guidelines in Seven Occupational Therapy Frames of Reference

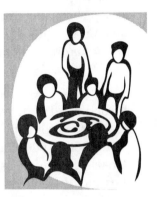

Humanistic

Structure—Loosely structured, discussion oriented
Time—1 hour or longer
Goals—Self-understanding, insight, self-actualization
Leadership—Facilitator/adviser
Activity Guidelines—Involve self-disclosure and interaction
1. *Introduction*—Members acknowledged, introduce ground rules
2. *Activity*—Explore meaning of life and personal values
3. *Sharing*—Feedback and mutual acceptance and empathy
4. *Processing*—Feelings explored thoroughly
5. *Generalizing*—Principles learned are elicited from members
6. *Application*—Members speak about how they will personally apply principles
7. *Summary*—Members contribute to summary

Psychoanalytic

Structure—Loosely structured, task oriented
Time—1 hour
Goals—Ego skill development and strengthening; gaining insight
Leadership—Facilitator
Activity Guidelines—Members project self through activities
1. *Introduction*—Purpose explained
2. *Activity*—Two types are appropriate
   a. Task-oriented group
   Phase 1: Planning a task
   Phase 2: Doing a task

b. Shared projective experience (i.e., group mural painting, role play exercise)

3. *Sharing*—All members choose and take part in task

4. *Processing*—
   Phase 3: Evaluating, feelings elicited and problems explored

5. *Generalizing*—Leader facilitates reflection of behavior and its consequences in the task group, evaluation is done at end of each session, possible interpretations of creative productions are explored

6. *Application*—Feedback is given to members to strengthen functions of ego or to gain insight

7. *Summary*—Therapist leads discussion with member input

Behavioral Cognitive Continuum

Structure—Highly structured with specific short-term goals based on cognitive deficit areas or need for coping strategies

Time—30 to 60 minutes based on member attention span

Goals—Specific, observable, measurable, focus on learning skills

Leadership—Director/educator, therapist instructs and assists throughout activity

Activity Guidelines—Should focus on alteration of thought process, attention, problem-solving, judgment, and metacognition

1. *Introduction*—Member names, no warm-up, short statement of purpose, focus on elaboration of specific goals and expectations for the session

2. *Activity*—Specific topics for learning and improving task performance or coping skills, goals often emphasized with worksheets and learning exercises, cognitive rehabilitation strategies applied in multiple contexts, activity takes most of session

3. *Sharing*—Minimal

4. *Processing*—Impact of feeling on thinking or learning is explored but not emphasized

5. *Generalizing*—Learning should coincide with group goals, therapist reviews principles learned, inductive reasoning is encouraged in higher level groups

6. *Application*—Members encouraged to anticipate applying new skills in future situations, homework is given for practice and elaboration in multiple real life contexts

7. *Summary*—Purpose is to reinforce learning

Cognitive Disabilities—Allen

Structure—Highly structured, minimal interaction, members work in parallel

Time—30 to 60 minutes

Goals—Specific, observable, measurable, patient has input, improve functional performance

Leadership—Directive, therapist instructs, assists, and provides cuing

Activity Guidelines—Use crafts from *Allen's Diagnostic Module* or other concrete tasks which meet Allen guidelines appropriate for member's cognitive level

1. *Introduction*—No warm-up, communicate specific expectations, and purpose geared to member understanding

2. *Activity*—Simple crafts or equivalent daily living tasks focusing on specific skills in a specific environment
3. *Sharing*—Materials not shared, results may be shared to learn from each other
4. *Processing*—Discuss feelings regarding task performance
5. *Generalizing*—Therapist assists members in generalizing skills from clinic environment to discharge environment
6. *Application*—Members discuss how they will apply learning, also communicated to caretakers
7. *Summary*—Reinforces learning

Developmental

Structure—Homogeneous groups work on specific age-appropriate skills in growth facilitating environment
Time—30 to 90 minutes, increases with maturity
Goals—Master skills needed to progress to next higher level of development
Leadership—Director, therapist sets up environment and plans activity
Activity Guidelines—Based on life tasks appropriate to age and stage of development in social, psychological, intellectual, or moral developmental theory
1. *Introduction*—Names, warm-up, structure and purpose explained
2. *Activity*—Graded to follow developmental guidelines matching stages of members
3. *Sharing*—Self-expression and feedback are encouraged
4. *Processing*—Feelings about both past and present experience are shared
5. *Generalizing*—Therapist guides discussion of general principles along developmental lines
6. *Application*—Each member applies new skills to his or her own life
7. *Summary*—Stress application of learning for growth

Sensory Motor

Structure—Highly structured sequence of sensory motor activities
Time—30 to 60 minutes
Goals—Stimulate development of central nervous system, adaptive functioning, and a sense of calm alertness
Leadership—Directive, role-modeling and imitation used to guide
Activity Guidelines—Movement oriented, according to specific theorist
1. *Introduction*—Acknowledge each member, always use warm-up to approach movement cautiously, therapist observes each member carefully to gauge tolerance for movement
2. *Activity*—Focus on movement and sensory stimulation
3. *Sharing*—Nonverbal interaction only, varies
4. *Processing*—Verbalize feelings about activity
5. *Generalizing*—Done by therapist in summary
6. *Application*—Spontaneous effects are noted by therapist
7. *Summary*—Therapist summarizes learning and expected outcomes

Model of Human Occupation

Structure—Members grouped by common/expected roles

Time—Wide range, 1 hour to several days

Goals—Restore order to daily occupation, re-establish occupational roles

Leadership—Facilitator/adviser, patient is given choices

Activity Guidelines—Normal daily activities: work, play, self-care at levels of exploration, competence, and achievement

1. *Introduction*—Names, warm-up optional, purpose discussed thoroughly with patient input
2. *Activity*—Work on tasks/skills needed to perform life roles of members
3. *Sharing*—Not necessary, varies
4. *Processing*—Acknowledge meaning of activity in context of personal causation
5. *Generalizing*—Meaning of activity with regard to system efficiency and meaningful occupational performance is discussed
6. *Application*—Individual performance is discussed and compared with demands of intended environment
7. *Summary*—Review goals and acknowledge individual achievement

Index

AAE, 73, 78
ACLS, 178
acting out, 112
activities
    Allen's task analysis, 195, 197–204
    behavioral cognitive continuum,
        160–161, 165–175
    developmental approach, 219, 223–237
    humanistic approach, 81-82, 85–97
    model of human occupational
        approach, 275–276, 279–290
    physical and mental capacities, 8
    psychoanalytic approach, 119–120,
        125–130
    sensory motor approaches, 252–256,
        258–265
activity analysis, 8–9
activity groups
    processing, 10–11
    seven-step format, 3–7
ADM, 178
advanced accurate empathy, 73, 78
adviser
    leadership style, 17
aggression, 103
Allen Diagnostic Module, 178
Allen's cognitive disabilities groups,
    177–204, 376–377
    assumptions, 179–187
    focus, 177–178
    group treatment, 189–194
Allen's Cognitive Levels Screen, 178
Allen's task analysis, 180–182
    activities, 195, 197–204
    change and motivation, 188–189
    function and dysfunction, 187–188
    group leadership, 194–195
anxiety, 63, 66, 103–104
application, 12
    Allen's task analysis, 195
    behavioral cognitive continuum,
        162–163

developmental approach, 222
humanistic approach, 83
model of human occupational
        approach, 277
sensory motor approaches, 257
attending, 69
attention, 108, 182
attention-getting behaviors, 50
authority
    leader
        group, 14–15
automatic actions, 183
automatic thoughts, 152–153
Ayers, A. J.
    sensory motor approaches, 243–244

behavioral cognitive concepts, 150–154
behavioral cognitive continuum, 131–175,
    376
    activities, 165–175
    assumptions, 132–133, 137–141
    change and motivation, 155–157
    focus, 132
    group leadership, 161–163
    group treatment, 157–160
behavioral concepts, 132–133, 137–141
behavioral goals, 132–137
    worksheet, 134–136
behavioral objectives, 132–133, 137
behaviors
    attention-getting, 50
biofeedback, 140–141
biomechanical approach, 141–145
Bion
    group development theory, 33
Bobaths
    sensory motor approaches, 241
body image, 107
brain conservation
    principle, 185
brain functions
    cognitive rehabilitation, 147f

Brunnstrom, S.
    sensory motor approaches, 241–242

chaining, 137–138
co-leadership, 18, 23–25
    advantages, 18, 23–24
    disadvantages, 24
    stages, 25
cognition
    dynamic nature, 150
cognitive disabilities, 179–187
    levels, 182–185
cognitive distortions, 152–153
Cognitive Performance Test, 178
cognitive rehabilitation
    brain functions, 147f
cognitive rehabilitation concepts, 145–150
complainer, 51
concepts
    humanistic approach, 63–66
concreteness, 69, 71
conditioning, 137
confrontation, 78, 81
conscious awareness, 183
content
    group, 28-29
counseling
    stages, 68
CPT, 178

DBT, 154
defense mechanisms, 104–113
    categories, 110
developmental approach, 205–238, 377
    activities, 219, 223–237
    assumptions, 206–216
    change and motivation, 217–218
    focus, 205–206
    function and dysfunction, 216–217
    group treatment, 218–219
    worksheets, 220–221
developmental groups, 355–360
    concepts, 355–356
    description, 356–357
    group interaction skill
        treatment, 357–359
    types, 355

dialectical behavior therapy, 154
directive leadership, 15–16

ego, 102
ego functions
    list, 101
ego psychology, 105–113
endurance, 142
Erikson
    developmental approach, 207
exploratory actions, 184–185
extrapolation
    Mosey's steps
        group theories, 58

facilitative leadership, 16–17
Fidler's lifestyle performance profile,
    144–145
Fidler's task-oriented group, 115
forms. See worksheet
frame of reference
    group leadership guidelines
        comparisons, 375–378
    selection procedure, 297–301
        worksheet, 298–299
freedom, 62
Freudian psychoanalytic theory, 101
Freud's psychosexual stages, 103t
functional performance, 143

generalization
    Allen's task analysis, 195
generalizing, 11–12
    behavioral cognitive continuum, 162
    developmental approach, 222
    humanistic approach, 83
    model of human occupational
        approach, 277
    sensory motor approaches, 257
genuineness, 63–64
Gilligan
    developmental approach, 215–216
goal-directed actions, 184
goals
    Allen's task analysis, 189–194
    behavioral cognitive continuum, 160
    humanistic approach, 81

model of human occupational
approach, 275
psychoanalytic approach, 119
sensory motor approaches, 252
group approaches
sensory motor approaches, 244–250
group development, 32–38
Schultz's stages, 37t
group development evaluation
worksheet, 39
group development theories, 32t
group dynamics, 27–56
forces, 27
group laboratory experience, 323–343
group leader
authority, 14–15
group leadership, 3–26
Allen's task analysis, 194–195
behavioral cognitive continuum,
161–163
model of human occupational
approach, 276–277
principles, 17
processing, 10–11
psychoanalytic approach, 121–124
sensory motor approaches, 256–257
group leadership guidelines
frame of reference
comparisons, 375–378
group motivation, 13–14
group norms, 38–43
group process, 347
group psychotherapy, 347
group roles, 42, 44–48
group session outline, 306–307
group stages
identification, 36–38
group termination, 52–53
group theories
Mosey's steps
extrapolation, 58
group therapies
Yalom's steps
clinical situations, 58
group treatment
Allen's cognitive disabilities groups,
189–194

behavioral cognitive continuum,
157–160
developmental approach, 218–219
humanistic approach, 67–81
model of human occupational
approach, 274–275
psychoanalytic approach, 117–120
sensory motor approaches, 251–256
group treatment plan outline, 301,
303–306
group treatment protocol
example, 323–343
preparation instructions, 307
writing, 294–322
group treatment protocol plan
worksheet, 308–322
groups
maturity, 35–36

habits, 137
habituation subsystem, 269–270
help-rejecting complainer, 51
humanistic approach, 61–98, 375
activities, 81-82, 85–97
assumptions, 62–63
change, 66–67
concepts, 63–66
focus, 61–62
function and dysfunction, 66
goals, 81
group treatment, 67–81
leadership, 82–84
motivation, 66
structure, 81
human occupation approach. *See* model
of human occupational approach
human open system, 268

id, 102
identification, 112–113
immediacy, 73
internal subsystems, 268–272
irrational beliefs, 153–154

judgment, 109–110
Jung
developmental approach, 206, 207t

King, L. J.
  sensory motor approaches, 244–247
Kohlberg and Wilcox
  developmental approach, 214–215

leader
  authority
    group, 14–15
leader responsibility, 13
leadership
  humanistic approach, 82–84
  task-oriented group, 351–352
leadership evaluation
  worksheet, 20–22
leadership roles
  Allen's task analysis, 189
  behavioral cognitive continuum, 160
  developmental approach, 218–219
  humanistic approach, 68–81
  model of human occupational
    approach, 275–276
  psychoanalytic approach, 118–119
  sensory motor approaches, 251–252
leadership styles, 15–17
  guidelines, 18t
learning, 109
Levinson
  developmental approach, 207–214
Levy, L.
  sensory motor approaches, 248–250
libido, 103
lifestyle performance profile, 144–145
Linehan's dialectical strategies, 154
logical thought, 109

manual actions, 184
Maslow's mountain, 65f
mastery/competence, 113
memory, 108–109
metacognition, 148–149
mind-brain-body performance subsystem,
    270–271
model of human occupational approach,
    267–290, 378
  assumptions, 268–272
  change and motivation, 273–274

components, 273
focus, 267
function and dysfunction, 272–273
group leadership, 276–277
group treatment, 274–275
MOHO. *See* model of human occupation-
    al approach
monopolists, 49
Mosey's adaptive skills, 361–362
  concept, 116–117
Mosey's role acquisition, 143–144
Mosey's steps
  group theories
    extrapolation, 58
motor action, 183
multicontextual approach, 146–148

narcissistic member, 51–52
non-judgemental acceptance, 64

object relationships, 104–105
occupational therapy
  ego oriented milieu, 116
  perspective, 114–117
  philosophy, 62
  uniform terminology, 363–374

PAE, 71, 73
patient population
  identification, 294, 297
  worksheet, 295–296
patient problems, 45, 49
perception/cognition
  areas, 146
performance areas, components, and con-
    texts
  worksheets, 302
performance subsystem, 270–271
personal group reaction outline
  worksheet, 55
planned actions, 185
PNF approach, 242–243
postural actions, 183–184
practice, 138–140
prevention, 142–143
primary accurate empathy, 71, 73
process

group, 30, 32
group dynamics, 28-29
processing
　activities, 10
　Allen's task analysis, 195
　behavioral cognitive continuum, 162
　developmental approach, 222
　humanistic approach, 83
　sensory motor approaches, 256–257
projection, 111
proprioceptive neuromuscular facilita-
　tion, 242–243
psychic energy, 103
psychoanalytic approach, 99–130, 375–376
　activities, 119–120, 125–130
　assumptions, 101–113
　change and motivation, 114
　focus, 99–100
　function and dysfunction, 113–114
　group leadership, 121–124
　group treatment, 117–120
psychoanalytic theory, 100–101
psychosexual stages, 102–103
psychotic patient behavior, 52

questionnaires. *See* worksheet

range of motions, 141–142
rational emotive therapy, 153
reality testing, 105–106
regression, 111–112
rehabilitative approach, 143
rehearsal, 138–140
reinforcement, 138
respect, 63
RET, 153
role acquisition, 143–144
role analysis
　worksheet, 46–47, 48
role playing, 140
ROM, 141–142
Rood, Margaret
　sensory motor approaches, 240–241
Ross' five stage groups, 254
Ross, M.
　sensory motor approaches, 247–248
Routine Task Inventory, 178

RTI, 178

schizophrenic
　task-oriented group, 352–354
Schultz
　group development theory, 33–35
Schultz's stages
　group development, 37t
self-actualization, 65–66
self-concept, 106–107
self-control, 110
self-deprecator, 50
self-esteem, 107–108
self-understanding, 64
sensory motor approaches, 239–265, 377
　assumptions, 239–244
　change and motivation, 250–251
　focus, 239
　function and dysfunction, 250
　group approaches, 244–250
　group treatment, 251–256
seven-step format
　activity groups, 3–7
shaping, 137
sharing
　activities, 9
　Allen's task analysis, 195
　behavioral cognitive continuum,
　　161–162
　developmental approach, 219, 222
　humanistic approach, 82–83
　sensory motor approaches, 256
silent member, 50
skill acquisition, 143
social learning theory, 151–152
strength, 142
structure
　humanistic approach, 81
sublimation, 111
superego, 102
systematic desensitization, 140–141

task analysis
　cognitive disabilities, 190t–191t
task equivalence
　principle, 186–187
task-oriented group, 115

context for treatment, 346–354
definition, 349
experimental studies, 347–349
occupational therapy, 349
purpose, 349–351
schizophrenic, 352–354
termination
groups, 52–53
theories
list, 58
therapeutic goals, 7–8
thought processes, 108–110
transfer of learning, 149–150
treatment aspects
selection procedure, 301
treatment guidelines, 59–60
Tuckman
group development theory, 32–33

usable task environment, 185–186

volitional subsystem, 268–269

worksheets
behavioral goals, 134–136
confrontation, 80

content-process reaction, 31
developmental approach, 220–221
empathy, 75-77, 79
feeling words, 74
first impressions, 70
group development evaluation, 39
group treatment protocol plan,
308–322
leadership evaluation, 20–22
monitoring norms, 43
open-ended questions, 72
patient population, 295–296
performance areas, components, and
contexts, 302
personal group reaction outline, 55
practice group plan, 19
role analysis, 46–48
selection procedure
frame of reference, 298–299
writing
group treatment protocol, 294–322

Yalom's self-reflective loop, 28f
Yalom's steps
clinical situations
group therapies, 58

*F*or your information

This book and many others on numerous different topics are available from SLACK Incorporated. For further information or a copy of our latest catalog, contact us at:

Professional Book Division
SLACK Incorporated
6900 Grove Road
Thorofare, NJ 08086 USA
Telephone: 1-609-848-1000
1-800-257-8290
Fax: 1-609-853-5991
E-mail: orders@slackinc.com
WWW: http://www.slackinc.com

We accept most major credit cards and checks or money orders in US dollars drawn on a US bank. Most orders are shipped within 72 hours.

Contact us for information on recent releases, forthcoming titles, and bestsellers. If you have a comment about this title or see a need for a new book, direct your correspondence to the Editorial Director at the above address.

If you are an instructor, we can be reached at the address listed above or on the Internet at educomps@slackinc.com for specific needs.

Thank you for your interest and we hope you found this work beneficial.

GROUP DYNAMICS
IN OCCUPATIONAL THERAPY

THE THEORETICAL BASIS AND PRACTICE
APPLICATION OF GROUP TREATMENT
SECOND EDITION